BACK PAIN –
An International Review

BACK PAIN
An International Review

Edited by
John K. Paterson, MB, BS, MRCGP

President of the British Association of Manipulative Medicine;
Member of the Scientific Advisory Committee and Chairman of
the Terminology Subcommittee of the Fédération Internationale
de Médecine Manuelle

and **Loïc Burn**, BA, MRCS, LRCP, DPhysMed
President of the Fédération Internationale de Médecine
Manuelle; Past President of the British Association of
Manipulative Medicine; Member Ex-Committee, Scientific
Section, British League against Rheumatism; Member, Council of
Management, National Back Pain Association

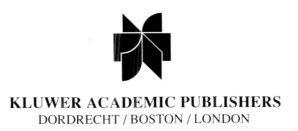

KLUWER ACADEMIC PUBLISHERS
DORDRECHT / BOSTON / LONDON

Distributors

for the United States and Canada: Kluwer Academic Publishers, PO Box 358, Accord Station, Hingham, MA 02018-0358, USA
for all other countries: Kluwer Academic Publishers Group, Distribution Center, PO Box 322, 3300 AH Dordrecht, The Netherlands

British Library Cataloguing in Publication Data

Back pain – an international review.
   1. Man. Back. Backache
   I. Paterson, John K. (John Kirkpatrick), *1921–*   II. Burn, Loic, *1936–*
   616.73

   ISBN 0-7923-8912-3

Copyright

Published in the United Kingdom by Kluwer Academic Publishers, PO Box 55, Lancaster, UK.

Kluwer Academic Publishers BV incorporates the publishing programmes of D. Reidel, Martinus Nijhoff, Dr W. Junk and MTP Press.

Printed and bound in Great Britain by Butler and Tanner Ltd., Frome and London.

Contents

CONTENTS

FREE PAPERS

List of contributors

G B J Andersson
Department of Orthopedic Surgery
Rush–Presbyterian–St Luke's
Medical Center
1653 West Congress Parkway, 1471J
Chicago
IL 60612
USA

A Arlen
Centre de Cure
Parc Albert Schweitzer
F-68140 Munster
France

J V Basmajian
Department of Medicine and
Anatomy
McMaster University
Hamilton
Ontario L8N 3Z5
Canada

G Berlinson
Nogent
F-52800 France

H Biedermann
Department of Surgery
Universitat Witten-Herdecke
Ev. Krankenhaus Schwerte
Schützenstr. 9
D-5840 Schwerte
FRG

G Brugnoni
Servicio di Riabilitazione
Case di Cura "S. Camillo"
Via M. Macchi 5
20124 Milano
Italy

L Burn
31 Wimpole Street
London W1
UK

A G Chila
College of Osteopathic Medicine
Ohio University
Grosvenor Hall
Athens, OH 45701
USA

I Colombo
Istituto di Terapia Fisica Ospedale
Ca'Grande Niguarda di Milano
Via Ghiberti 11
20149 Milano
Italy

F Combi
Istituto di Fisioterapia
Ospedale Bassini
Via M. Gorki 50
Cinisello Balsamo (Milano)
Italy

J-Y Cornu
CRF les Rosiers
45 rue Bazin
Dijon
F-21000 France

D R Dalley
St Albans Medical Centre
PO Box 21044
Christchurch 1
New Zealand

P Demma
10, rue Nicolas Charlet
75015 Paris
France

J P Duivon
Groupe d'Etude de Medecine
Manuelle Rhône Alpes
89 Cours Emile Zola
69100 Villeurbanne
France

K J Eiden
Rosenheimer Strasse 181
8000 München 80
FRG

R M Ellis
Wessex Regional Rehabilitation Unit
Odstock Hospital
Salisbury
Wilts. SP5 8BJ
UK

R T D FitzGerald
52 Shurland Avenue
Minster
Sheerness
Kent ME12 2RS
UK

J Fossgreen
Department of Rheumatology
Aarhus Amtssygehus
University Hospital
DK 8000 Aarhus C
Denmark

D M Fraser
Orthopedic Medicine Clinic
5147 Lewiston Road
Lewiston
NY 14092
USA

H H Gibson
Department of Psychology
The Hatfield Polytechnic
Hatfield
Herts. AL10 9AB
UK

P E Greenman
College of Osteopathic Medicine
Department of Biomechanics
Michigan State University
East Lansing
MI 48824
USA

M Hanna
Ludwig Boltzmann Institute and
Department for Conservative
Orthopaedics and Rehabilitation
Speisingerstr. 109
A-1134 Vienna
Austria

G Hellsing
Department of Clinical Oral
Physiology
Karolinska Institute
Box 4064
S-141 04 Huddinge
Sweden

K Hiemeyer
Rheumatologische Abteilung
Kreiskrankenhaus
D-8346 Simbach
FRG

M A Hutson
Orthopaedic Physician
Park Row Clinic
30 Park Row
Nottingham NG1 6GR
UK

V Janda
Department of Rehabilitation
Medicine
Postgraduate Medical Institute
Šrobárova 50
134 00 Prague 10
Czechoslovakia

J Jirout
Department of Neuroradiology
Neurologic Clinic
Charles University
120 00 Prague
Czechoslovakia

S Karagozian
Groupe d'Etude de Medecine
Manuelle Rhône Alpes
1, Avenue Victor Hugo
26000 Valence
France

M Kraemer
Centre de Cure
Parc A. Schweitzer
F-68140 Munster
France

P Lapsley
National Back Pain Association
31–33 Park Road
Teddington
TW11 0AB
UK

A H Laxton
Beechfield
Hookwood Lane
Ampfield
Romsey
Hants. SO51 9BZ
UK

C Leuci
Istituto Terapia Fisica Ospedale
Ca'Grande Niguarda di Milano
Residenza Mestieri – Milano 2
20090 Segrate (MI)
Italy

S M Levin
Potomac Back Center
5021 Seminary Road
Alexandria
VA 22311
USA

K Lewit
Department of Rehabilitation
Central Railway Health Institute
120 00 Praha 2 Vinohrady
Czechoslovakia

H Lohse-Busch
Centre de Cure
Parc Albert Schweitzer
F-68140 Munster
France

B Lynn
Department of Physiology
University College London
Gower Street
London WC1E 6BT
UK

S Lörincz
Ludwig Boltzmann Institute for
Conservative Orthopaedics and
Rehabilitation
Speisingerstr. 109
A-1134 Vienna
Austria

R Maigne
Chef de Service de Medecine
Orthopedique
Hopital Hotel-Dieu
75004 Paris
France

G Marx
Hochriesstrasse 6
8214 Hittenkirchen
FRG

S McMahon
Department of Physiology
St Thomas' Hospital Medical School
Lambeth Palace Road
London SE1 7EH
UK

M Mehta
King Edward VIIth Hospital
Midhurst
West Sussex GU29 0BL
UK

H Menninger
BRK Rheumazentrum Bad Abbach
I Med Klinik
D-8403 Bad Abbach, FRG

M C T Morrison
Orthopaedic Surgeon
Princess Margaret Hospital
Swindon
SN1 4JU
UK

M A Nelson
Department of Orthopaedics
General Infirmary at Leeds
Great George Street
Leeds LS1 3EX
UK

H-D Neumann
Buhlertalstrasse 45
7580 Bühl (Baden)
FRG

R Pastrana
Rehabilitation Service
Hospital 'Ramon y Cajal'
Carretera de Colmenar, km9,100
28034 Madrid
Spain

J K Paterson
31 Wimpole Street
London W1
UK

A Patris
Service d'Informatique Medicale
CHU de Nancy-Brabois
54500 Vandoeuvre les Nancy
France

G Piganiol
University of Dijon
49 rue de Dijon
Daix
F-21121 France

J P Randeria
28 Farm Close
Ickenham
Middx. UB10 8JB
UK

A E Reading
Department of Psychiatry and
Behavioral Sciences
UCLA School of Medicine
760 Westwood Plaza
Los Angeles
CA 90024
USA

K Rekola
Department of Physical Medicine and
Rehabilitation
Central Hospital Jyväskylä
SF-40620 Jyväskylä
Finland

J-F Renard
CRF les Rosiers
45 rue Bazin
Dijon
F-21000 France

E Rychlíková
Postgraduate Medical and
Pharmacological Institute
Department of Education and
Research of Manual Medicine
Prague
Czechoslovakia

M R Shah
St James' Health Centre
St James' St
London E17 7NH
UK

L Silverstolpe
Department of Clinical
Neurophysiology
Karolinska Hospital
S-104 01 Stockholm
Sweden

P Slatter
Ferry View Orthopaedic Clinic
Ferry View
Bath Road
Lymington
Hants SO41 9SE
UK

A Stevens
Department of Physical Medicine and
Rehabilitation
U.Z. Gasthuisberg, Herestraat 49
University of Leuven KUL
3000-Leuven
Belgium

A Stoddard
The Anchorage
Spinney Lane
Itchenor
W. Sussex PO20 7DJ
UK

I Swain
Wessex Regional Rehabilitation Unit
Odstock Hospital
Salisbury
Wilts. SP5 8BJ
UK

H Tilscher
Ludwig Boltzmann Institute and
Department for Conservative
Orthopaedics and Rehabilitation
Speisingerstr. 109
A-1134 Vienna
Austria

P Trouilloud
University of Dijon
1 Imp. Capit. Heim
Dijon
F-21000 France

D G Vivian
441 Bay Street
Brighton
Victoria 3186
Australia

C Weich
Ludwig Boltzmann Institute for
Conservative Orthopaedics and
Rehabilitation
Speisingerstr. 109
A-1134 Vienna
Austria

M Wisłowska
Rheumatological Outpatients
Department
Institute of Clinical Medicine
137 Komarowa St
Warsaw
Poland

H-D Wolff
Lehrbeauftragter für Manuelle Mediz
an der Universität des Saarlandes
(Homburg/Saar)
Gartenfeldstr. 6
D-5500 Trier
FRG

Preface

As we stated in our message in the book of abstracts for this congress, we have planned the programme over a long period with one clear objective: to present musculoskeletal medicine as an integral part of orthodox medical practice, rather than as something alternative or complementary. To this end we have based the plenary programme as far as possible on accepted epidemiological, anatomical, physiological and pathological phenomena. Scientifically well-validated material must surely be the base upon which any viable musculoskeletal medicine practice may be built.

While we have chosen the plenary programme to reflect musculoskeletal medicine as a part of orthodoxy, we realize and wish to emphasize that there is a wealth of original work that has been carried out within FIMM. For this reason our first innovation for the congress was to invite members of the scientific advisory committee to select for a 'directed' programme the three topics they felt were of greatest current importance. The results of this democratic procedure was the choice of the sacroiliac joint, a comparison of manual therapies and biomechanics. This illustrates the broad direction of present thinking within FIMM.

To our surprise and great encouragement, more free papers were offered than could be accommodated, which is a reflection of the keen and growing interest in this field of medicine. We have grouped these roughly according to the following themes: the pelvis, miscellaneous, assessment, innovation, imaging, and atlas therapy. Such grouping can only be approximate, on account of the extraordinary variety of topics addressed.

We have attempted to achieve this grouping without being too selective, in order that the wide range of professional interests displayed at the congress may be equitably represented.

We offer this second innovation, the congress book, expressly to reflect the current state of musculoskeletal medicine within FIMM, and only regret that it is not more complete, owing to a number of potential contributors not meeting the extended deadline.

John K. Paterson
Loïc Burn

London
October 1989

Introduction

Loïc BURN

We thought that you might be interested in how the programme for the FIMM congress, on which this book is based, came into being, and what this congress is about. First, FIMM congresses are organized by national societies, who have responsibility for the administration and for the programme. Therefore, every congress tends to have something of an individual flavour, because each will reflect the interests and concerns primarily of the organizing scientific committee. Nevertheless, of course, international opinion is sought from all quarters, as are contributions.

Most congresses are organized in plenary and free programmes. You will probably already have noticed that this is not so in the congress and in the book, and that we have introduced a novel category of 'directed' papers. The reason for this will become apparent, as it will for the order in which I address these three parts, beginning with the free papers.

We have over 60 free papers, which we regard as a very gratifying sign of the healthy interest in this subject internationally. In fact the volume has been so great that we have had to extend the time originally allocated for free papers, in order to accommodate them all. We would like to thank all those who contributed to this part of the programme.

With regard to the directed programme, this has a rather unusual history. The scientific committee first devised the plenary programme in the winter of 1985/1986, and we then circulated members of the Scientific Advisory Committee of FIMM, asking them for their comments. We did so, I have to say, in a mood of some complacency. However, it must also be said that our complacency was rather short-lived! The reason for this was that, although many people within FIMM thought the programme as proposed was acceptable, indeed praiseworthy, others had reservations.

A number of senior people from a variety of countries had a problem with it that was not difficult to define. Briefly, it was felt by some that insufficient emphasis was given to original work, which is of course continually going on in this field; that, in other words, as it stood, the congress was an inadequate showcase for original work. We felt this complaint to be perfectly legitimate and, after constructive discussion within FIMM, devised the following mechanism to meet it.

We circulated the Scientific Advisory Committee and asked its members to identify those issues they felt to be currently of the greatest importance in manual medicine. This procedure at least had the merit of being democratic. We selected from the replies the three topics most frequently suggested and allocated a programme of six papers to each session, equal in duration to the plenary papers.

The three issues chosen were the sacroiliac joint, muscle energy techniques and biomechanics. The first has always been a matter of concern and controversy, the latter two are relative newcomers to this arena. I am glad to tell you that all sessions are complete, and we now feel we have provided an adequate showcase for original work. We leave it to you to make your own judgement of these presentations.

FIMM, as befits so large an international organization, has several functions. A major function is, of course, that of bringing to the notice of our professional colleagues in other disciplines the problems and possibilities of manipulation as a treatment in many conditions. There are many treatments which must be assessed in the management of the universal scourge of back pain, but manipulation is certainly one of them.

FIMM has another extremely important function amongst the many. That is to bring to the notice of the medical profession as a whole the very unsatisfactory state regarding the management of vertebral problems. Despite the enormous scale of these troubles, medical education worldwide generally neglects them at both undergraduate and postgraduate level. Nobody, from whatever discipline, would regard the medical response to spinal pain as being adequate at the present time. Moreover this appreciation is not restricted to doctors. We are not the only people to say "Look, there is a great deal of back pain; should we not be doing more about it?" As Dr David Owen and Mr Peter Lapsley (of the NBPA) say, there is certainly in this country a growing interest among the public. Interested lay organizations make precisely the same point.

In the United Kingdom, we regard these endeavours as complementary. We think that the profession and responsible and distinguished members of the public and serious organizations together will achieve more than each separately. We warmly welcome such assistance, as it brings far greater hope of remedying what is universally identified as a lamentable situation, which regrettably is changing all too slowly.

How can FIMM best help to address this problem? Some of us were greatly impressed by the three masterly presentations of the Zurich congress in 1983 given by Professor Barry Wyke. He there gave a review of the field of articular neurology, which at that time had only been in existence for twenty years. He gave a remarkably clear and comprehensive account of the scientific bases which he demonstrated unequivocally to relate to the problems we have, and to the procedures we use as clinicians. Some of us were surprised at how much recent physiological work related to our practice. This raised the issue as to whether there were scientific data relating specifically to vertebral problems, and indeed there are; whether also there was scientific material relating to all clinicians involved in the treatment of pain, which, after all, is what the vast majority of our patients consult us about.

The worldwide flowering of the pain clinic popularized within the profession the idea of a multi-disciplinary approach to these problems, and to the consideration of any proposed therapy. It therefore seemed reasonable to provide not only a survey of the development of the basic aspects of musculoskeletal medicine, but we felt it also essential to consider the problems and contributions of the many other colleagues from different backgrounds dealing with pain. How much do our approaches differ? How much do they resemble one another? By the same token, it is not only relevant but necessary to consider the principal treatments that can be and are used in the treatment of back pain.

It is only by using terminology that is readily comprehensible to all doctors, and by identifying and comparing our bases with those of other colleagues, that we can translate a field which is currently widely regarded as being of marginal medicinal interest into being accepted (as we all believe it should be) as an integral part of the principles and practice of medicine. This, then is the theme of the plenary programme. I will now introduce a selection of the papers.

Dr Lynn, whose chapter in the *Textbook of Pain* many of us are familiar with, talks about the peripheral modulation of nociceptive input, with all the importance that has, not only diagnostically, but also relating specifically to some of the proven bases of the procedures that interest us particularly.

Professor Andersson talks about the intradiscal pressure changes, the estimation of which he has been associated with for many years in Gothenburg, and it is interesting to consider the current relationship between this work and the clinician.

Professor Basmajian discusses electromyography and its significance to the manipulator. Professor Basmajian is an international authority on this subject, which is one of prime importance to us. As students, we were all taught, and thereby knew, what muscles did, and it is fundamental that we now understand what the scientific reality is. Not only is muscle testing commonly used in diagnostic procedures, but exercises are probably the most commonly prescribed physical treatment worldwide at the present time. Therefore the proven facts about muscle function are of crucial relevance.

If physiology is making giant strides, so also is psychology becoming established as being of great importance to musculoskeletal problems. Professor Reading, again a world authority, rehearses with us the limitations of subject report, the value of the polymodal approach to history taking and the relevance of behaviour. None of us can afford to ignore these phenomena. Indeed, history taking that does not take cognizance of these factors must be diminished in validity.

Dr McMahon, of the Department of Physiology at St Thomas' Hospital, talks about the central modulation of nociceptive input, and in so doing, we have asked him and Dr Lynn to cooperate in providing a point-counter-point of their presentations of neurophysiology. Those who have read Melzack and Wall's *Textbook of Pain* will be very familiar with the repetition of the words 'connectivity' and 'plasticity' relating to central physiological problems, with the obvious implications they have for diagnosis and the presentation of an image of the continuous and continually varying 'hornet's nest' of physiological activity.

Mr Martin Nelson then discusses principles and problems of research in low back pain. He is particularly well qualified to do this, as he is Chairman of the Research Committee of the NBPA. However, the great problems in back pain research which he will discuss have often led me to feel that he was in a rather hot seat. This is because many people, insufficiently informed concerning these matters, who see funds available for research, are surprised and sometimes disconcerted at the extreme care that should be taken in order to ensure that these funds are not wasted on projects of dubious worth. Martin Nelson explains why and how this comes about.

The next two papers are devoted to diagnosis. This follows naturally on the basic aspects, some of which have already indicated diagnostic difficulties, to use an Anglo-Saxon understatement. We begin with an account of referred pain and tenderness, phenomena that bedevil the clinician.

In basic case analysis a presentation is made of a possible approach, based on existing knowledge which, given the present state of affairs, is of necessity tentative.

The next part of the plenary programme is devoted to manipulation. It begins with an overview of this therapy by one of the great authorities in this field. This is followed by the osteopathic approach to manipulation by a veteran of equal distinction. The consideration of the osteopathic approach is of historical relevance to the United Kingdom, because of the foundation of the London College of Osteopathic Medicine, which runs courses for doctors.

We include the thoracolumbar junction and the author who addresses it because this is one of the classics of medical manipulation for the identification of referred pain and referred tenderness, its elucidation and its management by a number of treatments, including manipulation.

Next we present an assessment of the Cyriax contribution. This is necessary in the United Kingdom, because of the remarkable impact that he made in this field, which is still a matter for discussion and debate.

We then include two subjects which we think are of particular relevance to members of FIMM, namely the sacroiliac joint and muscle energy techniques. It is of interest that we selected these topics before the directed programme was conceived, with its emphasis on the same themes. Perhaps, for once, we got something right! We did not include biomechanics for two reasons; first because of the limitations of time and space, and second because we wanted to confine ourselves to topics of direct clinical interest and, as many of us will well remember, Professor Panjabi (an acknowledged authority in this field) said to us in Madrid, 'I cannot see the relevance of this material to the work you people do'.

The last part of the plenary session is devoted to 'other therapies'. The constraints of time compel us to review only a few of these, there being of course many more. Firstly, injections, a great variety of them used routinely by us all.

Secondly, drug therapy, with its great ease of delivery for both patient and physician, but regrettably with the risk of serious side-effects, to some extent unpredictable. This makes the present universal use of this form of treatment, particularly in general practice, a matter for concern.

Thirdly, surgical results. This was not included as some kind of hostile move by clinicians using primarily conservative means; however it is a fact that only 50% of back pain is relieved by surgery and 70% of leg pain. The work of Mooney and Robertson and the emergence of the facet joint injection as a therapeutic option were in fact an orthopaedic response to the difficulties they contended with in surgery. I feel that the paper 'The causes of poor results of surgery in low back pain' in many ways might be better entitled, 'The causes of poor results in low back pain'.

We then consider psychological therapies in low back pain. I mentioned the importance of psychology from the point of view of case analysis. In therapy it has also emerged in the pain clinic, particularly in dealing with the patient who does not respond readily to any of the various physical treatments that can be deployed. What then to do with the patient? What is his concept of his situation, that of his family, what is his disability? How can this be assessed and attenuated? One is reminded here of the extraordinarily successful results of pure behavioural therapy in returning people to work that have been achieved by Fordyce and by Roberts and Reinhardt. The writer is Professor Michael Bond, again a world authority in these matters, and it is of interest that, as Professor of Psychological Medicine, he is in charge of a Pain Clinic in Glasgow.

Other treatments of particular interest are acupuncture and TNS, reviewed by Mark Mehta, a most distinguished consultant in pain relief and author of a book on pain published as early as 1973. He has always championed the use of what he calls the simple remedies in pain treatment, those which are simple to deploy, cheap and above all harmless. Those of us who do not use acupuncture and TNS should be familiar with them and consider them as viable alternatives to the treatments we use more often.

Finally, we have a contribution on hypnosis by Dr Gibson, again a multiple author on this subject. Hypnosis is a very good example of treatment at one time thought unorthodox, if not bizarre, which has been extensively studied and brought under review by many clinicians from many disciplines. An interesting account of this situation was given by Professor Orne in the *Textbook of Pain*.

This then was the programme that we created four years ago, and we thought produced a balanced view, placing low back pain as a central medical concern, and as a legitimate interest for clinicians of many different disciplines.

We hope you will agree the principal theme of this book is perhaps best summarized by Professor Wall, when he wrote "Each school of thought and training has reasonably tended to approach pain problems from a particular bias and to write articles and textbooks expressing that emphasis. It now seems apparent that all of these biases are both right and wrong and that the problems and the patient benefit from a multiple approach".

The economics of back pain

Peter LAPSLEY

INTRODUCTION

Back pain is amongst the commonest causes of absenteeism from work; it may well be the commonest. In the United Kingdom, Department of Health and Social Security (DHSS) figures show that 46.5 million working days were lost through back pain in the financial year 1987/1988 – 12% of all days lost through illness. The Offices of Health Economics estimate the cost to British industry at rather more than £2000 million.

The problem is an international one and is evident on similar scales elsewhere in the world. Figures published in an article in *The Lancet* in June this year suggest that the United States loses an estimated 217 million working days a year at a cost to that country's economy of as much as $11 billion.

THE BRITISH STATISTICS

The most recent British statistics on back pain, published by the DHSS earlier this year, are detailed in Table 1. They are quite startling.

Inter alia, they show:

(a)   that the 46.5 million days lost with spinal problems represents 12% of all incapacities;

(b)   that days lost by those diagnosed as suffering from spondylosis and allied disorders have increased significantly – up 74%, from 9.2 million in 1983 to 16 million in 1988;

(c)   that disc disorders represent 17% of all days lost through spinal problems and have risen by 28% since 1983;

(d)   that the number of days lost through ankylosing spondylitis have risen from 1.7 million in 1983 to 2.5 million in 1988 – an increase of 47%;

(e)   that unspecified sprain and strain disorders have risen by 26% over the five year period.

Table 1 Days of certified incapacity in the period 6 April 1987 to 2 April 1988 – analysed by cause of incapacity compared with those for 1982/83. Supplied by DHSS, Newcastle, Crown Copyright 1989

	1982/3	1987/88	% change
All incapacities (days)	361.0M	381.5M	+5.6%
Total of detailed list below	33.1M	46.5M	+40.0%
Spondylosis and allied disorders	9.2M	16.0M	+74.0%
Intervertebral disc disorders	6.0M	7.7M	+28.0%
Ankylosing spondylitis and other inflammatory spondylopathies	1.7M	2.5M	+47.0%
Other disorders (cervical region)	0.5M	0.5M	–
Sprains and strains (sacroiliac region)	0.5M	0.6M	+20.0%
Sprains and strains unspecified parts of back and unspecified back disorders	15.2M	19.1M	+26.0%

Very few employing organizations separate back pain from other ailments and afflictions in their own records and statistics. We strongly suspect that they are therefore largely unaware of the magnitude of the problem. It is interesting that one employer that does separate back pain out – the National Health Service – has found that the nursing profession loses 764 000 working days a year at an estimated cost of £160 million – figures which add credibility to the statistics for the country as a whole.

The medical professionals with whom we have discussed these figures do not disagree with them and tend (purely speculatively) to attribute the increases to:

(a)   the shift in employment from the production industries to service ones;

(b)   the increasing proportion of women in relatively sedentary employment (although there is no evidence to suggest that women are more susceptible to back pain *per se*), and;

(c)   increasingly sedentary lifestyles and consequent unfitness for occasional vigorous exercise.

THE PERSONAL COST

What these facts and figures conceal – and what the economists cannot assess – is the human misery caused by back pain and the economic downgrading of the individual sufferer.

The chronic back pain sufferer is very often quite unable to realize his or her full potential at work – either because he cannot travel, or because he cannot attend long meetings, or because he can only stand at a work bench for limited periods, or for whatever other reason. He may therefore be unable to compete for promotion and may well even lose his job. We at the National Back Pain Association receive many desperate letters each month from young, otherwise active people who have become unemployed because of their back pain.

Back pain in parents can have disastrous effects on children. When they are young, their father or mother may be unable to pick them up or to give them the cuddles that are so essential to their development. As they grow up, the parent may be unable to play energetic games of any sort with them.

Dr Geoff Lowe, of Hull University's Department of Psychology recently conducted a research programme to compare the behaviour and attitudes of school-age children of male lower-back pain patients with a group of children having healthy parents. The childrens' teachers monitored their behaviour for several weeks, and psychologists tested both parents and children for their attitudes towards health and feelings of personal control over it.

Children of back pain patients cried and whined, complained of sickness and were absent from school twice as often as children in the other group. They were also more likely to avoid stressful or unpleasant situations, such as participating in class. Like their fathers, these children felt excessively helpless about controlling their health.

Back pain creates very serious strains within marriages, often inhibiting proper relations between partners, limiting or preventing the development of social relationships with others and curtailing the ability to participate in sporting and other leisure activities. It frequently leads to marriage break-up. Occasionally, it leads to suicide.

For all these reasons, acute and chronic back pain sufferers are very likely go into a downward spiral – their handicap leading to economic and social disadvantage, which causes depression, which increases their consciousness of physical discomfort, and so on.

We in the National Back Pain Association have recognized this problem, and are addressing ourselves to the extraordinarily difficult task of encouraging the creation of multi-disciplinary research teams – to include orthopaedics, rheumatology, psychiatry and psychology. The work they must do is right on the fringes of knowledge in these fields. But if the cost to the individual, to the state and to the international community is to be drastically reduced – as it must be – the work must be done.

Section I
PLENARY PAPERS

1
The peripheral modulation of nociceptive input

Bruce LYNN

Inflamed and injured tissues are characteristically hyperalgesic, i.e. relatively minor stimuli become painful, sometimes very much so. Apart from cases where the injury has directly traumatized nerve trunks, the major process involved in causing hyperalgesia is the sensitization of nociceptive afferents by chemical agents released from inflamed tissues. The increased firing of nociceptors will itself make a major contribution to the hyperalgesia. In addition, the pathologically increased input triggers significant changes in the sensitivity of the centres in the central nervous system that process this input. Chapter 5 by McMahon will concentrate on these central changes; this article will deal with the peripheral effects.

The problem will be considered in three stages. Firstly, the normal properties of the nociceptive input from skin, muscle and joints will be briefly reviewed. Secondly, the way that nociceptors become sensitized in inflamed tissues and the key chemical factors in that sensitization will be discussed. Thirdly, neural factors, such as possible actions by sympathetic efferents, will be covered briefly.

NOCICEPTORS IN SKIN, MUSCLES AND JOINTS

The afferent innervation of these somatic tissues comprises subpopulations with specialized functions. Each particular class of receptors has axons in a particular size band, and afferent fibre type has been a key parameter in the classification of somatic afferents. The main classes and their fibre types are given in Table 1.1. Nociceptive afferents, those responding to damaging or potentially damaging stimuli, have A-δ (small myelinated) or C (unmyelinated) axons.

The nociceptive innervation of the skin has been studied extensively and two major classes of nociceptor have been identified. The properties of these are summarized in Table 1.2. As their name implies, *polymodal nociceptors* (PMNs) respond to a range of noxious stimuli, including strong pressure, heating and irritant chemicals. Examples of typical responses are shown in Figure 1.1. In all species examined, PMNs comprise at least 50% of the C-fibres in cutaneous nerves. Since there are more C-fibres than A-fibres, this makes them the single most numerous group of afferents. Innervation densities are correspondingly high, for example 800/cm^2 in the skin of the foot in rats. Although most PMNs have unmyelinated (C) axons, there are some similar afferents with A-δ axons. This clearly has to be the case in man, since reaction times on touching a hot object are shorter than would be possible if only slowly-conducting C-fibres carried information about noxious skin heating. *High threshold mechanoreceptors* (HTMs) comprise about one third of myelinated fibres and the great majority are in the slowly-conducting (A-δ) band. They respond well to strong mechanical stimuli, such as pressure with a needle. They are not responsive to heat or to irritant chemicals.

Table 1.1 Major classes of afferent fibre from skin, skeletal muscle and joints, by fibre size

Fibre type	A-αβ (Groups I & II)	A-δ (Group III)	C (Group IV)
Fibre morphology	Large myelinated	Small myelinated	Unmyelinated
Typical conduction velocities (m/sec)	30–100	6–24	0.5–1.5
Skin	Mechanoreceptors (e.g. Meissner's corpuscles; most hair follicle endings; Pacinian corpuscles)	Mechanoreceptors (e.g. D-hair follicle) Cold thermoreceptors Nociceptors (mostly mechanical nociceptors of HTM type)	Warm thermo-receptors Nociceptors (mostly polymodal type)
Muscle	Stretch receptors (Muscle spindles, Golgi tendon organs)	Nociceptors	Nociceptors
Joints	Proprioceptors	Proprioceptors Nociceptors	Nociceptors

In both muscles and joints there are some nociceptors that only respond to strong mechanical stresses, whilst others respond in addition to irritant chemicals. However, there is no clear subdivision into two distinct classes, one with C and one with A-δ axons[3,4].

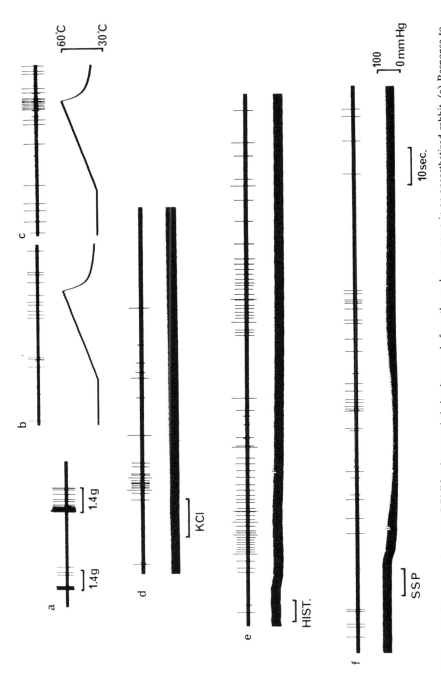

Figure 1.1 Responses from two C-PMN units recorded simultaneously from the saphenous nerve in an aneasthetized rabbit. (a) Response to vertical pressure on the skin using calibrated von Frey bristles, each field being tested in turn. Note that the action potential from the second unit tested is larger than that of the first unit, allowing the two units to be clearly distinguished. (b, c) Responses to linear increases in skin temperature, again each field tested in turn. (d, e, f) Unit responses and blood pressure changes following close arterial injections of (d) 0.7 ml of 140 mM KCl, (e) 200 μg histamine, and (f) 8 μg substance P. (From ref. 36)

Table 1.2 Properties of two widely distributed types of nociceptive afferent unit from mammalian skin

	High threshold mechanoreceptor (HTM)	Polymodal nociceptor (PMN)
Fibre type	A-δ	C
Response to strong pressure	+	+
Response to heat	0	+
Response to irritant chemicals	0	+
Receptive field	Multiple points	One small zone[a]

Key: +, responds well; 0, no response
[a]In primates some PMN units have larger receptive fields
(From ref. 2)

NOCICEPTOR SENSITIZATION

One of the earliest reports on the properties of afferents from the skin, that by Echlin and Propper in 1937[5], described how their sensitivity could be enhanced following minor injury. These workers were in fact studying small fibres from frog skin and they showed that, after scraping of the skin, afferent discharges were greatly increased. More recent studies have confirmed that nociceptors are also abnormally sensitive in inflamed skin.

Heat-induced sensitization has been much studied in the skin[6]. Typically C-fibre PMN units show reduced thresholds and increased suprathreshold firing following strong skin heating (e.g. to 50–55°C for several seconds). There is a good correspondence between the levels of heating required to produce PMN sensitization and those that cause hyperalgesia in man[7]. PMN units with A-δ axons also sensitize, and in glabrous skin appear to be the subpopulation whose pattern of changing sensitivity most closely corresponds to hyperalgesia in man[8]. A-δ HTM units do not respond to skin heating in normal skin. However, repeated skin heating can cause marked heat sensitivity to develop[9], a very remarkable form of sensitization indeed!

Sensitization following mechanical injury is less easy to study as it is difficult to avoid irreversible damage to afferents in the treated skin area. However, with care, sensitization of nociceptors by mild mechanical injury can be demonstrated[10]. In addition, nociceptors innervating the skin immediately adjacent to an area of mechanical trauma sometimes show enhanced responses[11], although this is not always the case. The enhanced responses seen in the sometimes extensive area of secondary hyperalgesia around a mechanical (or other) injury may depend in part on sensitization of afferents. However, these certainly always have a major central component (see Chapter 5 by McMahon).

The response of nociceptors, especially C-PMNs, in inflamed tissue have been extensively studied, and the perhaps not surprising finding is that thresholds are reduced and that suprathreshold responses are enhanced. Such findings have been reported for skin treated with formalin or carrageenin[12], for skeletal muscle inflamed with carrageenin[13] and for joints, either acutely inflamed with carrageenin and kaolin or chronically inflamed following adjuvant injections[14,15]. A typical example of nociceptor sensitization, in a joint A-δ unit, is shown in Figure 1.2.

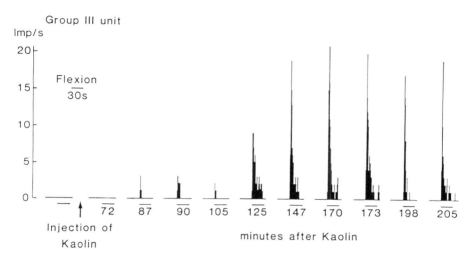

Figure 1.2 Sensitization of a high-threshold, presumably nociceptive, unit with A-δ (group III) axon from the knee joint of an anaesthetized cat. Initially the unit does not respond to a standard flexion stimulus covering the normal range of movement of the joint, although the unit did fire to extreme noxious joint rotations (not shown). An injection of kaolin was made at time zero, followed by a second injection of carrageenin (not marked). Over the next 3 hours a striking increase in sensitivity occurs, illustrated by the development of strong responses to the standard, previously ineffective, stimulus of joint flexion. Unit firing is graphed as spikes per second (impulses/sec) on the ordinate. (From ref. 37)

THE ENDOGENOUS CHEMICALS INVOLVED IN NOCICEPTOR SENSITIZATION

The crucial test for the involvement of a specific agent would be the blocking of nociceptor sensitization by a pharmacological antagonist of narrow and defined selectivity. Experiments attempting to investigate antagonists have proved tricky to carry out and to interpret, although some interesting positive results have emerged and will be discussed below. Before trying antagonists, however, it is necessary to show that putative mediators of sensitization can actually sensitize nociceptors. There is now a considerable literature on the immediate excitatory and sensitizing actions of putative mediators[16] and this will be considered next.

7

Bradykinin, a potent pain-producing agent in man, has been consistently found to activate nociceptive afferents. In skin there is a good degree of selectivity for C-PMN units[17]. Concentrations of bradykinin in the range 10 nM to 10 μM activate 50% of C-PMNs when applied to the inner surface of rat limb skin *in vitro*[18]. Close-arterial injection of bradykinin can activate many nociceptive afferents, both A-δ and C, from joints and skeletal muscle[19,20]. By this route it is more potent than serotonin or histamine. As well as exciting nociceptors, bradykinin also sensitizes them to other stimuli, including heat. Repeated application of bradykinin leads to marked reduction in responses (tachyphylaxis). However, the sensitization of heat responses show relatively little tachyphylaxis. Bradykinin responses are enhanced by pretreatment with serotonin. The tachykinin *substance P*, in contrast to bradykinin, is only a very weak excitant of C-fibre nociceptors (e.g. see Figure 1.1). Furthermore, brief application does not cause sensitization, although prolonged exposure to this agent may cause enhanced responses to other irritants.

The responses of cutaneous afferents to *histamine* are of interest, not just in relation to hyperalgesia, but also because histamine is an excellent itch-producing agent. As shown in Figure 1.1, some C-PMNs fire well to histamine. Histamine can also sensitize C-PMNs to skin heating, but not to pressure. Histamine, injected intradermally, excites C-PMNs in many species, including man[21]. Histamine is not as selective, or as potent, as bradykinin and excites a smaller proportion of nociceptors. The concentrations of histamine needed to fire C-PMNs have been found also to excite other classes of C-fibre and some slowly adapting mechanoreceptors with large A-$\alpha\beta$ axons. Another amine involved in tissue reactions to injury, *serotonin (5-HT)*, activates nociceptive afferents from skin, joints and skeletal muscle[22-24]. As mentioned above, it also sensitizes afferents to the excitatory actions of bradykinin.

The eicosanoids *prostaglandin E_2* and *leukotriene B_4* do not excite nociceptive afferents. However they can cause marked sensitization to heat and pressure stimuli in cutaneous nociceptors[25]. PGE_1 and PGE_2 have also been shown to sensitize nociceptive afferents from joints to mechanical stimuli[26].

Bradykinin is clearly a prime candidate as the endogenous agent causing enhanced nociceptor responses during inflammation. Recently, selective antagonists have become available for bradykinin. However, first attempts to use these to examine afferent responses have been unsuccessful, because agents that behaved as pure antagonists in other systems have proved, when applied to skin nociceptors, to be excellent agonists (i.e. they excited them almost as well as bradykinin itself!)[27]. Immediate heat-induced sensitization of cutaneous C-PMNs has been studied in the isolated perfused rabbit ear by Perl and colleagues[28,29]. Eicosanoid synthesis inhibitors (e.g. aspirin) have given conflicting results. Some studies have demonstrated a reduction in heat sensitization, with the most consistent results using an agent that blocks both major eicosanoid synthesis pathways[29]. There is thus some evidence for a role for prostaglandins and other eicosanoids in heat sensitization. Carrageenin-induced sensitization of muscle nociceptors and sensitization of nociceptors in inflamed joints have also been found to be partly reversed by aspirin[30,31]. Antihistamines, whether H_1 or H_2, do not affect heat sensitization of cutaneous C-PMNs[16].

Overall, the results from experiments on nociceptors have given results much as would be expected if, as is widely believed, their sensitization underlies the hyperalgesia and pain that occur in inflamed tissues. Substances known to be released in inflammation and to be capable of causing pain or hyperalgesia on injection in man have in turn been found to activate and/or sensitize nociceptors. Whether hyperalgesia following injury or inflammation can be explained by the actions of just one or two of these substances has yet to be established. The role of the most potent endogenous agent, bradykinin, is not clear because suitable antagonists are still not available.

NEURAL FACTORS AFFECTING NOCICEPTOR SENSITIVITY

In addition to mediators released by cells of the immune system or from precursors in plasma and extracellular fluid, the sensitivity of afferent fibres can also be modified by activating local nerves. Activating sympathetic nerves to normal skin has no affect on nociceptors, although it does change the sensitivity of some mechanoreceptors, exciting some subtypes (e.g. hair follicle endings)[32]. However, in skin subjected to mild heat injury, some A-δ nociceptors are now weakly activated by sympathetic stimulation[33]. This is interesting in that some chronic pain conditions in man are improved by sympathetic block. However, it seems likely that the sensitivity to catecholamines of fibres in damaged nerve trunks plays a more important part in the so-called reflex sympathetic dystrophies than does the sensitization of their terminals in the skin.

A particularly intriguing property of nociceptive C-fibres is their ability themselves to stimulate mild inflammation[34]. The best-known example of this is the vascular flare around focal skin injuries. In principle, therefore, it appears that C-fibres ought to be able to sensitize themselves. A test of this is to activate nerve trunks antidromically at C-fibre strength and look for C-PMN sensitization. Small effects have been found in rabbit skin[11], but no effects have been seen in monkey or rat. Therefore it would appear that, despite clear vasodilatation and increased microvascular permeability on antidromic stimulation, direct actions on nociceptors are limited. Nevertheless, the possibility needs to be considered[34,35] that under pathological conditions some inflammation and hyperalgesia are due to runaway activation of C-PMNs.

SUMMARY

Injury or inflammation of tissues leads to the sensitization of the specialized nociceptors that signal about potentially or actually damaging stimuli. In severe inflammation, many nociceptors fire to levels of stimulation that would be innocuous in normal tissue. The major mediators known to be released in damaged tissue all excite and/or sensitize nociceptors. Which of these mediators play dominant roles is not yet established. There are also possible neural factors involved at the nociceptor level, since both nociceptor activation itself, and activation of sympathetic efferents, have a degree of sensitizing action on subpopulations of nociceptive afferents.

REFERENCES

1. Burgess, P.R. and Perl, E.R. (1973). Cutaneous mechanoreceptors and nociceptors. In Iggo, A. (ed.) *Handbook of Sensory Physiology, Vol. 2, Somatosensory System*, pp. 29–78. (Berlin: Springer)
2. Lynn, B. (1983). Cutaneous sensation. In Goldsmith, L.A. (ed.) *Biochemistry and Physiology of the Skin*, pp. 654–684. (New York: Oxford University Press)
3. Mense, S. and Meyer, H. (1985). Different types of slowly-conducting afferent units in cat skeletal muscle and tendon. *J. Physiol.*, **363**, 403–417
4. Schaible, H.-G. and Schmidt, R.F. (1983). Activation of groups III and IV sensory units in medial articular nerve by local mechanical stimulation of knee joint. *J. Neurophysiol.*, **49**, 35–44
5. Echlin, F. and Propper, N. (1937). 'Sensitization' by injury of the cutaneous nerve endings in the frog. *J. Physiol.*, **88**, 388–400
6. Campbell, J.N. and Meyer, R.A. (1986). Primary afferents and hyperalgesia. In Yaksh, T.L. (ed.) *Spinal Afferent Processing*, pp. 59–81. (New York: Plenum)
7. LaMotte, R.H., Thallhammer, J.G., Torebjork, H.E. and Robinson, C.J. (1982). Peripheral neural mechanisms of cutaneous hyperalgesia following mild injury by heat. *J. Neuroscience*, **2**, 765–778
8. Meyer, R.A. and Campbell, J.N. (1981). Myelinated nociceptive afferents account for the hyperalgesia that follows burn to the hand. *Science*, **213**, 1527–1529
9. Fitzgerald, M. and Lynn, B. (1977). The sensitization of high threshold mechanoreceptors with myelinated axons by repeated heating. *J. Physiol.*, **265**, 549–560
10. Reeh, P.W., Bayer, J., Kocher, L. and Handwerker, H.O. (1987). Sensitization of nociceptive cutaneous nerve fibers from the rat's tail by noxious mechanical stimulation. *Exp. Brain Res.*, **65**, 505–512
11. Fitzgerald, M. (1979). The spread of sensitization of polymodal nociceptors in the rabbit from nearby injury and by antidromic nerve stimulation. *J. Physiol.*, **297**, 207–210
12. Kocher, L., Anton, F., Reeh, P.W. and Handwerker, H.O. (1987). The effect of carrageenin-induced inflammation on the sensitivity of unmyelinated skin nociceptors in the rat. *Pain*, **29**, 363–373
13. Berberich, P., Hoheisel, U. and Mense, S. (1988). Effects of a carrageenan-induced myositis on the discharge properties of group III and IV muscle receptors in the cat. *J. Neurophysiol.*, **59**, 1395–1409
14. Schaible, H.-G. and Schmidt, R.F. (1985). Effects of an experimental arthritis on the sensory properties of fine articular afferent units. *J. Neurophysiol.*, **54**, 1109–1122
15. Guilbaud, G., Iggo, A. and Tegner, R. (1985). Sensory receptors in ankle joint capsules of normal and arthritic rats. *Exp. Brain Res.*, **58**, 29–40
16. Lynn, B. (1989). Structure, function and control: Afferent nerve endings in the skin. In Greaves, M.W. and Schuster, S. (eds.) *Pharmacology of the Skin. Handbook of Experimental Pharmacology*, Vol. 87/1, pp. 175–192. (Berlin: Springer)

17. Szolcsanyi, J. (1987). Selective responsiveness of polymodal nociceptors of the rabbit ear to capsaicin, bradykinin and ultra-violet radiation. *J. Physiol.*, **388**, 9–28
18. Novak, A., Lang, E., Handwerker, H.O. and Reeh, P.W. (1987). Sensitivity of rat cutaneous C-fiber endings to bradykinin and interactions with other stimuli: an in vitro study. *Pain*, Suppl.4, R18
19. Mense, S. (1977). Nervous outflow from skeletal muscle following chemical noxious stimulation. *J. Physiol.*, **267**, 75–88
20. Kanaka, R., Schaible, H.-G. and Schmidt, R.F. (1985). Activation of fine articular afferent units by bradykinin. *Brain Res.*, **327**, 81–90
21. Torebjork, H.E. and Hallin, R.G. (1974). Identification of afferent C-units in intact human skin nerves. *Brain Res.*, **67**, 387–403
22. Beck, P.W. and Handwerker, H.O. (1974). Bradykinin and serotonin effects on various types of cutaneous nerve fibres. *Pflueger's Arch.*, **347**, 209–222
23. Fock, S. and Mense, S. (1976). Excitatory effects of 5-hydroxytryptamine, histamine and potassium ions on muscular group IV afferent units: a comparison with bradykinin. *Brain Res.*, **105**, 459–469
24. Herbert, M.K. and Schmidt, R.F. (1987). Effect of serotonin on groups III and IV afferent units from acutely inflamed cat knee joint. *Pflueger's Arch.*, **408**, Suppl. 1, R66
25. Martin, H.A., Basbaum, A.I., Goetzl, E.J. and Levine, J.D. (1988). Leukotriene B4 decreases the mechanical and thermal thresholds of C-fiber nociceptors in the hairy skin of the rat. *J. Neurophysiol.*, **60**, 438
26. Heppelmann, B., Schaible, H.-G. and Schmidt, R.F. (1985). Effects of prostaglandin E1 and E2 on the mechanosensitivity of group III afferents from normal and inflamed cat knee joints. In Fields. H.L., Dubner, R. and Cervero, F. (eds.) *Advances in Pain Research and Therapy*, pp. 91–101. (New York: Raven Press)
27. Khan, A.A., Raja, S.N., Meyer, R.A., Campbell, J.N. and Manning, D.C. (1988). C-fiber nociceptors in monkey are sensitized by bradykinin antagonists. *Soc. Neurosci. Abstr.*, **14**, 912
28. Perl, E.R., Kumazawa, T., Lynn, B. and Kenins, P. (1976). Sensitization of high threshold receptors with unmyelinated (C) afferent fibers. *Prog. Brain Res.*, **43**, 263–276
29. Cohen, R.H. and Perl, E.R. (1988). Chemical factors in the sensitization of cutaneous nociceptors. *Prog. Brain Res.*, **74**, 201–206
30. Diehl, B., Hoheisel, U. and Mense, S. (1988). Histological and neurophysiological changes induced by carrageenan in skeletal muscle of cat and rat. *Agents Actions*, **25**, 210–213
31. Guilbaud, G. and Iggo, A. (1985). The effect of lysine acetylsalicylate on joint capsule mechanoreceptors in rats with polyarthritis. *Exp. Brain Res.*, **61**, 164–168
32. Barasi, S. and Lynn, B. (1986). Effects of sympathetic stimulation on mechanoreceptive and nociceptive afferent units from the rabbit pinna. *Brain Res.*, **378**, 21–27
33. Roberts, W.J. and Elardo, S.M. (1985). Sympathetic activation of A-delta nociceptors. *Somatosensory Res.*, **3**, 33–44
34. Lynn, B. (1988). Neurogenic inflammation. *Skin Pharmacol.*, **1**, 217–224
35. Levine, J.D., Coderre, T.J. and Basbaum, A.I. (1988). The peripheral nervous system and the inflammatory process. In Dubner, R., Gebhart, G.F. and Bond, M.R. (eds.) *Proc. 5th World Congress on Pain*, pp. 33–43. (Amsterdam: Elsevier)
36. Lynn, B. (1984). The detection of injury and tissue damage. In Wall, P.D. and Melzack, R. (ed.) *Textbook of Pain*, pp. 19–33. (Edinburgh: Churchill Livingstone)
37. Schaible, H.-G. and Schmidt, R.F. (1988). Direct observation of the sensitization of articular afferents during an experimental arthritis. In Dubner, R., Gebhart, G.F. and Bond, M.R. (eds.) *Proceedings of the Vth World Congress on Pain*, pp. 44–50. (Amsterdam: Elsevier)

11

2

Intradiscal pressure changes and the clinician

Gunnar B.J. ANDERSSON

INTRODUCTION

Measurements of intradiscal pressures provide the most direct method of measuring loads on the lumbar spine. Following early examinations to measure disc expansions *in vitro*[10,19], Nachemson [12] proved that the disc was hydrostatic by measuring pressures while rotating a needle in the three principal directions of load. He estimated that the pressure in normal discs was about 1.3–1.6 times the applied compression load and increased linearly up to 2000 N. These findings were later confirmed by Tzivian and co-workers[21] who, however, found that the pressure response to compressive loads was non-linear in the higher load ranges.

Following these early measurements in which the load was applied in compression only, Berkson and co-workers[9] and Nachemson and co-workers[18] measured the intervertebral disc pressure under different external loading conditions. Pressure changes were comparatively small in torsion, extension and shear but quite large in compression, flexion and lateral bending. The relationship between the measured pressure and the externally applied load was found to decrease monotonically from about 2.5 at 100 N compression to 1.3 at 400 N compression. They concluded that pressure changes *in vivo* are mainly the result of compression loads.

IN VIVO MEASUREMENTS

In vivo measurements were first performed by Nachemson and Morris[16]. They measured pressures while subjects were standing, sitting, reclining, holding weights, performing a Valsalva manoeuver and wearing an inflatable corset. As illustrated in Table 2.1, the pressures when standing were 30% higher than when sitting, while pressures when reclining were 50% less than when sitting. The pressures were found to increase when the subjects performed the Valsalva manoeuver, while the use of an inflatable corset decreased the pressure. Nachemson subsequently performed specific studies of forward-leaning

12

postures[13,14]. These studies showed that when bending forward the pressure increased in proportion to the amount of forward flexion.

Table 2.1 Loads on the lumbar spine calculated from disc pressure (after ref.15)

Activity	Load (N)
Supine	300
Standing	700
Walking	850
Sitting (no support)	1000
Coughing	1100
Straining	1200
Laughing	1200
Bending 20°/holding 200 N	1850

In 1970, Nachemson and Elfstrom[15] published a comprehensive study of several common movements, manoeuvers and physical exercises. These pressure measurements were obtained using a piezoresistive semiconductor strain-guage needle that was smaller than the previously used needle and had an excellent dynamic response. A summary of main results is given in Table 2.1. One major conclusion from these studies was that isometrically performed physical exercises yielded significantly lower pressures than dynamic exercises (Figure 2.1).

Studies by Andersson[1] and co-workers[6,7] of sitting postures indicated the importance of various chair supports to the pressure within the lumbar discs, and therefore to the load on the lumbar spine. As illustrated by Figure 2.2, the pressure was found to increase when sitting unsupported in agreement with the previous results by Nachemson and Morris. When using a back support, however, the pressure was found to decrease both when the backrest was inclined backward and when a lumbar support was fitted to the backrest (Figure 2.3). When rising from a chair, pressure increases occurred up to more than twice the resting (sitting) pressure[4]. The use of arm support when rising was found to significantly reduce the maximum pressure measured.

Following these studies of sitting postures, Andersson, Ortengren and Nachemson[5] performed studies of different degrees of forward flexion and of holding different weights in defined angles of forward flexion (Figures 2.4 and 2.5). These studies indicated linear relationships between the angle of flexion and the disc pressure, and between the amount of external load and the disc pressure. Rotation of the trunk was found to increase the pressure further, particularly in postures of forward flexion.

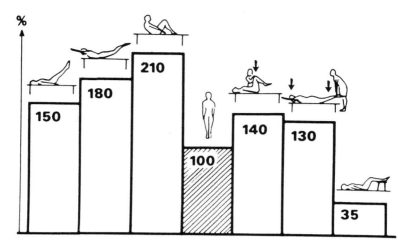

Figure 2.1 Disc pressure measurements obtained during physical exercises. Note the low pressures when isometric exercises are performed. (After ref. 15)

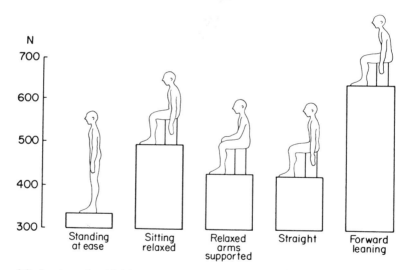

Figure 2.2 Load on the third lumbar disc (calculated from disc pressure measurements) when standing and sitting unsupported. (After ref. 1)

14

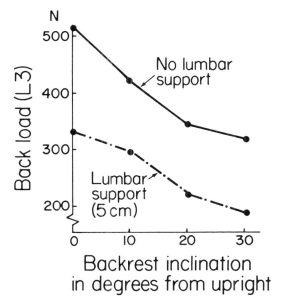

Figure 2.3 When a backrest is used, the load on the lumbar spine decreases the more the backrest is inclined. A lumbar support reduces the load further. (After ref. 7)

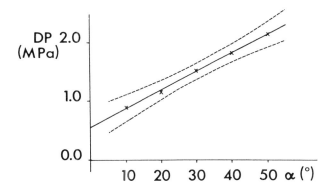

Figure 2.4 The disc pressure increases when the angle of flexion of the trunk increases. Measurements obtained when standing. (After ref. 5)

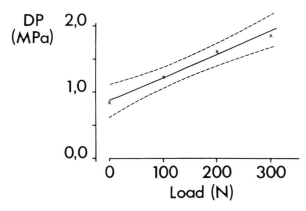

Figure 2.5 The disc pressure increases when an increased load is held by the hands. Measurements obtained at 30° of forward flexion. (After ref. 5)

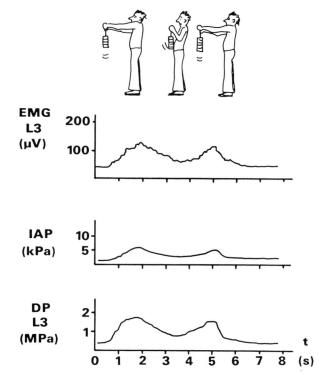

Figure 2.6 The disc pressure changes (DP L3) with a change in moment arm. The weight is lifted with straight arms, brought in close to the chest, and then out again. Myoelectric back muscle activity (EMG L3) and intra-abdominal pressures (IAP) were measured at the same time. (After ref. 3)

Studies of pulling and lifting have also been published[2,3]. When lifting, similar peak pressures were found regardless of whether the lift was performed using the back-lift technique or the leg-lift method, as long as the moment arm to the load was kept constant. The importance of the moment arm was also determined in these studies by moving the weight from far away, in toward the body and then out again (Figure 2.6). The use of the Valsalva manoeuver was not found to have a marked effect on the disc pressure when lifting, but did of course result in high intra-abdominal pressures.

Hein-Sorensen and co-workers[11] used disc pressure measurements to study post-traumatically paralysed patients, and developed a mobilization programme based on these studies. Quite vigorous activities can be permitted early after the injury.

The *in vivo* studies all indicated that the disc pressure responded to moments acting on the upper body in a predictable fashion. This lead to the development of a biomechanical model and to its validation using disc pressure[20]. In these studies, several tasks were performed under well-controlled conditions imposing compression loads on the spine up to about 2400 N. The intradiscal pressure was found to be highly correlated with the predicted spine compression (Figure 2.7). This lends credibility to the use of biomechanical models.

In addition to the previously mentioned study of physical therapy manoeuvers, disc pressure measurements have also been used to measure the mechanical effect of other treatment modalities. The effect of five different orthoses of three principal types was studied by Nachemson and co-workers[17]. Wearing a brace was found to significantly reduce the pressure in some situations, while it actually increased it in others (Table 2.2). None of the orthoses was found to be clearly superior. The best effect seemed to occur in forward-bending postures. Andersson, and co-workers[8] studied the effect of traction. Active traction (performed by the patients) resulted in an increase in pressure, while passive traction under some circumstances did result in a small reduction in pressure. A negative pressure was never recorded.

DISCUSSION

It is important to remember that the measurement of disc pressures is *not* a method of measuring back pain, but rather a method of indirectly measuring loads on the lumbar spine. This information can be used to improve workplaces, advise on safe work practices and leisure-time activities, and to determine the mechanical effects of different treatment methods.

Although intradiscal pressure measurement is the most direct and reliable method for assessing loads on the spine presently available, it has the disadvantage of being invasive and, therefore, is limited in use to laboratory settings. The risk of fracture of the needle precludes studies of large and rapid movements and the requirement of a hydrostatic disc medium limits the use of pressure measurements to studies of young healthy volunteers. The validation of biomechanical models lends support to their use in evaluating loads on the spine. In this way, spine loads can be predicted under circumstances in which the use of a measurement technique is prohibited or impractical.

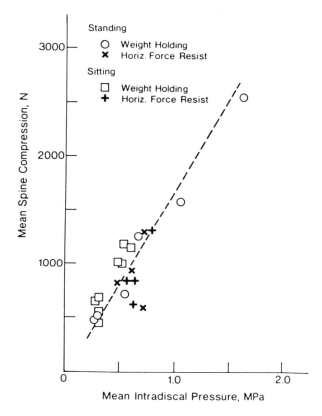

Figure 2.7 Correlation of measured disc pressures and calculated spine compression forces. An excellent agreement was obtained. (After ref. 20)

CONCLUSIONS

(1) The load on the lumbar spine is low when lying down, higher (but still low) when standing, and higher still when sitting without support.

(2) Forward bending increases the load on the spine in proportion to the angle of flexion.

(3)   Torsion increases the load further.

(4)   Forward bending and particularly twisting should be avoided.

(5)   When sitting, the chair should have a backrest with a lumbar support, and where applicable, armrests.

(6)   Isometric exercises are preferable in patients with acute low back pain.

(7)   The mechanical effect of a corset is moderate, occurring primarily in forward flexion.

(8)   When lifting, the trunk should be upright and the load held as close to the body as possible.

Table 2.2 Intradiscal pressures without orthoses and percentage of no-orthosis pressure with orthosis (from ref. 7)

Exercise	Pressure (kPa) no orthosis	Percentage of no-orthosis pressure		
		Camp	Raney	Brace
Relaxed standing	275	83	103	83
Resist flexion	685	104	108	106
Resist extension	690	83	90	84
Resist twisting	490	75	100	84
Resist lateral bending	570	102	104	95
Bending 30°/holding 80 N	1685	83	75	68

REFERENCES

1. Andersson, G.B.J. (1974). On myoelectric back muscle activity and lumbar disc pressure in sitting postures. *Thesis*, Goteborg, Gotab.
2. Andersson, G.B.J., Herberts, P. and Ortengren, R. (1976). Myoelectric back muscle activity in standardized lifting postures. In Komi, P.V. (ed.) *Biomechanics* **5-A**, pp. 520–529. (Baltimore: University Park Press)
3. Andersson, G.B.J., Ortengren, R. and Nachemson, A. (1976). Quantitative studies of back loads in lifting. *Spine*, **1**, 178–185
4. Andersson, G.B.J., Ortengren, R. and Nachemson, A. (1982). Disc pressure measurements when rising and sitting down on a chair. *Eng. Med.*, **11**, 189–190
5. Andersson, G.B.J., Ortengren, R. and Nachemson, A. (1977). Intradiscal pressure, intra-abdominal pressure and myoelectric back muscle activity related to posture and loading. *Clin. Orthop.*, **129**, 156–164
6. Andersson, G., Ortengren, R., Nachemson, A. and Elfstrom, G. (1974). Lumbar disc pressure and myoelectric back muscle activity during sitting. Part I: Studies on an experimental chair. *Scand. J. Rehabil. Med.*, **6**, 104–114
7. Andersson, G., Ortengren, R., Nachemson, A. and Elfstrom, G. (1974). Lumbar disc pressure and myoelectric back muscle activity during sitting. Part IV: Studies on a car driver's seat. *Scand. J. Rehabil. Med.*, **6**, 128–133

8. Andersson, G.B.J., Schultz, A.B. and Nachemson, A.L. (1985). Intervertebral disc pressure during traction. *Scand. J. Rehabil. Med. Suppl.*, **9**, 88–91
9. Berkson, M.H., Nachemson, A. and Schultz, A.B. (1979). Mechanical properties of human lumbar spine motion segments. Part II: Responses in compression and shear; influence of gross morphology. *J. Biomech. Eng.*, **101**, 53–57
10. Charnley, J. (1952). The imbibition of fluid as a cause of herniation of the nucleus pulposus. *Lancet*, **1**, 124
11. Hein-Sorensen, O., Elfstrom, G. and Nachemson, A. (1979). Disc pressure measurements in para- and tetraplegic patients. A study of mobilization and exercises in para- and tetraplegic patients. *Scand. J. Rehabil. Med.*, **11**, 1–11
12. Nachemson, A. (1960). Lumbar intradiscal pressure. *Acta Orthop. Scand.*, **43** (Suppl.), 1–104
13. Nachemson, A. (1963). The influence of spinal movements on the lumbar intradiscal pressure and on the tensile stresses in the annulus fibrosus. *Acta Orthop. Scand.*, **33**, 183–207
14. Nachemson, A. (1965). The effect of forward leaning on lumbar intradiscal pressure. *Acta Orthop. Scand.*, **35**, 314–328
15. Nachemson, A. and Elfstrom, G. (1970). Intravital dynamic pressure measurements in lumbar discs. A study of common movements, maneuvres and exercises. *Scand. J. Rehabil. Med.*, **1** (Suppl.), 1–40
16. Nachemson, A. and Morris, J. (1964). In vivo measurements of intradiscal pressure. *J. Bone Joint Surg.*, **46-A**, 1077–1092
17. Nachemson, A., Schultz, A. and Andersson, G.B.J. (1983). Mechanical effectiveness studies of lumbar orthoses. *Scand. J. Rehabil. Med.*, Suppl. **9**, 139–149
18. Nachemson, A., Schultz, A.B. and Berkson, M.H. (1979). Mechanical properties of human lumbar spine motion segments. Influences of age, sex, disc level and degeneration. *Spine*, **4**, 1–8
19. Petter, C.K. (1933). Methods of measuring the pressure of the intervertebral disc. *J. Bone Joint Surg.*, **15**, 365
20. Schultz, A.B., Andersson, G.B.J., Ortengren, R., Nachemson, A. and Haderspeck, K. (1982). Loads on the lumbar spine: Validation of a biomechanical analysis by measurements of intradiscal pressures and myoelectric signals. *J. Bone Joint Surg.*, **64A**, 713–720
21. Tzivian, I.L., Rayhinstein, V.H., Mosolova, M.D. and Ovseychik, J.G. (1970). Mechanical properties of the nucleus pulposus of the lumbar intervertebral discs. *Ortopedija Traumatologija*, **1**, 55 (in Russian)

3
Electromyography – its significance to the manipulator

John V. BASMAJIAN

Controversy persists about the role of paravertebral muscles both in normal kinesiology and in the aetiology and management of back programmes. However, electromyography reveals the true state of affairs ignored by those who prefer to build their clinical hypotheses on nineteenth-century conjecture. Modern research with both intramuscular and surface electrodes clearly defines the levels of activity in normal and painful and/or spasming muscles, and it offers more surprises than comfort to clinicians who have failed to keep informed. The need for research and validation is great for any treatments that bear a cost of money, time and human hopes. Because many of the indications for manipulation are often couched in exotic language usually unknown to the medical scientist, the problem of research becomes almost – but not completely – impossible. In fact, the frequent use of glib, fallacious or irrelevant pathomechanics to the medical problem may pose a threat that is greater to progress in research than an absence of truly scientific explanations.

PLACEBO EFFECTS

The old definition of placebos was 'anything given to please the patient with a strong suggestion that the inert substance given has a powerful therapeutic effect'. The therapist or physician knew that the treatment was inert but gave a strong suggestion that it was an effective treatment, possibly even a powerful treatment. When the patient recovered from the symptom rapidly, apparently as a result of the treatment, then it was said that a 'placebo response' had occurred. My more useful and contemporary definition of the placebo response would be 'a response in a conscious patient to the treatment of a symptom, sign, disease and/or condition when there is no scientific basis in demonstrated fact that the treatment has a specific effect'. It is not deception; it is a non-specific effect.

Even though much of what physicians did for many centuries is now known to

21

be absolutely contrary to physiology and scientific management, nevertheless they were credited with many cures and substantial improvements due to non-specific effects. Much of what they did was inert by scientific standards, and yet it worked! Intensive research to determine the specific effects of everything we do is essential. While we may advocate and admire some non-specific effects, science and plain honesty demand that we learn as much about specific effects as possible.

Physical agents other than ingested chemicals might have the same influence as a placebo response, as difficult as it may be for those in manual medicine to accept. In my research study on the treatment of back problems[1], I found the electronic gear of the recording devices (inserted electrodes, EMG equipment, various electronic devices and a computer) raised the placebo response in almost 200 patients with back problems from the usual 30% (or so) for sugar pills to about 50%.

The therapist's role

The therapist – whether a physical therapist, manual therapist, or physician – is vital. It is the human being, surrounded by the mystique of a profession, who has the strongest influence. If that therapist is knowledgeable about the procedures employed, is confident, and, above all, comes into close contact with the patient, success of almost any treatment occurs in 30–50% of patients. If the therapist touches and manipulates the patient with confidence, this greatly enhances the effectiveness, regardless of whether the technique is carried out accurately. Hence, many patients will recover from disabilities of the musculoskeletal system by having an 'improper' procedure rather than the 'proper' one advocated by some charismatic healer. It does not seem to matter whether transcutaneous electrical nerve stimulation or acupuncture are done absolutely 'correctly' – a large number of patients will achieve substantial success or cure. The important element seems to be a close contact between the patient and the therapist. This is at least as important as the specific effect of the treatment.

NORMATIVE DATA

Floyd and Silver[2] examined the function of the erector spinae in certain postures and movements and during weight-lifting. They used both surface and confirmatory needle electrodes for the thoracolumbar parts of the erector spinae. Posture was recorded by photography, direct measurements and radiography.

Most subjects standing in a relaxed erect posture showed a 'low level of discharge' in the erector spinae. Small adjustments of the position of the head, shoulders or hands could be made that would abolish the activity of the muscle,

22

i.e. an equilibrium or balance could be achieved.

From the easy upright posture, Floyd and Silver found that extension (hypertension) of the trunk is initiated, as a rule, by a short burst of activity.

While standing upright, flexion of the trunk to one side is accompanied by activity of the erector spinae of the opposite side, i.e. the muscle is not a prime mover but an 'antagonist'. However, if the back is already arched in extension (hypertension), not even this sort of activity occurs.

Floyd and Silver state that erectores spinae contract (apparently vigorously) during coughing and straining. This occurs even in the midst of their normal silence, whether the subject is erect or 'full-flexed'. The clinical implications of this last observation have not been, from our point of view, adequately explored by orthopaedic specialists.

In the initial stages of flexion of the trunk in bending forward, the movement is controlled by the intrinsic muscles of the back. The ligaments take over and are quite sufficient in the fully flexed position. A reflex inhibitory mechanism explains the complete relaxation of erector spinae in full flexion. Finally, they suggested that this relaxation of the muscle and the dependence on the ligaments, including the intervertebral disc, had implicit dangers, including injuries to the disc.

With the subject standing, the activity in erector spinae ceases earlier during forward bending than it does when the subject is seated. In some patients they found complete relaxation in the sitting but not the standing posture.

Finally, Floyd and Silver reported that the erector spinae remained relaxed during the initial movement of lifting weights of up to 28.5 kg (56 lb). They proved that it is movement at the hip joint that accounts for the earliest phase of apparent extension of the trunk. However, the ligaments of the back were required to carry the added weight without help from the adjacent muscles. Most of these findings were confirmed by Morris et al.[3] and Waters and Morris[4], who investigated the activity of different layers and parts of the spinal musculature – iliocostalis in the thoracic and lumbar parts, longissimus and rotatores in the region of the 9th and 10th ribs, and multifidus abreast of the 5th lumbar spine.

During the performance of various trunk movements, muscles showed patterns of activity that clearly showed two functions – sometimes they initiate movement and at other times they stabilize the trunk. Almost all the movements recruit all the muscles of the back in a variety of patterns, although the predominance of certain muscles is also obvious.

In compound movements, when subjects are not trying to relax, there is constantly more activity than when the movement is carried out deliberately and with conscious effort to avoid unnecessary activity of muscles. Complete relaxation and lower levels of contraction are the 'ideal' rather than the rule for normal bending movements. Morris et al. found that muscles that might be expected to return the spine to the vertical position often remain quiet; they suggest that such factors as ligaments and passive muscle elasticity play an important role.

In almost all vigorous exercises performed from the orthograde position, Pauly[5] found that the most active muscle is spinalis; next in order is longissimus, and least active is iliocostalis lumborum. Nevertheless, all three muscles and the main mass of erector spinae act powerfully during strong arching of the back in the prone posture. During push-ups, there is considerable individual variation but, typically, the lower back muscles remain relaxed.

Deep muscles

Donisch and Basmajian[6] investigated the deep layers of the transversospinal muscles in 25 healthy subjects, with bipolar wire electrodes inserted bilaterally at the level of the sixth thoracic and the third lumbar spinous processes. Activity was registered simultaneously in sitting and standing, and during movements while in these positions. The same muscle group displayed different patterns of activity in the thoracic, as compared to the lumbar level. Variations in the pattern of activity during forward flexion, extension, and axial rotation suggest that the transversospinal muscles adjust the motion between individual vertebrae. The experimental evidence confirms the anatomical hypothesis that the multifidi are stabilizers rather than prime movers of the whole vertebral column.

In their efforts to relate paravertebral muscle function to disc pressures, Andersson et al.[7] found that the amplitude of the EMG signal and pressure increased both with angles of forward flexion and with increasing static loads in flexion. During asymmetric loading, pressure values and myoelectric activity increased, being greater on the contralateral side of the lumbar region and ipsilateral side of the thoracic region. The disc pressure, intra-abdominal pressure, and semi-integrated rectified EMG signal were higher throughout when the trunk was loaded in rotation, rather than in lateral flexion.

Forward flexion in sitting and standing positions

Donisch and Basmajian found spontaneous electrical silence of the lumbar muscles in extreme flexion in most subjects, but only half of them showed spontaneous inactivity of their thoracic muscles in both seated and standing postures.

During the Valsalva manoeuver with increased intrathoracic and abdominal pressure while holding a sandbag of 11.25 kg, all thoracic and a number of lumbar muscles showed activity instead of electrical silence. This might be explained partly by the fact that most subjects were no longer in extreme flexion and might have reached the 'critical point' of activity.

Kumar's study[8] clarified some of the physiological responses to weight-lifting. A weight of 10 kg was lifted by 11 normal male volunteers (mean age 34.2 years) from ground to knee, hip, and shoulder levels in the sagittal, lateral, and oblique planes. During these lifting manoeuvers, intra-abdominal pressure was measured by telemetry, and the activity of erector spinae and external obliques were recorded by electromyography. The values obtained for peak and sustained intra-abdominal pressure and the averaged electromyographic activities of erectores spinae and external obliques were subjected to analysis of variance and correlation analysis. A significant difference between the responses in these three planes was found: the sagittal plane activities evoke least response. Intra-abdominal pressures, erector spinae activity, and the external oblique activity were highly significantly correlated in each of the three planes.

Axial trunk rotation

In the Donisch–Basmajian experiment, all subjects showed bilateral activity in the thoracic level; in more than half, this activity did not appear to be related to the direction of rotatory movement. In the lumbar region the muscular activity seemed more often to support the theory of rotatory function. On the other hand, the position of articular facets in relation to the direction of muscle pull casts doubt on the anatomical feasibility of such a function.

Perhaps the designation of specific muscular function is almost impossible in the back, where we have a complex arrangement of muscle bundles acting on a multitude of equally complex joints. Those who insist on finding prime movers, antagonists, and synergists in the genuine musculature of the back will be always disappointed.

Asymmetry

There are some differences in activity of the transversospinal muscles at the same levels. This asymmetrical activity occurred during quiet sitting and standing but was also noted with movements in the sagittal plane. Wolf and Basmajian[9] and Wolf et al.[10] assembled and analysed quantified lumbar EMG data correlating normal back movements with the EMG activity in 121 adult subjects who reported no history of low-back discomfort. All results in relation to the mechanical advantage, centre and line of gravity, and the possible axis of movement confirm the idea that the transversospinal muscles act as dynamic ligaments[11,12]. These adjust small movements between individual vertebrae, while movements of the vertebral column are probably performed by muscles with better leverage and mechanical advantage.

Spasms

My EMG studies have demonstrated a profound reduction of low-back and cervical EMG activity during painful muscle spasms[1]. With clinical improvement, myoelectric activity increases to normal during prescribed stressful movements. A painful back inhibits muscular activity.

REFERENCES

1. Basmajian, J.V. (1978). Cyclobenzaprine hydrochloride effect on skeletal muscle spasm in the lumbar region and neck: two double-blind controlled clinical and laboratory studies. *Arch. Rehabil. Med. Rehabil.*, **59**, 58–63
2. Floyd, W.F. and Silver, P.H.S. (1955). The function of the erectores spinae muscles in certain movements and postures in men. *J. Physiol.*, **129**, 184–203
3. Morris, J.M., Benner, G. and Lucus, D.B. (1962). An electromyographic study of the intrinsic muscles of the back in men. *J. Anat.*, **96**, 509–520
4. Waters, R.L. and Morris, J.M. (1972). Electrical activity of muscles of the trunk during walking. *J. Anat.*, **111**, 191–199
5. Pauly, J.E. (1966). An electromyographic analysis of certain movements and exercises. Part I. Some deep muscles of the back. *Anat. Rec.*, **155**, 223–234
6. Donisch, E.W. and Basmajian, J.V. (1972). Electromyography of deep back muscles in men. *Am. J. Anat.*, **133**, 25–36
7. Andersson, J.G., Ortengren, R., Nachemson, A.L., Elfstrom, G. and Broman, H. (1975). The sitting posture: an electromyographic and discometric study. *Orthop. Clin. N. Am.*, **6**, 105–120
8. Kumar, S. (1980). Physiologic responses to weight lifting in different planes. *Ergonomics*, **23**, 987–993
9. Wolf, S.L. and Basmajian, J.V. (1980). Assessment of paraspinal electromyographic activity in normal subjects and in chronic back pain patients using muscle biofeedback device. In: Amussen, E. and Jørgensen, K. (eds.) *Biomechanics VI-B.* (Baltimore: University Park Press)
10. Wolf, S.L., Basmajian, J.V., Russe, C.T.C. and Kutner, M. (1979). Normative data in low back mobility and activity levels: implications for neuromuscular re-education. *Am. J. Phys. Med.*, **58**, 217–229
11. Basmajian, J.V. (1989). *Muscles and Movements: A Basis for Human Kinesiology* (Melbourne, Fl.: Robert Krieger)
12. Basmajian, J.V. and De Luca, C.J. (1985). *Muscles Alive: Their Functions Revealed by Electromyography, 5th Edn.* (Baltimore: Williams & Wilkins)

4
The clinical testing of pain

Anthony E. READING

Evaluation of the patient in pain requires an appreciation of pain mechanisms. Pain comes about via stimulation of a noxious nature, whereby the sensation is transmitted from nerve cell to nerve cell via a complex electrochemical process, then to the spinal cord and ultimately to the brain. These messages may be blocked, superseded or occasionally lost. Such models work reasonably well for acute pain, although there are conditions involving body damage where there is no pain stimulus at all and others where pain stimuli are fired without being registered cortically. As a result, models of pain as a sensation have serious deficiencies and it is now accepted that pain, whether acute or chronic, is a complex experience, with evidence confirming that it involves variation on several dimensions, depending upon ever-changing states, continuously influenced by a multitude of extrinsic and intrinsic stimuli.

Attempting to define pain as psychogenic or organic becomes academic, because psychological factors may exert a lesser or greater role irrespective of the organic pathology. A hierarchical model of pain, consisting of four levels, has been described: namely, nociception, sensation, suffering and behaviour. Such a model discards the notion of a straightforward relationship between the amount of noxious input and pain experience and is able to accommodate the possibility of pain behaviour being present, possibly maintained by the reinforcement contingencies available in the patient's social or physical environment, even when the nociceptive input has become quiescent.

This four-level model of pain distinguishes pain sensation from suffering, although there is an implicit assumption that the greater the pain the more it is believed to cause suffering. However, there may be some exceptions to this. The temporal dimension may be important, in that less suffering may arise from pains that are known to be short-lived or time-limited. Conversely, pains that are associated with dire consequences, those accompanied by uncertainty as to their cause, or fear as to being uncontrollable, are likely to give rise to increased suffering. Melzack et al.[13] illustrated the way in which individuals in acute pain assume that it will continue to increase, thereby giving rise to increasing levels of anxiety. It follows therefore, that under certain circumstances, by changing the individual's degree of control, removing uncertainty or other such interventions, suffering may be relieved, despite continued pain. However, pain and suffering tend to evoke comparable behaviours, leading to a difficulty in differentiating pain behaviours from suffering behaviours.

Similarly, with the persistence of pain over time, its potential to influence behaviour becomes great. It is important to appreciate that pain behaviours may be occurring for reasons other than in response to nociceptive input, possibly maintained by the reinforcement contingencies in the environment. Similarly, discrepancies may exist between what people say and what they do. Therefore, measurement in all settings, and in particular in the study of chronic conditions, cannot rely solely on verbal statements. As a result, behavioural indicators need to be assessed in parallel with verbal reports and any discrepancies pursued in order both to understand controlling factors and to delineate the various routes of expression. Actions may be generally a more reliable reflection of an individual's functioning and are always more amenable to independent study.

Such a framework demonstrates the limitations imposed by the biomedical model of disease. Such a model relies upon the identification of causal mechanisms of disease with molecular biology as its basic scientific discipline. This view of disease, suggests the host or recipient as a passive victim with little opportunity for control. While this system has heuristic and practical value for acute illness, it has many limitations when applied to chronic diseases, because their causes may be multifactorial. Psychological and behavioural factors may affect the onset, course and outcome of disease through a number of mechansims. The course and outcome of disease may be influenced by a host of psychological factors that affect recovery through interfering with steps necessary for rehabilitation, such as reluctance to engage in exercises or take medications, or psychological states that focus on loss and lead to a progressive withdrawal of functioning.

It is evident, therefore, that the manifestations, course and outcome of disease is influenced by a variety of individual differences that involve both constitutional and psychosocial processes. The latter involve personality differences, psychological state and reinforcement contingencies. These may act both as risk factors, in that when present they increase the likelihood of an acute condition becoming chronic, as well as affect the course of a disease once established. As a result of these limitations, the biomedical model has evolved into a biopsychosocial framework, recognizing that the outcome of a disease process is dependent upon both biological as well as psychosocial processes. Such a framework presents a challenge from the standpoint of measurement. It indicates the necessity of our assessments reflecting functioning in each of the areas of sensation, suffering and behaviour.

From a measurement standpoint, it is necessary to draw a distinction between acute and chronic pain because their presentation, impact and management will differ. Acute pain is defined as pain arising in response to an acute event, such as infection, trauma and surgery, and by definition it runs a finite time course. This pain requires immediate treatment, whether by the individuals in pain themselves or by medical agencies, and will be selflimiting or will resolve once the underlying pathology has been treated. Chronic pain refers to pain that is enduring, refractory to medical treatment and shows little change in status. The goals of management have changed from eradicating the problem to assisting the patient in making the best possible adjustment to the condition. Pain may persist under a number of conditions. It may be continuous or occur intermittently. Intermittent pain may vary as a function of endogenous factors, such as pain related to the female menstrual cycle, or affected by exogenous factors, such as activity. It may also occur in the absence of obvious precipitants or pattern. Both continuous and intermittent pain may be associated with obvious pathology, as in the case of cancer, or be associated with benign disease or disease that is not readily identifiable.

The distinction between acute and chronic pain is important from a number of reasons. One is the nature of treatment provided, in that the study of pain behaviour in chronic conditions has demonstrated that the principles of management for acute pain may be contraindicated for pain problems that persist. Examples consist of p.r.n. medication, withdrawal from activities and social attention being given contingent on the pain report. All of these may entrench the individual even further in the sick role, remove them from potential sources of distraction, thereby amplifying attention on the pain. For the chronic-pain patient, time-contingent medication, distraction from pain and contingent attention on non-pain behaviour may be more effective and appropriate. A second reason is the emphasis given to the different aspects of the pain under study. In acute conditions, there has been greater emphasis given to subjective report, whereas the emphasis in the case of chronic pain may be on behaviour: what the person is able to do, as well as their report of what it feels like while doing it. This is not to imply that individuals in acute pain are more accurate reporters of their experience, rather it reflects the different treatment focus. In the chronic condition, the emphasis may be on behaviour change, becaues the patient's pain report may have been influenced by the prevailing reinforcement contingencies. This means that the report of pain may be amplified by the attention that it demands.

Within a measurement framework, a similar distinction may be drawn between three main components or response channels: subjective report of sensation, behaviour and concomitant suffering. Nociception or physiological measures will not be discussed. With the exception of verbal report, taken to reflect subjective experience, the content of these responses are not unique to pain, since their meaning is inferred from the context in which they occur. By drawing a distinction between the different components of the pain experience, the question of the level of association or concordance among them is introduced. Early thinking proposed a direct, one-to-one relationship between the level of sensory input, however defined, and the amount of pain expressed subjectively and behaviourally. Such a view assumed concordance between subjective processing and expression of pain, as well as behavioural manifestations. This model has been generally discarded to be replaced by a dynamic view, accepting that concordance will vary to differing degrees, depending upon the circumstances. In the light of these considerations, assessment methods in each of these areas will be considered in turn.

MEASUREMENT: SENSORY EXPERIENCE

Pain is a private experience, not open to verification by another. There are no methodologies for directly measuring pain because pain is inherently a subjective, personal experience. In acute pain settings, attempts at measurement have met with some success, in terms of being able to establish reliability and validity. Most notably, the use of cross-modality matching methods have shown that volunteers can reliably use verbal descriptor scales to report both pain arising from clinical procedures and experimentally induced pain[3], and differential patterns of response have corresponded to the pharmacological properties of drugs studied[4,5]. Less consistency has been found in magnitude estimation judgements obtained from chronic pain patients[19]. While acute pain studies may be able to focus on a narrow range of measures concerned with pain, it is evident that chronic pain is a more complex entity, with additional social and psychological influences, requiring a multidimensional approach to measurement.

No satisfactory diagnostic test or procedure exists that is capable of establishing the extent or quality of pain experienced by patients. As Lasagna stated[10]: 'The investigator who would study pain is at the mercy of the patient, upon whose ability and willingness to communicate he is dependent'. Advances in diagnostic tests and analgesic efficacy have enabled acute pain to be diagnosed and treated. In chronic pain, well-defined causes are seldom isolated. In such cases it is necessary to refrain from invoking concepts of conversion hysteria, psychogenic pain, depressive equivalents or malingering, or recommend psychiatric treatment. It is necessary to acknowledge there can be real psychological and physical events that do interact.

Assessing the subjective report of pain provides important information and is of interest, providing this is not relied upon in isolation, nor is assumed to be a literal index of pain state. In addition to semantic and linguistic difficulties, implicit personalities, theories and reinforcement contingencies, numerous other factors operate to distort and confound the information obtained by self-report.

Specific problems with self-report methods include the following:
(a) They must be subject to response bias or falsification.
(b) The report of pain may not be uniformly related to the severity of the noxious input.
(c) Verbal report may be discordant with other indices.
(d) Assessments may have a reactive effect – in terms of sensitizing the patient to the pain and so affecting the rating given.

These considerations notwithstanding, self-report remains the most acceptable means of assessing functioning in population-based research. Subjective report of pain experience may reflect an overall evaluation, drawing upon processing of sensory input, the accompanying level of distress and resultant emotional state, as well as motivational factors. The clinical interview is a vital component of the evaluation. It should include a description of the current problem and background, the intensity, duration, frequency, antecedents and consequences of the target behaviour, avoidance and escape behaviours, body-image concerns, expectations and goals of treatment[2], as well as resources and assets. Related problems such as substance or medication abuse, depression, anxiety, marital, social and occupational functioning should be addressed.

Rating scales have been used in order to assess the intensity of pain. These vary from category scales, visual analogue scales, to more elaborate descriptor scales, such as the McGill Pain Questionnaire[12]. A common distinction is between ratings of sensation and unpleasantness[4]. An extension of self-ratings is to require patients to complete diary cards, on which pain occurrence, intensity and duration may be rated. Such methods have been used extensively in the study of headache, but less commonly reported in other pain types. One problem with such scales, over and above that of the failure to complete them altogether, is the need to control for the possibility that they may be completed retrospectively. Requiring patients to rate their pain at specified times, such as meal times, may decrease the likelihood of retrospective reporting. Even in the absence of any objective criteria by which to judge these self-reports, it may be reasonable to assume that daily records kept on a prospective basis would be less subject to the distortions of memory and therefore more accurate than periodic retrospective reports, suggesting a degree of information loss using retrospective methods.

MEASUREMENT: BEHAVIOUR

It is evident that the patient in pain will engage in behaviour indicative of this state, which is potentially observable and therefore amenable to objective measurement strategies. This category of assessment will be discussed, even though it is recognized that such measures will rarely be feasible in epidemiologic research. Three categories of pain behaviour may be distinguished: (a) somatic interventions, such as taking medication, seeking surgery or nerve blocks; (b) impaired functioning in terms of reduced motility or range of movement, avoidance of occupational commitments or impaired personal relationships; and (c) pain complaints in the form of moaning, contortions or facial expressions. For example, from a behavioural standpoint, the content of verbal expressions would be ignored but recording of their cumulative frequency per unit of time would be made. Such indices lend themselves to well-established methods of measurement, in terms of recording the number of sit-ups that can be performed or the number of drugs taken, with recently reported attempts to automate the recording of such activity levels. The importance of direct behavioural counts of this kind has been demonstrated in a series of studies by Fordyce[1]. He showed that performance in a rehabilitation setting was influenced by reinforcement contingencies, as opposed to nociceptive input. This emerged from studies demonstrating that numbers of repetitions on exercise tasks were not randomly distributed, but were more likely to cluster around multiples of 5 or 10, and that when rehabilitation behaviours increased, pain complaint decreased, which is the opposite of expectations, had pain complaint been directly related to nociceptive input.

While reference may be made to behavioural records, it is necessary to acknowledge that many studies have collected information on behavioural parameters only indirectly, through patient self-report, rather than by direct observation. The emphasis in such approaches has been to define in a very clear way the behaviour under study. The differences between this and subjective report is that, with the latter, patients are asked to evaluate their subjective experience, while with the former they are asked to indicate whether a particular behaviour has occurred or not. Studies have examined the correspondence between self-reported activity levels, or medication use and independent report. Kremer et al.[9] studied four patients and compared staff and patient logs of physical activity and social behaviour. While the results were variable, some patients did report significantly lower levels of physical activity and social behaviour than observed by staff, despite reporting decreased levels of pain. Similarly, Ready et al.[16] studied pain medication use prior to hospital admission, by self-report, and compared this to medication requirement upon hospital-ization. The trend, as a whole, was for patients to report less narcotic and sedative intake prior to admission than actually requested during hospitalization.

Objective measurements can be obtained by direct observation of behaviour. This endeavours to reduce subjectivity in obtaining a functional assessment by standardizing instructions and scoring. Among the commonly reported variables are: activity; measure of the amount of time spent standing, sitting or reclining; sleep pattern; sexual activity; performance on a specified task such as joint movement, walking, stair climbing or sit-ups; medication demand or intake; food intake; normal household activities such as meal preparation and gardening; and engagement in recreational activities. Most measures can be reduced to frequency or range counts. Keefe and Block[6] attempted to validate a number of behaviours (guarded movement, bracing, rubbing, grimacing and sighing) during observation of assignments undertaken by low back pain patients. They found these indices could be reliably observed and their frequency correlated with pain ratings. The discriminant validity of these indices was investigated by comparing frequency in low back pain patients with a group of normal controls and a group of depressed psychiatric patients. The pain behaviours were found to be distinctive for the low back pain group.

Keefe *et al.*[7] have extended their behavioural evaluations of pain to samples of head and neck cancer patients and osteoarthritic patients. In the former study, they found behavioural measures taken before treatment to be highly predictive of behavioural dysfunction scores at completion of the cancer treatment. Naliboff *et al.*[14] described a comprehensive functional evaluation for low back pain patients. This included measures from four domains: physical abilities, level of activities, psychological adjustment and pain perceptions. Their analysis demonstrated a strong relationship between objective disability and psychological and psychosocial adjustment but little relationship between level of pain and other disability variables.

Although it is ideal to include an observational or functional assessment, this may not always be possible. An alternative is to assess functioning via the use of specific, behaviourally referenced self-report questions that specify a number of tasks or activities. Such questions need to emphasize what the respondent does, rather than their evaluation of discomfort or their belief as to what they could do. Similarly, a behavioural account of pain-management methods currently and formerly being utilized can be obtained in this way. Even though ongoing diaries may not be feasible, a behavioural review can be made of the preceeding 24 hours, as a representative time sample of functioning. Wherever possible, direct functional and observational assessment during a number of specified tasks is desirable.

MEASUREMENT: SUFFERING

It is evident that chronic pain can only be understood by assessing the emotional, familial and socio-economic context in which it is being experienced and expressed. Understanding individual differences may help to address the question of why pain persists or becomes so debilitating in some cases but not in others. In the absence of premorbid measures, it is difficult to distinguish between changes resulting from the disability and those that were pre-existing. A further distinction can be drawn between changes resulting from disability in general, in other words, disruption in functioning resulting from chronic conditions, compared with those unique to a pain problem.

To return to the four-level model of pain presented earlier, it is evident that the subjective report of pain may reflect processing of information at any of these levels. It may be dominated by sensation or the degree of suffering or be a reflection or response to the limitations in functioning that have become established. Between the processing of sensory input and its expression via complaints and behaviour is an appraisal stage that reflects numerous influences. It is at this point that distorting processes may operate. These distorting influences, or individual differences, may operate as pre-existing risk factors, in that if pain develops they predispose towards impaired recovery or entrenchment in the sick role. These include the following:

Personality. Objective personality measures have been used extensively with chronic pain patients, in order to describe the type and severity of psychological disturbance, as well as to predict the treatment outcome. The results indicate that chronic pain patients exhibit increased emotional disturbance when compared to controls, a medical control group or an acute pain group. Chronic pain patients typically show elevations on scales 1, 2 and 3 of the MMPI. Naliboff et al.[15] compared chronic back pain patients and migraine patients with two other patient groups (hypertensive and diabetic patients). The results showed that in general, the MMPI pain group subscale elevations could be accounted for by individual self-rated functional limitations. They did not support attempts at finding a low back pain or chronic pain personality profile, as distinct from the emotional disturbances associated with chronic limitations and disruption of activity.

Constitutional differences affect both the processing of sensory information (in terms of threshold levels) and, perhaps more significantly, the expression or manifestation of pain behaviour. Personality may have other contributions in terms of influencing conditionability, in that pain sensation may become established as a conditioned response to triggering or eliciting stimuli. Additionally, personality may affect the coping styles habitually used by the individuals, with certain constitutional factors, such as high neuroticism, predisposing toward less adaptive coping styles.

Mood. A number of studies have found depression to be common in chronic pain patients[11]. Depression appears to be a risk factor for impaired response to treatment for chronic pain and antidepressant medication may decrease pain in many patients. Fordyce has suggested that depression may develop and persist when the patient's customary reinforcing activities are disrupted because of pain.

Pain threshold and tolerance will be affected by mood, with the relationship being bidirectional in that pain may intensify dysphoric feelings, either directly or indirectly through a withdrawal from reinforcing and rewarding activities and stimuli. Mood will also influence cognitive processing, with depressed mood associated with greater accessibility of negative cognitions and memories. These distorting influences may affect selection of behavioural responses as well as influence future perception. Depression has been associated with an attributional framework emphasizing global, stable and external attributions. Such appraisals are likely to magnify further the individual's distress and suffering.

Reinforcement. Although verbal processing and report may be reinforced directly through contingent attention, pain report may reflect behaviour, in that the individuals may evaluate pain in terms of what they can do, which then has an effect on how they feel. Behaviour may be influenced by reinforcement contingencies and at a secondary level, determine subjective report.

Coping style. Recent attention has been given to intrapersonal resources in terms of ways of coping and the possibility of stable individual differences in coping styles. There have been attempts to survey systematically ways of coping with pain amongst different chronic pain populations[17]. Research in other settings has emphasized the individual difference of hardiness made up of the dimensions of control, involvement, and commitment.

Stress. Related to coping style or appraisal may be the concomitant level of stress, as indexed by exposure to stressors or sources of stress. The importance of emotions and pain has emerged from surveys in which a higher prevalence of back pain has been found in those who lost a spouse through divorce, death or separation within the previous year. Back pain has also been associated with increased work stress. Social climate has also been associated with pain, in that spouses of chronic pain patients have been shown to have higher levels of psychological distress.

CONCLUSIONS

Pain assessment is a multidimensional enterprise. There needs to be attention to the patient's subjective experience, behaviour, functioning and the psychosocial context. Multidimensional assessment approaches have been described (e.g. Kerns *et al.*[8], Turk *et al.*[18]). Desynchrony between different dimensions need not be taken as invalidating measures but rather as affording important diagnostic information. Systematic information permits the practitioner to treat the different components and to chart progress on each of the target dimensions under study.

REFERENCES

1. Fordyce, W.E. (1976). *Behavioural Methods for Chronic Pain and Illness*. (St Louis: Mosby)
2. Gotestam, K.G. and Linton, S.J. (1985). Pain. In Hersen, M. and Bellack, A.S. (eds.) *Handbook of Clinical Behaviour Therapy with Adults*, pp. 353–379. (New York: Plenum Press)
3. Gracely, R.H. (1983). Ideal properties of pain assessment. In Melzack, R. (ed.) *Pain Measurement*. (New York: Raven Press)
4. Gracely, R.H. and Dubner, R. (1987). Reliability and validity of verbal description of scales of painfulness. *Pain*, **29**, 175–185
5. Gracely, R.H., McGrath, P. and Dubner, R. (1979). Narcotic analgesia: fentanyl reduces the intensity but not the unpleasantness of painful tooth pulp sensation. *Science*, **203**, 1361–1379
6. Keefe, F.J. and Block, A.R. (1982). Development of an observation method for assessing pain behaviour in chronic low back pain patients. *Behav. Ther.*, **13**, 363–375
7. Keefe, F.J., Brantley, A., Manuel, E. and Crisson, J.E. (1985). Behavioural measures of head and neck cancer pain. *Pain*, **23**, 327–336
8. Kerns, R.D., Turk, D.C. and Rudy, T.E. (1985). The West Haven–Yale Multidimensional Pain Inventory (WHYMPI). *Pain*, **23**, 345–356
9. Kremer, E.F., Block, A. and Gaylor, M.S. (1981). Behavioural approaches to treatment of chronic pain: the inaccuracy of patient self-report measures. *Arch. Phys. Med. Rehabil.*, **62**, 188–191

10. Lasagna, L. (1960). Clinical measurement of pain. *Ann. N.Y. Acad. Sci.*, **86**, 28–37
11. Magni, G. (1987). On the relationship between chronic pain and depression when there is no organic lesion. *Pain*, **31**, 1–21
12. Melzack, R. (1975). The McGill Pain Questionnaire: Major properties and scoring methods. *Pain*, **1**, 277–299
13. Melzack, L., Weisz, A.Z. and Spague, L.T. (1963). Strategems for controlling pain: contributions of auditory stimulation and suggestion. *Exp. Neurol.*, **8**, 239–247
14. Naliboff, B.D., Cohen, M.J., Swanson, G.A., Bonebakker, A.D. and McArthur, D.L. (1985). Comprehensive assessment of chronic low back pain patients and controls: physical abilities, level of activity, psychological adjustment and pain perception. *Pain*, **23**, 121–134
15. Naliboff, B.D., Cohen, M.J. and Yellen, A.N. (1982). Does the MMPI differentiate chronic illness from chronic pain? *Pain*, **13**, 333–361
16. Ready, L.B., Sarkis, E. and Turner, S.A. (1982). Self-reported versus actual use of medications in chronic pain patients. *Pain*, **12**, 285–294
17. Rosenstiel, A.K. and Keefe, F.J. (1983). The use of coping strategies in chronic low back pain patients: Relationship to patient characteristics and current adjustment. *Pain*, **17**, 33–44
18. Turk, D.C., Rudy, T.E. and Stieg, R.L. (1988). The disability determination dilemma: toward a multiaxial solution. *Pain*, **34**, 217–229
19. Urban, B.J., Keefe, F.J. and France, R.D. (1986). A study of psychological scaling in chronic pain patients. *Pain*, **20**, 157–168

5
The spinal modulation of pain

Stephen McMAHON

INTRODUCTION

Chapter 1 describes how noxious stimuli and tissue injury are encoded as signals in particular groups of afferent fibres. Here we will consider the fate of these signals when they enter the spinal cord. Firstly, we will examine how they are processed and routed through spinal circuitry, and how they are finally transmitted to supraspinal structures. Secondly, we will consider the powerful processes that can modulate the transmitted signals. It is important to realize that somatosensory systems are not 'hard-wired' or immutable, but have dynamic properties that integrate present and past circumstances to control the quality and measure of transmitted information. Such neuronal plasticity is likely to be of particular relevance to our understanding of the physiological processes underlying persistent or chronic pain states, and indeed neuroscientists have recently begun to turn their attention in this direction.

THE SPINAL PROCESSING OF NOCICEPTIVE SIGNALS

The spinal termination of nociceptors

Fine-diameter afferent fibres (A-δ and C fibres) that encode noxious stimuli travel mainly in the dorsal roots to pierce the spinal cord at the root entry zone. In some spinal segments, notably sacral ones, many unmyelinated afferents are present in the ventral root. However, the functional role of these branches in the ventral roots is unclear since there is no good evidence that they penetrate into the spinal cord or are capable of exciting spinal neurones.

Nociceptive afferents in the dorsal root clearly do penetrate into the substance of the cord. Within the cord these afferents may run rostrally or caudally for one or more segments in the dorsally placed tract of Lissauer or dorsal columns. Collaterals from these axons turn ventrally and terminate in specific loci in the dorsal horn. The sites of these terminations have been studied by a number of methods. Many histochemical markers have been identified that are located within subsets of primary afferent neurones. The enzyme fluoride-resistant acid phosphatase (FRAP) and the peptides substance P and CGRP (calcitonin gene-related peptide) have been most intensively studied as they occur predominantly in small-diameter neurones that are the cell bodies of nociceptive afferents. The highest concentration of these markers is found in the superficial dorsal horn in the laminae designated I and II by Rexed; see Figure 5.1. A weaker projection of small afferent fibres is seen in the deeper dorsal horn in lamina V. Since CGRP and FRAP do not occur in intrinsic dorsal horn neurones, this distribution marks the termination of the small primary afferents containing them. Direct injection of markers into single nociceptive fibres has confirmed this interpretation. However, fine afferents innervating different peripheral targets do not show identical termination patterns. Fine visceral afferent terminals are concentrated in laminae I and V, whilst cutaneous afferents are most dense in lamina II. The situation for muscle afferents is less clear, but there is evidence for terminations in I and II.

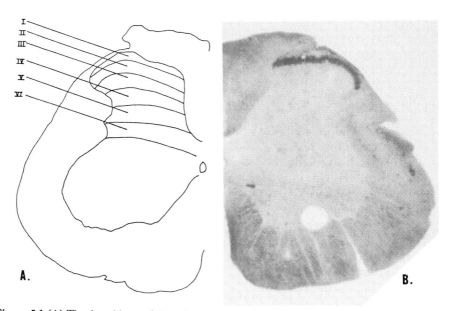

A.   B.

Figure 5.1 (A) The dorsal horn of the spinal cord can be subdivided on anatomical grounds into a series of roughly horizontal layers or laminae. The laminae are conventionally numbered I to VI, with the most dorsal or posterior being lamina I. (B) Different types of primary afferent fibres terminate in different laminae. This photograph shows a transverse section of rat spinal cord stained for the enzyme fluoride-resistant acid phosphatase, which is contained only in unmyelinated afferent fibres. The cutaneous C-fibre terminals shown here are heavily concentrated in lamina II of the dorsal horn. There is another type of organization in afferent terminals in that the labelling in the most medial part of this section occurs in afferents supplying the foot and toes, whilst that in the lateral dorsal horn occurs in afferents innervating more proximal skin areas of the leg.

These projection patterns are markedly different from those seen for low-threshold mechanosensitive afferents, which have the great majority of their terminations in laminae III, IV and V, and frequently an additional branch projecting directly to the dorsal column nuclei, lying in the brainstem.

Both nociceptive and low-threshold mechanoreceptive afferent fibres show an additional form of organization, and that is a highly ordered somatotopy, with projections from each part of the body surface having a limited rostro-caudal and medio-lateral projection area.

Response properties of dorsal horn neurones

The termination patterns described above might lead one to suppose that messages relating to noxious and innocuous stimuli are processed separately within the dorsal horn. However, it must be remembered that dorsal horn neurones usually have profuse dendritic arbors that receive inputs from a wide area. Moreover, it is known that direct, monosynaptic inputs from primary afferent fibres constitute only a small fraction of the total input, and indirect, polysynaptic inputs are likely to significantly increase the convergence onto a particular neurone.

It is not surprising, therefore, that dorsal horn neurones have receptive fields that are larger than those of primary afferents, and frequently complex, responding to activation of different fibre types. Whilst there are many neurones that only encode information from tactile receptors, there are additionally two classes of neurone that respond to noxious stimuli. The first and most common type is the so-called wide dynamic range neurone (also known as convergent or multireceptive). This type of cell is particularly common in the deeper laminae of the dorsal horn (IV and V). As the name suggests, these cells are activated by both noxious and innocuous stimuli. The receptive field as studied in animals typically has several components consisting of a central zone extending over perhaps 2 or 3 digits, where tactile stimuli will excite the cell. This zone sits in a larger area, perhaps the whole of a paw, where noxious stimuli will excite the cell. Finally, there may be an even larger surrounding zone where noxious stimuli inhibit the firing of the cell. Despite the apparent difficulties the brain might have in decoding the firing of such a cell, the available evidence suggests that this type of cell plays a central role in signalling information about injurious stimuli. The intensity, location and time course of noxious stimuli are all well encoded in this class of neurone.

The second type of cell responding to noxious stimuli is the so-called noxious-specific type. These cells are less common than the wide dynamic range type, but are more frequently found in the superficial layers of the dorsal horn. As their name suggests, they are excited by noxious but not innocuous stimuli. These cells can, however, also have inhibitory surrounds. At first sight it might seem that this class is much better suited to signalling information about injury.

In fact there are various reasons to question the idea that they are the sole signallers of noxious events, such as their limited ability to encode the intensity of a noxious stimulus. There is also some direct evidence that activation of the axons of wide dynamic range neurones, rather than noxious-specific neurones, is sufficient to produce pain.

Processing of information from deep tissue

Most of the above description, and indeed most of the experimental work that has been done, relates to processing of information from cutaneous structures. From a clinical perspective it is of course of great importance to know whether similar mechanisms operate for inputs from deep structures. In muscle and joint there are clear groups of afferent fibres that respond exclusively to strong mechanical stimuli and algesic chemicals. For the viscera it is generally less clear what constitutes a noxious stimulus. Whereas the function of the skin is to interact with the environment of the organism, afferents from within the body are more apt to signal the internal milieu of the body. Thus, stimuli such as crushing are exquisitely painful in skin, but may not be perceived in some viscera such as the bowel. One has to remember that the neurones are not only involved in the signalling of consciously perceived sensations, but are essential for the co-ordinated reflex function of most viscera such as continence and voiding. It has long been recognized that many forms of trauma applied to normal healthy visceral tissue in man do not give rise to pain. For the hollow viscera it is apparent that distension may produce pain and there is some evidence that a minority of afferents can specifically encode such stimuli. A large number of afferents, however, show a graded response to distension, encoding stimuli in the innocuous as well as the noxious range.

In the dorsal horn a minority of cells respond to stimulation of deep structures. These are found in the most superficial lamina (lamina I) and in the deep dorsal horn, and are absent from the intermediate laminae. The viscera do not have a private line to the brain: cells responding to visceral inputs are invariably also activated by somatic inputs. This somato-visceral convergence has formed the basis of several theories of referred pain. It has now been fully realized that the convergence–projection theory, described below, is the most likely explanation for this phenomenon. Disease or injury to the viscera sometimes produce pain that is perceived as deep, usually poorly localized, and often has a distinct nauseating quality. But such stimuli can also produce pain that is perceived as arising in more superficial structures, distant from the afflicted viscus. This referred pain is typically felt at a somatic locus that is innervated by the same spinal segments that innervate the viscus. The most common explanation is that visceral inputs activate circuits that are more frequently activated by noxious events in somatic tissue, and the brain incorrectly interprets the source of the signal.

40

Transmission to supraspinal centres

The perceptual experience of peripheral events requires the rostral transmission of signals processed in the dorsal horn. There are a number of ways in which this might occur. Tactile stimuli from the skin are likely to be processed by a fast conducting system with high fidelity through the relay nuclei of the dorsal column nuclei of the brainstem and the thalamus to end in the somatosensory cortex. The processing of noxious information appears to be less straightforward and hence is more liable to modulation at several levels of its ascent to the brain. There is some evidence for the existence of a multisynaptic chain of neurones, with each link projecting a short distance rostrally, and with the entire network being diffusely localized throughout the spinal cord. In addition, it is clear that there are several pathways that originate in the dorsal horn and have long ascending axons that ascend directly in specific white-matter tracts to terminate in supraspinal nuclei.

There is a long-standing body of literature dating back about a century that describes the sensory deficits resulting from lesions of different spinal tracts in man and animals. The cardinal findings of these studies are that (i) lesions of the antero-lateral white matter consistently result in an analgesia or hypalgesia in body areas contralateral and caudal to the lesion; (ii) lesions to the posterior columns or posterio-lateral white matter do not produce analgesia or hypalgesia. More recent experimental evidence has confirmed that there are indeed many neurones in the deeper laminae of the dorsal horn that have long axonal projections in the contralateral antero-lateral quadrant. Most of these cells are of the noxious specific or wide dynamic range type. They project to a number of brainstem targets but the direct projection to thalamus has been strongly emphasized. Whilst this scheme has the important advantage of being conceptually simple, it is clearly an over-simplification. Firstly, approximately one half of patients who have antero-lateral cordotomies (for intractable pain problems), and who survive for more than a year, experience a recurrence of their pain and sensitivity to noxious stimuli. Since the lesioned pathways do not regenerate, some other system of neurones must now be signalling the noxious events. Secondly, a number of anomalies are associated with the lesion data, such as the fact that small lesions of the antero-lateral columns are reported to produce a more persistent and profound analgesia than large lesions. Finally, basic anatomical and physiological studies have identified a plethora of other long ascending pathways which travel outside the antero-lateral quadrant and which encode signals from injured tissue. Perhaps the most perplexing of these is the output system that originates in lamina I of the dorsal horn. As we have said, neurones in lamina I lie amongst the densest terminations of nociceptors, and the majority of these cells are noxious-specific. Whilst many of these cells do have long ascending axons, the vast majority of these ascend not in the antero-lateral but in the contralateral dorso-lateral white matter. The role of these highly specialized projection cells remains obscure, but it is unlikely to be one of a simple relay in a nociceptive transmission system.

THE MODULATION OF INJURY SIGNALS

In the preceding sections we have considered the basic organization of the spinal systems that are activated by signals arising from nociceptors and that transmit that information to the brain. We will now consider some of the modulatory influences that can modify this basic transmission system, and which may be particularly important in the genesis or treatment of chronic pain states.

Sensitization of spinal cord neurones

A particular problem for experimental neuroscientists is the extent to which the mechanisms of acute and chronic pain are equivalent. On the one hand, scientists have generally utilized transient, near-threshold noxious stimuli in their studies; on the other hand, the painful conditions that patients complain of are generally long-lasting and severe. If the mechanisms of chronic pain are not simple reiterations of acute phenomena, an understanding of the patient's problem and the therapies that are offered may be severely deficient. In fact, the management of acute pain in patients is rarely a therapeutic problem and most symptoms will resolve spontaneously after some time. However, the frequent failure of adequate pain relief in more chronic states raises the possibility that the neural substrate of both states is not identical. In the past five years there has been a growing awareness of this problem amongst neuroscientists, and there are an increasing number of attempts to study the longer-term processes associated with tissue injury in experimental animals. There is an emerging picture of a dynamically organized nervous system the properties of which can be substantially altered following tissue damage.

The receptive field properties of dorsal horn cells have been studied before and after the creation of localized cutaneous burns or small skin incisions. These cells, which initially had small receptive fields and high thresholds, became more active and more responsive to peripheral stimuli in the tens of minutes after the injury was made. This increased responsiveness was seen as an expansion of the receptive field areas, and a decrease in the threshold necessary to excite the cells. Figure 5.2 shows an example of the changes seen for one neurone. One might predict that one consequence of this increased state of excitability in somato-sensory transmission systems would signify a hyperalgesic state, and indeed it is a common experience that even slight injuries are associated with tenderness and pain at the site and surrounding injury. Whilst there is evidence that this type of injury may make some primary afferent nociceptors more responsive, Figure 5.2 shows that there are also important changes within the spinal cord. Electrical transcutaneous stimulation, which elicits a constant volley of afferent impulses, can be seen (Figure 5.2B) to produce an augmented response in the central neurone following the tissue injury. These central changes appear to be triggered by signals in unmyelinated afferents at the site of injury, and are long-lasting. Once they have become established, they may be independent of the peripheral inputs that initiate them.

Similar sensitizations of spinal somatosensory systems have been observed following the injection of inflammatory substances into muscle and joint. Under these conditions, central neurones also become responsive to new inputs and show decreased thresholds for activation. More widespread inflammatory states, such as polyarthritis induced by injections of Freud's adjuvant, also lead to sensitization of central neurones that persist for weeks. Taken together, these studies suggest that unmyelinated afferents from a variety of peripheral targets not only signal, on a second-to-second basis, the presence or absence of strong mechanical or thermal stimuli, but also continuously report the status of the chemical environment of the tissues. In this context unmyelinated afferents may be particularly adapted to signal the presence of inflammation. Direct evidence has recently been obtained in the case of the urinary bladder. Recordings from unmyelinated afferent fibres running in the pelvic nerves to this organ have shown that most of these afferents are not activated by distensions of the viscus in the physiological or supraphysiological range. Some of these afferents do respond, however, to chemical inflammatory agents instilled into the lumen of the bladder. Moreover, recordings in the dorsal horn have shown that inflammation of the urinary bladder can also induce a slow sensitization (Figure 5.3). This sensitization includes a facilitation of dorsal horn cell responses to convergent somatic inputs, and this may be an important contributor to conditions of referred pain and tenderness. Similar mechanisms may also apply for the inflamed joint.

In addition to these altered physiological inputs, peripheral injury has also been found capable of altering other aspects of dorsal horn function. For instance, adjuvant-induced arthritis causes an increased expression of the peptide dynorphin in many dorsal horn cells, including some projection neurones, and this may affect the second-order cell's postsynaptic effectiveness. Similarly, signals from injured tissue can alter other forms of gene expression in dorsal horn cells, and hence potentially alter the machinery controlling all aspects of the cells' function.

The pharmacological basis for these slow changes in somatosensory processing is unclear. One possibility is that neuropeptides, so prevalent in unmyelinated afferent fibres, initiate these changes.

Segmental inhibitory controls

In 1965 Melzack and Wall proposed a model – the gate control theory – that attempted to account for many experimental observations on the dorsal horn processing of nociceptive information. Since that time a number of the details of the model have been challenged and of course much more information has become available. However, the central concepts of the gate control theory have

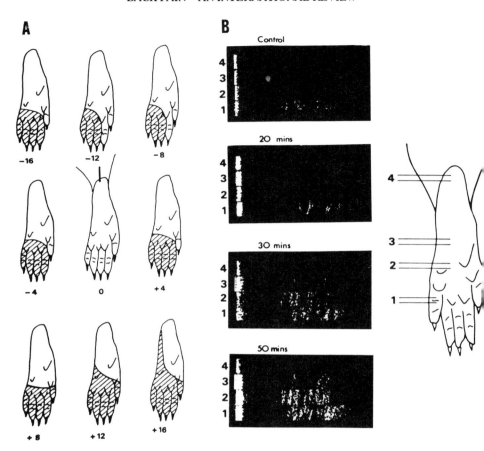

Figure 5.2 (A) The effects of a nearby injury on the receptive field properties of a single projection neurone. The shaded regions show the areas of skin where noxious stimulation excited this neurone. The receptive field was determined every few minutes before (shown as negative times) and after (shown as positive times) the creation of a small skin incision on the ankle. Note that the receptive field is relatively stable before the injury, but slowly expands in area starting about 10 min after the injury. (B) The increased excitability of the neurone is at least partly a central phenomenon. Transcutaneous stimuli were given at four sites on the foot (1,2,3,4). At each site the response of the cell was recorded as a 'raster' display, which was collected before and 20, 30 and 50 min after the creation of the injury shown in (A). In the raster display, each dot represents the firing of the cell following an electrical stimulus that was given transcutaneously at the beginning of the oscilloscope trace. Later responses to the stimulus are seen displaced to the right, the extreme right-hand edge of the display representing 500 msec after the stimulus. Responses to successive stimuli are shown higher and higher in the display. Note that in the control raster, stimulation at all four sites produced an early burst of firing whilst stimulation only at site 1 (inside the receptive field) also produced a late burst of firing due to activity in primary afferent C-fibres. After the injury (and as the receptive field expanded – see A), the responsiveness of the cell increased. The early and late responses are augmented, and new late responses start to occur to stimulation of sites 2 and 3. Since the transcutaneous stimulus evokes a constant afferent volley, the increased responsiveness represents an increased excitability occurring within the spinal cord.

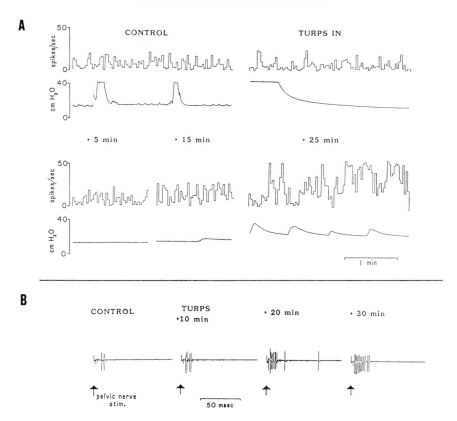

Figure 5.3 The effects of urinary bladder inflammation on the responses of dorsal horn cells. (A). The firing rate of a single cell is shown before and after the urinary bladder was inflamed with a chemical agent (turpentine). Initially the cell fires spontaneously but is unaffected by contractions of the urinary bladder (intravesical pressure is shown below the firing record). After the inflammatory stimulus, the spontaneous firing rate slowly increases and at 25 min after the inflammation, a novel mechanosensitivity occurs, and the neurone is now inhibited by the spontaneous bladder contractions. (B) The response of another dorsal horn to electrical stimulation of the pelvic nerves before and after urinary bladder inflammation. Note that in the control state only a few action potentials are elicited by the nerve stimulus, whilst after inflammation the excitability of the neurone increases and the same afferent volley induces a greater discharge.

been supported by experimental observations, it has provided several successful therapies, and it has been particularly useful in providing a framework for the assessment of patients.

The central premise of the gate control theory is that the output neurones of the dorsal horn that signal nociceptive events constitute a dynamic system whose activity is increased by input from small-diameter nociceptive afferents, and decreased by repetitive inputs from large-diameter low-threshold afferents. This system is segmental, which is to say that inputs from the same body regions show

45

the greatest interactions. The electrophysiological basis for the interaction has been studied extensively. A single supramaximal electrical shock to a peripheral nerve most commonly evokes two bursts of activity in dorsal horn transmission cells. The first one is associated with the arrival at the cord of impulses carried by fast-conducting myelinated fibres, and the second from unmyelinated afferents. But following the initial burst of activity, there occurs a period of inhibition, typically lasting a few hundred milliseconds. The second excitatory response is superimposed on this inhibition. The interneurones generating the A-fibre-mediated inhibitions were located by Melzack and Wall in the substantia gelatinosa of the dorsal horn (lamina II). If the A fibres are repetitively activated either by electrical stimulation of the peripheral nerve trunk or tactile stimulation of the receptive endings in the skin, the inhibition generated by the activity accumulates and the responsiveness of the central cell is depressed.

A second possible electrophysiological mechanism for the effects of the A-fibre stimulation is presynaptic inhibition. If the central terminals of nociceptive afferents are partially depolarized, action potentials invading these terminals release less neurotransmitter and consequently the post-synaptic effect is reduced. Presynaptic inhibition has a prolonged time course, and repetitive activation of the system would also induce a strong, maintained reduction in the effectiveness of C-fibre inputs.

The normal processing of nociceptive information depends critically on the balance of inhibitory and excitatory inputs. For example, in microneurographic experiments the activity of individual afferent C fibres can be recorded in conscious man, and compared with the sensory experiences evoked by peripheral stimulation. When the skin is heated above about 40°C a subject reports pain at a time when C-fibre afferents are firing at very low levels, less than 0.5 impulses/sec. However, if the same area of skin is subjected to a strong mechanical stimulus, pain is not reported until the same C-fibres are firing at much higher frequencies, of some 10 impulses/sec. The difference between these two experiments is that in the latter low-threshold tactile afferents are activated in addition to the C fibres, and this results in a reduced effectiveness of C-fibre activity.

It is also likely that some of the abnormal pain states seen in patients may result from a disturbance of these inhibitory processes. A-fibre-mediated inhibitions are reduced, for instance, following damage to peripheral nerves.

The gate control theory has generated an important therapy for the relief of pain. This aims to exacerbate the A-fibre-mediated inhibitions by the high-frequency electrical stimulation of myelinated afferent nerve fibres. Such stimulation can be performed in the periphery, by means of transcutaneous nerve stimulation (TINS), or by means of implanted electrodes in the dorsal columns, to backfire the central branches of myelinated primary afferent fibres, but produce the same activation of dorsal horn inhibitory systems. Dorsal column stimulation may additionally activate neurones other than primary afferents, and this may contribute to the antinociceptive effect.

Supraspinal control of spinal cord function

In 1969, Reynold's observed that electrical stimulation delivered to the midbrain caused analgesia in rats. More detailed searches have produced reports of analgesia from stimulation of a large number of brainstem sites, including sites in the medulla, midbrain, diencephalon, and even sensory cortex. The specificity of effect is somewhat uncertain, since at most of the sites electrical stimulation has been found capable of inducing other behaviours, such as alterations in posture, locomotion, vocalization, and pressor responses.

Microinjection of opiates, rather than electrical stimulation, into some areas can also elicit analgesia; there is a rough but not exact correspondence between the most effective sites with the two methods.

It is proposed that these brain areas exert actions at a spinal level and do so by activating pathways that project down to the spinal cord. However, it is probably wrong to regard the analgesia as the action of 'antinociceptive pathways', but rather as one element of a profuse number of descending control pathways that act to modulate or control many different functions of the spinal cord.

In the last 10 years or so there have been extensive investigations of the anatomy, physiology and pharmacology of descending pathways.

Neuroanatomical tracing techniques have shown that the dorsal horn receives heavy projections from a number of brainstem sites. The best-described system originates in the medullary n. raphe magnus and adjoining n. gigantocelularis. The projections descend in the white matter of the dorso-lateral funiculus, and are bilateral with a predominant ipsilateral component. These descending axons terminate throughout the dorsal horn, but are most dense in the superficial laminae. Some connections are made directly on to output neurones of the dorsal horn, but the major influence is exerted via interneurones. The n. raphe magnus and gigantocellularis themselves receive heavy projections from the more rostral midbrain periaqueductal grey and n. cuneiformis (although these latter also have some direct projections to the spinal cord).

The hypothalamus also sends direct projections to the dorsal horn, again descending through the dorsolateral funiculus and terminating heavily in superficial laminae. The projection is reportedly mainly ipsilateral. The cortex of course has a direct spinal projection, and some of this terminates in the dorsal horn and presumably has a sensory rather than a motor role.

Not all areas where stimulation produces analgesia have direct spinal projections, and stimulation at one site may produce effects other than by activating a direct projection.

There have of course been extensive efforts to identify the physiological mechanisms that might underlie the behavioural analgesia seen with brainstem stimulation. When descending pathways are acutely lesioned or the spinal cord is blocked, many cells caudal to the block become more excitable, suggesting that the net effect of tonically active descending pathways is usually inhibitory. Many studies have examined the response properties of dorsal horn neurones whilst electrically stimulating different brainstem regions. The first reports found that most dorsal horn cells were inhibited. Responses to noxious peripheral stimulation were found to be especially inhibited, although it is clear that innocuous inputs can also be modulated. Activation of all the pathways described above has been found to be effective. A variety of stimulating regimes have been tested, from single shocks to long periods of high-frequency pulses. The inhibitions from the former generally last from a few tens to a few hundreds of milliseconds; those from the latter, for the period of stimulation and sometimes for seconds or minutes following it. Thus, at first sight, there would appear to be a good match between the behaviour and electrophysiological findings. However, a number of electrophysiological studies have also reported excitatory components in responses. In a minority of cells, excitation was the only or predominant response, but most commonly a short-duration excitatory response was followed and perhaps truncated by a more prolonged inhibitory response. These excitatory responses are particularly marked in cells in the superficial dorsal horn.

The pharmacology of these descending systems has also been studied extensively: some studies have identified the neurotransmitters or putative neurotransmitters present in cells that have descending spinal projections; others have applied agonists or antagonists directly to the spinal cord to interfere with or mimic transmission in descending systems.

Enkephalin is found in descending neurones originating in various brainstem sites including the midbrain periaqueductal grey and cells of the medullary n. raphe magnus and adjoining reticular formation. Serotonin is also present in the periaqueductal grey matter and is extremely common in the descending projections from the medulla. Noradrenaline-containing projections are much more restricted in the brainstem, but none the less these neurones probably mediate, indirectly, the effects of stimulation at a number of sites. The peptides substance P, TRH and CCK are also found in subpopulations of the descending pathways.

The role played by these different transmitters has been tested by eliciting analgesia by brainstem stimulation (or microinjections of opiates) and applying antagonists directly to the spinal cord. Antagonists to enkephalin, noradrenaline and serotonin can all attenuate brainstem-evoked analgesia. Since noradrenaline and serotonin are not contained within intrinsic neurones in the cord, the antagonism can be attributed to descending pathways. Enkephalin is found in spinal neurones, and release of enkephalin from both descending projection and spinal interneurones is likely to be capable of producing analgesic effects.

Opiate and noradrenergic receptors are both found on primary afferent terminals and some of the effects of descending pathways are likely to be mediated by presynaptic inhibition. It is clear that postsynaptic actions also occur, and may be more significant.

The study of these descending control pathways has already produced one new form of treatment for some painful conditions. Pharmacological agents are administered locally and directly to the spinal cord by an epidural injection. To date, opiates have been the most widely used, but there are possibilities for the use of other agents that mimic the effects of activating descending pathways. This treatment has the advantage of restricting the distribution of the drug, and therefore minimizing side-effects, whilst allowing relatively high concentrations to be achieved at the site of action.

The demonstration of the existence of these powerful descending controls also raises questions about the physiological role of these systems and the conditions under which they are activated. Several answers to these questions have been suggested. The phenomenon of counter-irritation is well described and readily appreciated. Painful stimuli to one body region are capable of suppressing the appreciation of a second painful stimulus at a different site. There is a wealth of electrophysiological evidence that noxious peripheral stimulation activates ascending spinal pathways that in turn activate some of the descending pathways described above. In this way noxious stimulation at one site can lead to a suppression of the ability of other parts of the spinal cord to encode noxious stimuli. The consequence is to exaggerate the difference between the firing of the ascending neurones excited by the noxious stimulus and those in other spinal segments. Thus the 'contrast' within the whole population of ascending cells is enhanced. Some people have also tried to include acupuncture as a pain-relief therapy in this scheme. The idea is that the acupuncture stimuli (usually at a body site distant from the source of pain) will similarly activate the inhibitory descending pathways and reduce transmission in spinal neurones signalling some ongoing noxious event. Whilst this may appear to provide a rationale for one perplexing aspect of acupuncture, action at a distance, it should be recognized that traditional acupuncture is not itself noxious (and noxious stimuli are necessary to activate the descending controls) and, further, that the ability to activate these descending controls is not restricted to particular meridians or special points on the body surface. The issue has become confused because of the tendency of many western adherents of acupuncture to use a fundamentally different form of stimulus – severely noxious electro-acupuncture applied locally to the site of some chronic pain.

A second and entirely different role for these descending systems has been suggested on the basis of recordings made from the cells themselves. In the lightly anaesthetized rat, heating of the tail to about 45°C produces a protective reflex in which the tail flicks away from the source of the heat, with a somewhat variable latency. Cells at the origin of important descending pathways in the medulla often have one of two distinct firing properties in relation to such tail heating. Some cells, normally quiescent, are excited by the tail heating. Another group show ongoing activity that stops just before the tail flick occurs, and these cells have been called 'off-cells'. Because the latency of the tail flick is somewhat variable, one can show that the inhibition of the tonically active cells is correlated much more with the occurrence of the reflex response than with the temperature of the tail. A number of experiments suggest that the ongoing activity in these cells is sufficient to prevent the occurrence of a tail flick and that it is the pause in the firing of the cells that then 'permits' spinal circuitry to execute the response. One important action of opiates may be to block the input to these off-cells and so result in them firing continuously with the consequence that spinal reflex responses continue to be inhibited. This view of the action of a descending pathway, that the system 'gives permission' to the spinal cord to process information in one particular way, marks an important shift in thinking about the possible ways in which the brain can modify the activity of the spinal cord. Yet more fundamentally different forms of control undoubtedly remain to be discovered.

FURTHER READING

Basbaum, A.I. and Fields, H.L. (1984). Endogenous pain control systems. Brainstem pathways and endorphin circuitry. *Ann. Rev. Neurosci.*, 7, 309–338

Casey, K.L. and Morrow, T.J. (1988). Supraspinal nocifensive responses of cats: spinal cord pathways, monoamines and modulation. *J. Comp. Neurol.*, 270, 591–605

Cervero, F. (1988). Visceral pain. In Dubner, R., Grebhart, G.F. and Bond, M.R. (eds.) *Pain Research and Clinical Management*, Vol.3, pp. 216–226. (Amsterdam: Elsevier)

Cook, A.J., Woolf, C.J., Wall, P.D. and McMahon, S.B. (1987). Dynamic receptive field plasticity in rat spinal cord dorsal horn following C-primary afferent input. *Nature*, 325, 151–153

Devor, M. (1988). Central changes mediating neuropathic pain. In Dubner, R., Grebhart, G.F. and Bond, M.R. (eds.) *Pain Research and Clinical Management*, Vol.3, pp. 114–128. (Amsterdam: Elsevier)

Gibson, S.J. and Polak, J.M. (1986). Neurochemistry of the spinal cord. In Polak, J.M. and van Noorden, S. (eds.) *Immunocytochemistry, Modern Methods and Applications*, pp. 360–389. (Bristol: Wright)

Guilbaud, G. (1986). Peripheral and central electrophysiological mechanisms of joint and muscle pain. In Dubner, R., Gebhart, G.F. and Bond, M.R. (eds.) *Pain Research and Clinical Management*, Vol. 3, pp. 201–215. (Amsterdam: Elsevier)

Fields, H.L. and Basbaum, A.I. (1989). Endogenous pain control mechanisms. In Wall, P.D. and Melzack, R. (eds.) *Textbook of Pain*, 2nd edn., pp. 206–219. (Edinburgh: Churchill Livingstone)

Fields, H.L. and Heinricher, M.M. (1985). Anatomy and physiology of a nociceptive modulatory system. *Phil. Trans. R. Soc. B.*, 308, 361–374

Fitzgerald, M. (1989). The course and terminations of primary afferent fibres. In Wall, P.D. and Melzack, R. (eds.) *Textbook of Pain*, 2nd edn., pp. 45–62. (Edinburgh: Churchill Livingstone)

Hunt, S.P., Pini, A. and Evan, G. (1987). Induction of c-fos-like protein in spinal cord neurones following sensory stimulation. *Nature*, 328, 632–634

Le Bars, D., Dickenson, A.H., Besson, J.M. and Villanueva, L. (1986). Aspects of sensory processing through convergent neurones. In Yaksh, T.L. (ed.) *Spinal Afferent Processing*, pp. 467–508. (New York: Plenum Press)

Lewis, T. (1942). *Pain*. (London: Macmillan)

McMahon, S.B. (1988). Neuronal and behavioural consequences of chemical inflammation of rat urinary bladder. *Agents and Actions*, 25, 321–324

McMahon, S.B. and Abel, C. (1987). A model for the study of visceral pain states: Chronic inflammation of rat urinary bladder by irritant chemicals. *Pain*, 28, 109–129

McMahon, S.B. and Wall, P.D. (1989). The significance of plastic changes in lamina I systems. In Cervero, F., Bennett, G. and Headley, P. (eds.), *Processing of Information in the Superficial Dorsal Horn of the Spinal Cord*. (New York: Plenum)

Melzack, R. and Wall, P.D. (1965). Pain mechanisms: a new theory. *Science*, 150, 971–979

Noordenbos, W. (1969). *Pain*. (Amsterdam: Elsevier)

Price, D.D. (1986). The question of how the dorsal horn encodes sensory information. In Yaksh, T.L. (ed.) *Spinal Afferent Processing*, pp. 445–466. (New York: Plenum Press)

Reynolds, D.V. (1969). Surgery in the rat during electrical analgesia induced by focal brain stimulation. *Science*, **164**, 444–445

Rexed, B. (1952). The cytoarchitectonic organization of the spinal cord of the cat. *J. Comp. Neurol.*, **96**, 415–495

Ruda, M.A. (1986). The pattern and place of nociceptive modulation in the dorsal horn. In Yaksh, T.L. (ed.) *Spinal Afferent Processing*, pp. 141–164. (New York: Plenum Press)

van Hees, J. and Gybels, J.M. (1981). Pain related to single afferent C-fibres from human skin. *J. Neurol. Neurosurg. Psychiatr.*, **44**, 600–607

Wall, P.D. (1973). Dorsal horn electrophysiology. In Iggo, A. (ed.) *Handbook of Sensory Physiology*, Vol. II. (Berlin: Springer)

Woolf, C.J. (1983). Evidence for a central component of post-injury pain sensitivity. *Nature*, **306**, 686–688

Willis, W.D. (1982). Control of nociceptive transmission in the spinal cord. *Progress in Sensory Physiology 3*. (Berlin: Springer)

Willis, W.D. and Coggeshall, R.E. (1978). *Sensory Mechanisms in the Spinal Cord*. (New York: Plenum Press)

Yaksh, T.L. (1986). The effects of intrathecally administered opioid and adrenergic agents on spinal function. In Yaksh, T.L. (ed.) *Spinal Afferent Processing*, pp. 505–539. (New York: Plenum Press)

6
Principles and problems in clinical research in low back pain

M.A. NELSON

"Man can learn nothing except by going from the known to the unknown" Anon

Sir Robert Platt[1] wrote in 1963 that "a conclusion based on a badly conceived experiment is usually further from the truth than one based on clinical observation".

Most clinical research begins with an observation, usually noted in disease rather than in health as nature more closely guards her secrets in the healthy body and reveals them in disease. It may be conducted at many different levels from the sub-molecular to the cellular, from system to organism, seeking to discover new information.

In the clinical area of back pain information is sought to improve our understanding of the natural history, diagnosis, treatment, complication and prevention of this common problem.

However, back pain presents special problems to the researchers. It is a symptom of a wide range of dissimilar conditions. Furthermore, the patient with back pain is a patient in pain which happens to be in the back and in this way he or she behaves no differently than the patient with pain elsewhere.

Pain is an abnormal affective state in which a nociceptive receptor is stimulated and messages are sent to the brain which are coded, assessed and modified within the thalamus. Many factors determine how the pain will be perceived[2-4].

A number of these factors have been studied in normal and mentally disturbed patients. It was found that factors such as the individual's past experience of pain or painful situations, the effect of pain as a threatening influence on lifestyle, work and pleasure determine how the individual reacted to the situation in which he found himself[5]. Litigation and compensation may further modify and alter an individual's response.

Those working in the field of low back pain need to remember these widespread, ill-defined and almost immeasurable factors in order to design research projects which can reach some conclusions upon which an hypothesis can be based.

A project may analyse the effect of a certain treatment but unless the natural history of back pain is understood with its wide fluctuation in severity and its very intermittent presentation over a long period, an inaccurate conclusion may be reached.

In 1987 a Task Force based in Quebec[6] reviewed the world literature on research in back pain and concluded that 95% of the studies failed to fulfil strict scientific criteria.

Before expressing surprise or criticism, it is essential to consider the difficulties facing the clinical researcher in back pain.

TERMINOLOGY AND NOSOLOGY

In recent years, there have been significant and important studies in the problem of language in clinical research.

As patients we use many words to describe pain. It is apparent that each of us selects the descriptive term on the basis of our experience in other areas of our lives. Mersky quotes Brain (1962): "Our vocabulary for the description of pain is relatively poor and we tend to fall back on terms which portray the pain by describing the way in which it might be produced, thus we speak of pricking pains, stabbing pain, bursting pain and so on. We use metaphores of violence tending to talk about how we think it occurred rather than what it actually feels like. Thus the descriptions of burning and cutting are related to heat and sharpness. Other words like agonising, terrifying denote introspective components which are always present in any chronic or longstanding period of pain"[7].

Even simple words like back pain require definition and when we talk of leg pain, where does the leg begin? Does it include the buttock? Acute and chronic are terms commonly used but are we agreed as to their meaning? Clearly words like sciatica, lumbago, fibrositis are widely in use by members of this audience but their meaning is not agreed. Another example is a word like paraesthesiae which covers a very wide range of unusual feelings and clinicians when listening to a history do not necessarily agree when to use this word as a description. The problem of semantics has been recognized in the many clinical descriptions of syndromes[8].

At a recent pain meeting in Birmingham for the Society of Back Pain Research, the problem was again highlighted. At this meeting a number of different disciplines dealing with back pain were asked to present their clinical syndromes. These were based on a very wide range of parameters including clinical, radiological, the response of the pain to examination, the response of pain to treatment and finally the clinical history and findings were subjected to computer analysis and cluster suggesting that groups of symptoms and signs occurring more frequently in a population may indicate some defineable disorders[9].

UNRELIABLE NATURE OF INFORMATION OBTAINED

Inter- and intra-observer error

If we agree that terminology is confused, then observer reliability is in an even more chaotic situation.

Reliability studies in a wide range of clinical areas have established the high rate of error both in the individual and between individuals dealing with the same patients: these studies include observer error in medical history taking[10,11] and errors in leg length measurements[12]. More recent work using computer studies on abdominal pain have attempted to address the problem of inter- and intra-observer error[13].

All confirm the importance of inter- and intra-observer error in the accuracy of clinical information. Any clinical study therefore must include a study of the inter- and intra-observer error within the study in order to eliminate this factor as a bias in a result. This is particularly so in any study in which measurement of X-rays is included. Not only are the X-rays often not of the same density or taken at the precise angle but the observer himself has an error in his own measurement of an angle and two observers clearly introduce further inaccuracies. Despite this obvious problem there continue to be many studies in the literature failing to recognize the importance of these reasons for error and bias in the results.

My own work in 1979[14] and more recent work by Fairbank[9] highlighted the problems in history and examination which, briefly stated, conclude that the more precisely we try to define the item of history and examination, the more commonly the two observers will disagree. One could conclude that perhaps one way forward is to define the clinical history and examination on those features which are reliable and to simplify rather than make the history more complicated.

THE FREQUENT OCCURRENCE OF PAIN-FREE PATHOLOGICAL PROCESSES

The ageing process seen so clearly in the face and skin as wrinkles and grey hair and in the body as loss of firmness and sagging frame is also reflected in the spine, facet joints and soft tissues.

Fundamental observations have been carried out on the natural incidence of degenerative changes which were unrelated to the incidence of symptoms[19].

Population studies have shown that when we correlate osteoarthritic symptoms and X-rays, we find that in a large number of patients a well recognized pathological process is not associated with symptoms[20].

Recently CAT-scan technology has further confirmed the many common age-related changes.

The clinician must clearly show that the abnormality that he has identified is in fact producing the pain of which the patient complains. While there is no doubt that with age there are increasing pathological changes, there is at present no definite evidence that this increase is associated with an increased incidence of back pain. Furthermore the finding of pathological changes in the spine of a patient with back pain does not necessarily relate one to the other[21-24].

NATURAL HISTORY

There is a dearth of studies on the long-term natural history of back pain and the absence of this information threatens the whole validity of studies into the effect of treatment of back pain.

Badley[15] reports that while back pain appears to occur with increasing frequency in adults until middle age, there is a lessening in frequency as you get older. The peak incidence is 45 to 64 and thereafter back pain becomes a less frequent problem. This is similar to studies carried out on neck and knee symptoms and other joint problems which suggests there is a very real lessening of experience of back pain as one gets older. This has to be balanced against the undoubted increase and frequency of pathological changes with age[16,17].

Back pain is not associated with an increased mortality and therefore the statistics would suggest a real rather than apparent improvement.

In 1983, a prospective study established a one-year new incidence of first attacks of back pain of 11% in 30-year-olds and only 6% in the older decades[18].

There is a paucity of studies on the incidence of back pain in patients with known spondylolisthesis, disc degeneration etc. A cohort of 500 children was followed for 25 years. By the time they reached adulthood, 5.8% were found radiologically to have spondylolisthesis. Back pain was found not to be associated[25]!

Patients seeking medical help for back pain are a highly selected group and do not reflect the true incidence of the radiological abnormality in the population.

STATISTICS[26]

Statistics are a central tool of any research study. The nature of the biological model in back pain is such that there are a wide number of uncontrolled variables which cannot be fully assessed.

A statistical analysis of the data is essential to try and smooth out the biological variables which exist. Furthermore in any field in which the clinical problems has a variable natural history, including a propensity to recover, it is essential to eliminate chance as a factor in any optimistic result.

A statistician or someone trained in statistics is essential to plan the study from the outset in order to ensure that adequate numbers of patients and adequate data observations are made to permit statistical analysis. Failure to do so can lead to an abortive study when it becomes obvious that insufficient data has been collected for analysis.

Furthermore it is important to choose the correct statistical model for the appropriate study. It is important to note that the data can be analysed from a number of difference approaches. Choosing the best method requires experience and knowledge. Whereas the basic scientist can design a study to eliminate variables, the clinical researcher must resort to statistics to balance out those many variables over which he can have no control.

THE IDEAL EXPERIMENT

Bearing these many factors in mind, it is clear why well constructed studies to investigate back pain are so extraordinarily difficult to design[27]. The following minimal requirements for a satisfactory study should be fulfilled.

1. Prospective

The study should be prospective. A question should be posed and the study designed to answer it.

2. Controls

The characteristics of the study group should be well defined so that a matched control group can be identified. Factors such as age, sex, weight, height, occupation, racial groups, social class, litigation, physical activities, etc. must be considered. If one is comparing treatment, three groups are required, the study group, the placebo group and the untreated group (control).

3. Non-specific back pain

The recognized difficulties in establishing a diagnosis has prompted the use of a group of non-specific back pain patients. It is suggested that this group is more or less homogeneous and can be used as a trial group. There are serious flaws in this thinking.

Non-specific back pain can include undiagnosed back pain such as:
(1) Early ankylosing spondylitis.
(2) Lumbar disc derangement before the nerve root involvement has developed.

(3) Soft tissue injury associated with certain occupations and sports.

(4) Missed spondylolysis because oblique X-rays are not requested.

4. Adequate follow-up

The follow-up period must be adequate to allow for the natural recovery period of back pain. A two-year but ideally a five-year study is required to eliminate natural recovery.

5. Assessment of patients

This should be carried out by someone not involved in the study. Ideally all patients should be examined clinically according to an agreed protocol. Postal questionnaires are notoriously unreliable and ideally should be discarded. Any patients lost to review must be included in the results. It is unacceptable to start the study with 500 patients, lose 300 and report the findings in the 200 remaining. One cannot assume that those lost to follow-up will behave the same as those seen at review.

Clinical research covers a wide range of problems including, diagnosis, treatment and prevention.

Diagnosis

This will include an analysis of the features of the history and examination, their reliability and validity. The delineation of the clinical syndromes, the value of investigations and their reliability.

Treatment

In any evaluation of treatment, the features of the study group must be very carefully defined. Back pain is a symptom. One cannot design the study to evaluate the effect of a certain treatment of back pain without very carefully defining the features of the group. It is important to define clearly what are the parameters which indicate improvement: return to work, patient's assessment, clinician's assessment, etc.

The problems are enormous. Large numbers of patients are required and this usually means a multi-centre study. Alternatively, studies should be department based so that a long-term prospective project can be undertaken by successive generations of researchers each one contributing one to two years.

Recently the MRC supported a project looking at manipulation versus physiotherapy for a defined type of back pain in a multi-centre trial under the supervision of Dr Tom Meade of Northwick Park. We took part in this study and found that even in our limited group the chiropracter and myself did not agree which patients should be included. One anecdote comes to mind: a patient who was sent to me as suitable for the trial was found to have gross nerve root compression and came to surgery within a week. Needless to say the protocol had excluded this type of patient. Somehow the clinical findings had changed dramatically in the two weeks which elapsed between the chiropracter seeing the patient and myself.

At present clinical research into back pain has reached an impasse. On the one hand there is increasing sophistication of investigations to identify and localize the pathological process deemed to be the cause of the symptoms, and on the other increasing information to show that patients with widespread pathological processes may not necessarily have back pain. Perhaps we need to alter the whole emphasis of our research and move away from the present accepted concepts to a new perception of the problem. I would contend that the return to reliable descriptions of clinical syndromes represent one such avenue despite the very real difficulties which will face us.

If this all seems very negative and depressing, I'm sorry.

I would like to end on a more optimistic note, namely that progress in any field of endeavour depends on knowledge and knowledge is based on observation and well defined studies. If we continue to look at small areas of the problem, limiting the question to a simple one and then building on that information, I feel sure that as time passes we will make positive inroads into our understanding and treatment of this challenging clinical problem.

REFERENCES

1. Sir Robert Platt (1963). Reflections on medicine and humanism – Linacre Lecture. *University's Quarterly*, 17, 327–340
2. Wyke, B. (1987). In Jayson, M. (ed.) *The Lumbar Spine and Back Pain*, 3rd edn. (Churchill Livingstone)
3. Huskisson, E.C. (1974). Measurement of pain. *Lancet*, 2, 1127–1128
4. Downie, W.W., Leatham, P.A., Rhind, V.M., Wright, V., Bianco, J.A. and Anderson, J.A. (1978). Studies with pain rating scales. *Ann. Rheum. Dis.*, 37, 378–381
5. Mersky, H. and Spear, F.G. (1967). *Pain, Psychological and Psychiatric Aspects*, (London: Balliere Tindall)
6. Spitzer, W.O., LeBlac, F.E., Dupuis, M. *et al.* (1987). Scientific approach to the assessment and management of activity-related spinal disorders. *Spine*, 12, 4–5
7. Mersky, H. (1968). Psychological aspects of pain. *Postgrad. Med.*, 44, 297–306
8. Anderson, J.A.D. (1977). Problems of classification of back pain. *Rheum. Rehab.*, 16, 34–36
9. Fairbank, J.A. Personal communication
10. Cochrane, A.L., Chapman, P.J. and Oldham, P.D. (1951). Observer's error in medical histories. *Lancet*, 1, 1007–1009
11. Johnson, M.L. (1955). Observer error – it's bearing on teaching. *Lancet*, 2, 422–424
12. Nichols, P.J.R. and Bailey, N.T.J. (1955). The accuracy of measuring leg length differences... an observer error experiment. *Br. Med. J.*, 2, 1247–1248

13. Gill, P.W., Leaper, D.J., Guillou, P.J., Staniland, J.R., Horrocks, J.C. and De Dombal, F.T. (1973). Observer variation in clinical diagnosis. A computer-aided assessment of its magnitude and importance in 522 patients with abdominal pain. *Meth. Med.*, **12**, 108–111
14. Nelson, M.A., Allen, P., Clamp, S.E. and De Dombal, F.T. (1979). Reliability and reproducibility of clinical findings in low back pain. *Spine*, **4**, 979–1013
15. Badley, E.M. (1987). Epidemiological aspects of the ageing spine. In Hukins, D.W.L. and Nelson, M.A. (eds.) *The Ageing Spine*, pp. 1–17. (Manchester University Press)
16. Mitchie, L. (1972). Radiological changes and their significance in older men. *Geront. Clin.*, **14**, 310–316
17. Calliet, R. (1975). Lumbar discogenic disease. Why the elderly are more vulnerable? *Geriatrics*, **30**, 73–76
18. Biering-Sorensen, F. (1983). A prospective study of low back pain in a general population, occurrence, recurrence and aetiology. *Scand. J. Rehab. Med.*, **15**, 71–79
19. Kellgren, J.H. and Lawrence, J.S. (1957). Radiological assessment of osteoarthroses. *Ann. Rheum. Dis.*, **16**, 494–502
20. Lawrence, J.S., Bremner, J.M. and Bier, F. (1966). Osteoarthrosis, prevalence in the population and relationship between symptoms and X-ray changes. *Ann. Rheum. Dis.*, **25**, 1–24
21. Allander, E. (1974). Prevalence, incidence and remission rates of some common rheumatic diseases or syndromes. *Scand. J. Rheum.*, **3**, 145–153
22. Torgerson, W.R. and Dotter, W.E. (1976). Comparative roentgenographic study of the asymptomatic lumbar spine. *J. Bone Joint Surg.*, **58A**, 850–853
23. Magora, A. and Schwartz, A. (1978). Relation between the low back pain syndrome and X-ray findings. 2. Transitional vertebra (mainly sacralization), *Scand. J. Rehab. Med.*, **10**, 135–145
24. Magora, A. and Schwartz, A. (1980). Relationship between the low back syndrome and X-ray findings. 3. Spina bifida occulta. *Scand. J. Rehab. Med.*, **12**, 9–15
25. Fredrickson, B.E., Baker, D., McHolick, W.J., Yuan, H.A. and Lubicky, J.P. (1984). The natural history of spondylolysis and spondylolisthesis. *J. Bone Joint Surg.*, **66A**, 699–707
26. Bradford-Hill, A., Sir (1984). *Principles of Medical Statistics*, 11th edn. (London: Hodder & Stoughton)
27. Hamilton, M. (1958). Measurement in medicine. *Lancet*, **1**, 977–982

7
Referred pain and tenderness

J. FOSSGREEN

From clinical observations it has been known for a long time that visceral diseases are frequently accompanied by referred pain to definite areas of the body surface. Typical examples are pain in the right shoulder during a gallstone attack and pain in the left shoulder and arm in connection with angina pectoris.

However, nociceptive and other afferent input from the viscera may not only cause referred pain but may give rise to alterations in the dermatomes, myotomes and sclerotomes that are segmentally linked to the diseased organ[1-3]. In the dermatomes, hyperaesthetic areas may appear and vasomotoric, pilomotoric and sudomotoric changes can be observed[4]. In the myotomes, tenderness and hypertonicity of certain muscles may occur and in the sclerotomes tenderness of the periosteum[3,5-7]. Regarding the spine, there may occur segmental restricted mobility corresponding to the segments related to the diseased internal organ, probably due to contraction of the deep muscles of the spine resulting in movement restriction of two or more adjacent segments[8].

SEGMENTAL PAIN SYNDROMES OF THE SPINE

Referred pain, segmental hyperaesthesia and tenderness can also be caused by nociception from spinal ligaments[9], muscles[10,11], intervertebral joints[12,13], and pericapsular tissue of the intervertebral joints[12].

In human experiments, hypertonic saline solution has been injected into spinal muscles and ligaments[4,9,10,]. The injections provoked two types of pain. The first appeared within a few seconds and had a sharp and stinging quality. This pain disappeared after a few minutes. The other type was a referred pain with roughly segmental distribution. This pain sensation arose about 30 sec after the injection and lasted for several minutes and even hours. With a delay of about 5 min, hyperaesthesia and hyperalgesia could occur in distant areas. Reddening of the skin and muscle spasm could also be observed. McCall et al.[12] investigated the referred pain pattern on intra-articular and pericapsular injection of hypertonic saline solution. In both localizations an aching, cramp-like, deep-pain sensation was reported.

There are clinical observations which make it probable that pain syndromes very similar to pain arising from visceral organs may originate from structures of the spine. Glover described the 'hyperaesthesia syndrome' which he found extremely common in back pain cases[14]. The syndrome may occur at any level from the occiput to the coccyx.

Chest pain is often considered as a sign of disease in the internal organs in the chest as well as in the abdomen. However, there are several references to the fact that chest pain could emanate from the thoracic spine and/or the chest wall[15-20]. The condition is called thoracic segmental pain syndrome or thoracic facet syndrome, assuming that the facet joints most likely are involved.

The syndrome has the following symptomatology[21]. The onset is often acute and related to small uncontrolled movements of the spine. The pain may be severe and be described as a stabbing in the back. Gradual onset may occur. The pain is localized to the segment and in typical cases, pain radiation occurs. Painfully restricted movements of the spine in one or more directions can be observed. Movements in other directions are pain-free or pain-relieving. This is an important sign from the differential point of view.

Often there is pain exaggeration on deep breathing. In the paravertebral muscles corresponding to the involved segments, tightness and tenderness can be found. Furthermore, areas of hyperaesthesia or dysaesthesia can be demonstrated.

All paraclinical tests are normal and the diagnosis has to be based on a thorough clinical examination and exclusion of other diseases.

The frequency of the thoracic facet syndrome appears to be relatively high. In a study from a cardiac hospital unit a thoracic segmental pain syndrome was found in 13% of 1097 patients who were admitted because of chest pain during a period of two years[21]. In another study from general practice comprising 162 patients, a thoracic facet syndrome occurred in 23%[22]. Elsborg treated 30 patients with abdominal pain caused by a thoracic facet syndrome[23]. The treatment was either manipulative or injection with local anaesthetics; 83% of the patients became painfree. After an observation period of 6 months to 5 years, 57% of the patients were still pain free. Relapsing thoracic facet syndrome was observed in 25% of the patients.

Ashby found during a 1-year period 53 patients with abdominal pain of spinal origin[24]. The segments Th XI–XII were most often affected. The patients were treated with intercostal injections of local anaesthetics; 61% of the patients became symptom free.

Maigne found in a group of 350 patients with low back pain that the thoracolumbar junction between Th XI and LI was most often the site of origin[25]. Treatment with manipulation or local injection was used and excellent improvement obtained in 62% of the patients.

SOME NEUROPHYSIOLOGICAL MECHANISMS

Pain from the viscera is often diffuse, dull and aching. Frequently it is accompanied by referred pain to cutaneous and other somatic structures innervated by the same spinal segments that receive input from the internal organs[2,26,27]. Pain from deep somatic structures such as muscles, ligaments, joints and periosteum is essentially similar to visceral pain[5].

Regardless of the primary site of the pain focus, changes as tenderness and hypertonicity may occur in segmental muscles, especially in long-lasting sympathicotonia[5,6]. In clinical experiments it has been shown that patients after more than one attack of renal or uretral calculosis had lowered pain thresholds on selective electrical stimulation of the muscles, subcutaneous tissue and skin at the first lumbar segment on the side of the calculosis[7].

Cervero[5] stated that visceral pain from the upper abdominal viscera is mediated by the activation of few visceral fibres. The spinal cord projection of these fibres converges onto neurons that are viscero-somatic since they are also activated by inputs from the skin and from other somatic structures such as muscles, tendons and ligaments. These observations are considered to be in favour of the 'convergence–projection theory' of Ruch[28], which explains some of the characteristics of referred pain from visceral organs.

Some of the viscero-somatic neurons project their neurons to supraspinal levels. On the other side, the sensory neurons are subjected to supraspinal control of descending signals that comprise both tonic inhibition and phasic excitation.

The sympathetic nervous system has a widespread distribution throughout the body, innervating not only visceral organs, but also peripheral blood vessels, sweat glands and hair follicles. Even the muscle spindles are subjected to sympathetic influence[29,30].

CONCLUSION

In conclusion it appears from clinical and experimental observations that referred pain and segmental tenderness and hyperaesthesia of the back may be brought about from different sources as diseases of the visceral organs, dysfunction of structures of the spine and probably other pain conditions as well.

The mechanisms behind referred pain and segmental tenderness are still not fully explained.

REFERENCES

1. Beal, M.C. (1983). Palpatory testing for somatic dysfunction in patients with cardiovascular disease. *J. Am. Osteopath. Assoc.*, **82**, 822–831
2. Brodal, A. (1981). *Neurological Anatomy in Relation to Clinical Medicine*, 3rd edn., pp. 773–776. (New York: Oxford University Press)

3. Hansen, K. and Schliack, H. (1962). Segmentale Innervation. *Ihre Bedeutung für Klinik und Praxis*. (Stuttgart: Georg Thieme)
4. Lewis, T. and Kellgren, J.H. (1939). Observations related to referred pain, visceromotor reflexes and other associated phenomena. *Clin. Sci.*, 1, 47–71
5. Cervero, F. (1987). Fine afferent fibres from viscera and visceral pain. Anatomy and physiology of viscero-somatic convergence. In Schmidt, R.F., Schaible, H.-G. and Vahle-Hinz, C. (eds.) *Fine Afferent Nerve Fibres and Pain*, pp. 321–331. (Weinheim: VCH Verlagsgesellschaft)
6. Korr, I.M. (1978). Sustained sympathiconia as a factor in disease. In Korr, I.M. *The Neurobiologic Mechanisms in Manipulative Therapy*, pp. 229–268. (New York: Plenum Press)
7. Vecchiet, L., Giamberardino, M.A., Dragani, L. and Able-Fessard, D. (1989). Pain from renal/ureteral calculosis: evaluation of sensory thresholds in the lumbar area. *Pain*, 36, 289–295
8. Beal, M.C. (1985). Viscerosomatic reflexes: a review. *J. Am. Osteopath. Assoc.*, 85, 786–801
9. Hockaday, J.M. and Whitty, C.W. (1987). Patterns of referred pain in the normal subject. *Brain*, 9, 481–496
10. Feinstein, B. (1977). Referred pain from paravertebral structures. In Buerger, A.A. and Tobis, J.S. *Approaches to the Validation of Manipulative Therapy*, pp. 134–174. (Springfield, Ill: Charles E. Thomas)
11. Kellgren, J.H. (1938). Observations on referred pain arising from muscle. *Clin. Sci.*, 3, 175–190
12. McCall, I.W., Park, W.M. and O'Brien, J.P. (1979). Induced pain referral from posterior lumbar elements in normal subjects. *Spine*, 4, 441–446
13. Mooney, V. and Robertson, J. (1976). The facet syndrome. *Clin. Orthop.*, 115, 149–156
14. Glover, J.R. (1977). Characterization of localized back pain. In Buerger, A.A. and Tobis, J.S. *Approaches to the Validation of Manipulative Therapy*, pp. 175–186. (Springfield, Ill: Charles E. Thomas)
15. Cyriax, J. (1962). *Textbook of Orthopaedic Medicine*, Vol.I, 4th edn., p. 331. (London: Cassell)
16. Epstein, S.E., Gerber, L.H. and Borer, J.S. (1979). Chest wall syndrome. *J. Am. Med. Assoc.*, 241, 2793–2797
17. Grieve, G.P. (1986). Thoracic joint problems and simulated visceral diseases. In Grieve, G.P. *Modern Manual Therapy of the Vertebral Column*, pp. 377–404. (Edinburgh: Churchill Livingstone)
18. Ollie, J.A. (1937). Chest pain. *Can. Med. Assoc.*, 37, 209
19. Raney, F.L., Jr. (1966). Costovertebral-costotransverse joint complex as source of local or referred pain. *J. Bone Joint Surg.*, 48A, 1451–1452
20. Travell, J. and Simons, D.G. (1983). *Myofascial Pain and Dysfunction*, p. 46. (Baltimore: Williams & Wilkins)
21. Bechgaard, P. and Fossgreen, J. (1980). Das thoracale Segmentschmerz-syndrom. *Münch. Med. Wschr.*, 122, 759
22. Schmidt, H., Hansen, J.G., Bitsch, N. and Steinmetz, E. (1984). Brystsmerter i almen praksis. *Ugeskr. Laeger*, 146, 2008–2011
23. Elsborg, L. (1982). Abdominale smerter ved thorakalt facetsyndrom. *Ugeskr. Laeger*, 144, 16–18
24. Ashby, E.C. (1977). Abdominal pain of spinal origin. *Ann. R. Coll. Surg. Engl.*, 59, 242–246
25. Maigne, R. (1980). Low back pain of thoracolumbar origin. *Arch. Phys. Med. Rehabil.*, 61, 389–395
26. Appenzeller, O. (1982). *The Autonomic Nervous System*, 3rd edn., pp. 314–317. (Amsterdam: Elsevier)
27. Willis, W.D. (1985). *The Pain System*, pp. 63–65. (Basel: S. Karger)
28. Ruch, T.C. (1946). Visceral sensation and referred pain. In Fulton, J.F. *Howell's Textbook of Physiology*, 15th edn. pp. 385–401. (Philadelphia: Saunders)
29. Hunt, C.C. (1960). The effect of sympathetic stimulation on mammalian muscle spindles. *J. Physiol.*, 151, 332–341
30. Kieschke, J., Mense, S. and Pralhakur, N.R. (1988). Influence of adrenaline and hypoxia on rat muscle receptors in vitro. In Hamann, W. and Iggo, A. *Transduction and Cellular Mechanisms in Sensory Receptors, Progress in Brain Research, Vol. 74*, pp. 91–97. (Amsterdam: Elsevier)

8

Basic case analysis

Loïc BURN and John K. PATERSON

We use the term case analysis rather than diagnosis because of the unpredictability of the phenomena of referred pain and referred tenderness, and because nociceptor systems are present at many sites, and therefore, 'in the great majority of cases we do not know the tissue or tissues from which back pain is originating, or the cause of that pain'[1].

From the historical point of view, the problem of referred pain results in the site of perception of pain not necessarily being of diagnostic significance and frequently being misleading. Further, the 'hornet's nest' of physiological activity to be found at all levels of the neuraxis, periphery, dorsal horn, EMAS and cortex, means that symptoms are inevitably subject to modification on this count alone, and are thereby unreliable.

When it comes to clinical examination, the phenomenon of referred tenderness mirrors that of referred pain, and the 'hornet's nest' we have mentioned in respect of history is as applicable to physical signs as it is to symptoms. However, the physiological phenomena that may or may not accompany pain can, within certain limits, be used in case analysis. But it must be remembered that, on scientific grounds, physiological parameters cannot be used in case analysis as a means of measuring pain.

It will be appreciated that any clinician dealing with the chronic pain patient who is unaware of the complexities of these problems, as of the possibilities and limitations of the methods of their assessment, is at a substantial disadvantage in effective case analysis, as he is likely to rely upon features that do not have the advantage of scientific validation.

We allocate primacy to behavioural indices in case analysis because these are objective and may therefore be agreed by all clinicians, whatever their discipline. This greatly simplifies the complex question of patient assessment and avoids the difficulties inherent in subject report, which is notoriously unreliable. We choose to use these criteria in the knowledge that no single response channel can ever provide the perfect method of evaluation, but that they afford the clinician a practical base for case analysis. We do not favour this to the exclusion of all else, but 'if it is pushed too far, it [behavioural assessment] results in a rather farcical situation, where patients say, "They will treat me, but they will not listen to me about my pain", and that is no good'[2].

It will be seen from the case analysis record sheet (Figure 8.1) that other administrative and historical data are familiar to the clinician and need no description. Of particular interest to musculoskeletal practice are disturbances of gait (raising the question of myelopathy), saddle anaesthesia and problems with micturition (raising the possibility of sacral root compression) and symptoms of basilar artery insufficiency.

The traditional methods of examination of the back and its investigation are well known to all within FIMM, and we mention them only to emphasize that they are essential to the proper evaluation of musculoskeletal problems. They do, however, have their limitations.

With regard to the cervical spine, 'we early came to the conclusion, reinforced by long experience, that, contrary to the statements of many physicians on this topic, but in agreement with Brain *et al.* (1952), neurological findings are of extremely limited use in the assessment of the precise level of cord and root involvement and may be misleading'[3]. 'In a series of 500 patients surgically treated for disc disease, correct preoperative clinical localization was achieved in only 39.2%'[4].

Local examination of the spine is traditionally medically unorthodox. There are perhaps two exceptions to this: the search for trigger points and, more recently, the emergence of the 'facet joint syndrome'. However, local examination is an integral part of osteopathic and chiropractic practice: for both of them, mobility is of prime importance. For the chiropractor, 'the first characteristic of the manipulative lesion is restricted joint motion. This is the so-called fixation or blockage. The diagnosis of restricted motion is through palpation of movement between vertebrae or by motion X-ray. For example, the palpation of flexion/extension motion can be achieved by placing the fingers between the spinous processes and having the patient flex and extend the spine'[5]. The chiropractor seeks to find by palpation tissue changes, and in particular changes in mobility, at the segmental level assumed to be at fault.

For the osteopath, the keystone of his practice is the osteopathic spinal lesion, which is a condition of impaired mobility in an intervertebral joint. To quote Colin Dove, 'what the osteopath aims to do is to restore the normal functions of tissues, particularly movement, where it is perceived to be lacking. Even if his assessment leads him to assume that the symptoms are arising at the level of hypermobility, he will seek to improve mobility elsewhere'[6].

Mobility tests

We have three reservations regarding the use of mobility tests in local examination.

MUSCULOSKELETAL CASE ANALYSIS SHEET

Patient's name..Serial No:.........
Address..Insurance..........
....Phone..............
Date of birth   / /   Male.... Female....

Family doctor's name...........................
Address..
.................................Phone...............NHS/Private......

HISTORY - Present episode.

Subject report

	/ /		/ /		/ /	
	L	R	L	R	L	R
Pain – Site						
Radiation						
Intensity						
Duration						
Worsened by						
Improved by						

Altered sensation

	L	R	L	R	L	R
P & N						
Numbness						

Activities of daily living

Hoovering			
Bedmaking			
Ablutions			
Cooking			
Ironing			
Putting on socks			
Shopping			
Gardening			
Sports			
Sitting at desk			
Other work			
Road/rail travel			
Air travel			

Pain behaviour

Pill taking habit			
Other treatments			
Hours in bed per 24			
Forced absenteeism			
Litigation pending			

Previous episodes

         Year...... Site.......... Duration Days... Weeks... Months....
         Therapy.......................... Outcome..................
         Year...... Site.......... Duration Days... Weeks... Months....
         Therapy.......................Outcome..................

Relevant medical history..

Investigations...

Figure 8.1 Obverse of data sheet

(1)   They are entirely subjective, so that the sceptical of our colleagues will
        remain for ever fully entitled to their scepticism.

(2)   The 'normal' range of vertebral movement varies enormously, making its
        positive identification very difficult[7,8].

(3)   Despite a great deal of work worldwide, 'vertebral mobility is not fully
        understood'[9].

It is for these reasons that we prefer to confine ourselves to other undisputed
physiological phenomena. These are detailed as follows.

Reflex phenomena

(1)   Referred deep tenderness

(2)   Muscular reflex

(3)   Reflex skin tenderness

These are reflex phenomena that may or may not accompany pain, but they are
not quantifiable indices of the severity of that pain, nor are they reliable
indicators of its site of origin. For these reasons, the use of physiological changes
to measure pain has invariably failed. 'In general there would seem to be little
basis for discrete physiological changes related to the pain experience'[10].
Because of referred pain and referred tenderness, these signs cannot be used to
identify a specific site of origin of that pain.
        What, then, is the point of seeking these signs? The answers are two.

Value of local signs

(1)   As an indication of segmental level or levels to which local therapy may
        best be directed.

(2)   As a monitor of therapeutic progress, (like global movements, or the SLR
        test).

For these reasons, and for these reasons alone, they have clinical relevance. They
have *no* diagnostic validity.
        These signs have been known to clinicians for a very long time. They have
been described in many varied and at times eccentric ways. For example, Korr[10],
in 1948, described the 'spinal lesion' as being associated with:

(a)   Tenderness
(b)   Muscular changes
(c)   Autonomic changes
(d)   Pain that may be referred

Items (a) and (b) are clearly relevant to our present discussion: item (c) is a matter for separate consideration which will be found in ref. 11; while (d), as we have already said, suffers from all the unreliability of subject report.

Within the body of orthodox medicine, many authors from different countries have seen fit to make use of these signs (for example, Brügger[12] and Sutter[13]). In fact, many doctors may share scientific bases to a greater extent than some realise. This is a fact from which bodies such as FIMM might well profit.

More than 20 years ago, Maigne[14] (amongst others) made two major contributions; the first was to translate the description of these signs into terms both intelligible and acceptable to the medical profession in his country, the second was to use diagnostically the term that translates most readily into English as the 'painful segmental disorder'. By this means he avoided the pitfall of making a specific diagnosis that, in the light of subsequent modifications of understanding, would of necessity at some stage become untenable. This showed remarkable prescience, and has indeed stood the test of time.

The six local tests we use are all unoriginal and, in order to appeal to the medical profession as a whole, are here presented in terms as explicit and orthodox as possible. It is essential that these be sought anteriorly as well as posteriorly (it must be remembered that spinal pain and tenderness, for example, can be referred to the anterior chest or abdominal wall). In view of the difficulties we have already emphasized, local examination must be comprehensive – the whole spine must be examined.

1. Skin pinching

This is a test for tenderness of the skin and subcutaneous tissues. The examiner raises a fold of skin at paired sites either side of the midline and pinches as nearly symmetrically as he can. Because of the phenomenon of referred tenderness, this must be done widely, both posteriorly and anteriorly. Not infrequently the examiner will observe a difference in thickness of the skinfold between the two sides at the level the patient reports tenderness. This difference may be eliminated on resolution of the tenderness. There is currently no valid explanation for this phenomenon. A positive finding does *not* indicate the segmental level of dysfunction.

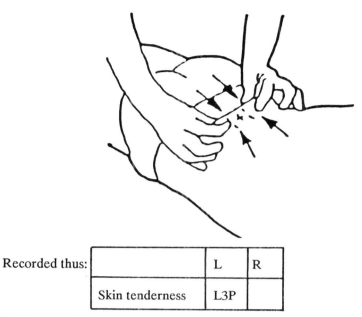

Recorded thus:		L	R
	Skin tenderness	L3P	

Figure 8.2 This patient has a positive sign posteriorly on the left at L3

2. Muscle guarding

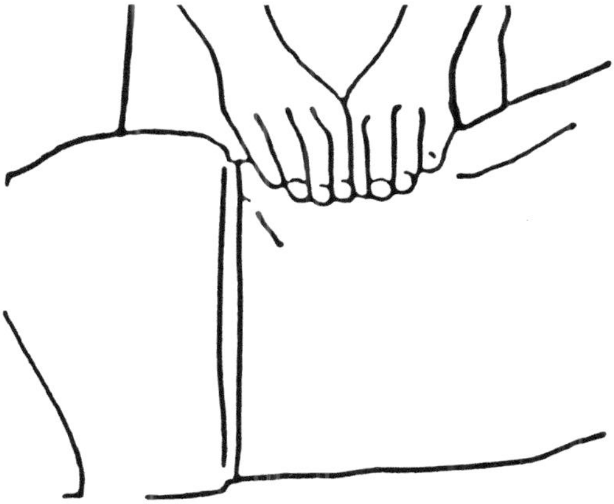

Recorded thus:		L	R
	Local guarding	L2–4	

Figure 8.3 This patient shows increased tone on the left from L2 to L4

This test seeks to identify segmental levels at which there is a difference in muscle tone between the two sides. A positive finding, while clearly subjective, is well known to physicians and generally accepted by them, as in the case of guarding in acute abdominal pathology. This finding is commonly associated with tenderness.

3. Trigger points

Owing to the wide distribution of trigger points, it is not profitable to illustrate trigger points, other than by defining their site using the crude criterion of the dermatomes.

Recorded thus:

	L	R
Trigger points	L2P	

This patient has a trigger point on the left in the distribution of L2, posteriorly.

Deep palpation seeks to elicit tenderness in trigger points. Since these may be found widely, they must be sought equally widely.

4. Segmental sagittal pressure

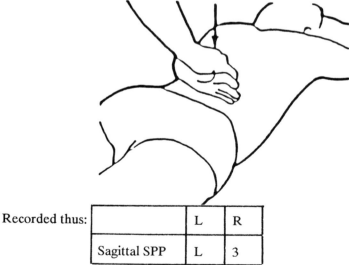

Recorded thus:

	L	R
Sagittal SPP	L	3

Figure 8.4 This patient suffers pain on pressure at the third segmental level

This test seeks to elicit pain on applying a midline sagittal force to the spinous processes at successive segmental levels. It serves to implicate either the vertebra to which it is applied, or the various joints above and below. Since the spinous processes in the cervical spine are (except for that of C7) so deep and small as to be in practice impalpable, this test is inapplicable to the cervical region. Of course, many more joints are moved by this test than those immediately adjacent to the vertebra pressed upon, but the force and resultant movement are concentrated in sequence at each segmental level.

5. Lateral spinous process pressure

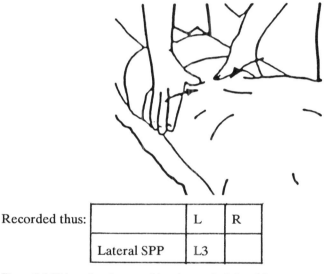

Recorded thus:

	L	R
Lateral SPP	L3	

Figure 8.5 This patient has a positive sign on the left at L3

This test produces a passive rotation of successive vertebrae, performed by pressing with the thumbs on the lateral aspect of each spinous process, alternately to the left and the right. Once more, it involves a *minimum* of *all* the joints between the vertebrae pressed upon and its two neighbours, but many more joints must be affected, so rendering it pretty non-specific.

6. Zygoapophyseal tenderness

This test seeks to reveal any tenderness there may be of the zygoapophyseal joint capsules and adjacent structures, in an attempt to locate the site of origin of the symptoms. The examiner presses firmly over the joints at each segmental level in

71

turn and asks the patient to report tenderness at any site. Apart from its use in determining a possible site of dysfunction, this test is of value in that it may reveal the potentially most suitable site for local treatment (e.g. injection). It is more specific than the previous two tests, in that it gives some indication of the side as well as the segmental level.

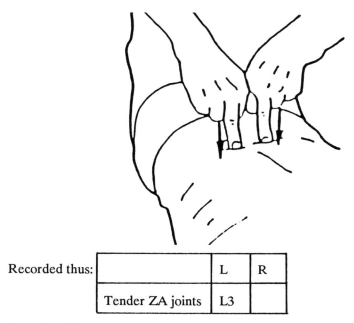

Recorded thus:

	L	R
Tender ZA joints	L3	

Figure 8.6 This patient has tenderness over the left L3 joint

CONCLUSION

The practical features of this system of case analysis are as follows (see Figure 8.7).

(1)   It is based on the relevant anatomical, physiological, psychological and pathological facts, as they are currently understood.

(2)   Whatever its acknowledged shortcomings, it provides a rational basis for clinical assessment and management.

(3)   It is brief enough to be of use to every clinician.

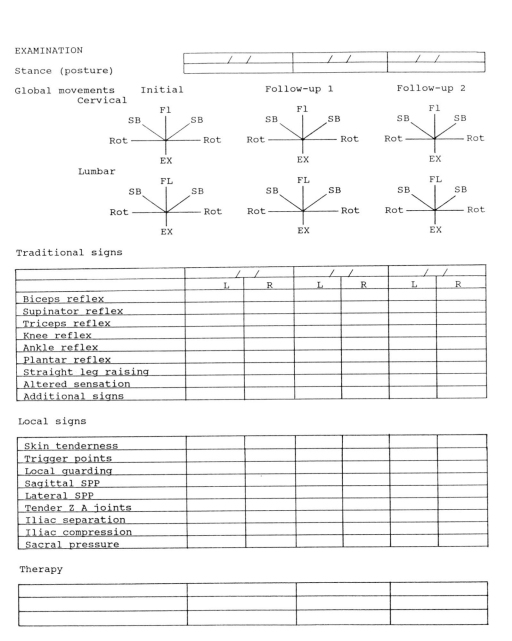

Figure 8.7 Reverse of data sheet

73

(4)   To this scientifically oriented basis, physicians may add whatever further symptoms and signs they may find useful in their individual practices (e.g. spinal joint mobility).

(5)   Because it is founded on scientific considerations, it will inevitably be subject to modification in the light of further knowledge and understanding.

(5)   It thereby avoids dogma, as baneful an influence in musculoskeletal medicine as in other fields.

(7)   The case analysis sheet provides a check list for the clinician, which aims at:
        (a)   Being comprehensive,
        (b)   Affording comparability of data from different observers.

REFERENCES

1. Wyke (1983). *Presentation at 7th FIMM Congress, Zürich*
2. Merskey (1982). *Proceedings of the International symposium organized by the National Back Pain Association, London*
3. Phillips (1975). Upper limb involvement in cervical spondylosis. *J. Neurol. Neurosurg. Psychiatr.*, **38**, 386
4. Lansche (1960). Correlation of the myelogram with clinical and operative findings in lumbar disc lesions. *J. Bone Joint Surg.*, **48**, 193
5. Haldeman (1982). *Presentation at the Colt symposium, London*
6. Dove (1982). *Presentation at the Colt symposium, London*
7. Hilton (1980). In Jayson (ed.) *The Lumbar Spine and Back Pain*, 2nd edn.
8. Moll and Wright (1980). In Jayson (ed.) *The Lumbar Spine and Back Pain*, 2nd edn.
9. Reading (1983). In Wall and Melzack (eds.) *Textbook of Pain*, p. 202
10. Korr (1948). The emerging concept of the osteopathic lesion. *The Collected Papers of Irvin M. Korr*, p. 128. (Colorado Springs: American Academy of Osteopathy)
11. Burn and Paterson (1989). *Musculoskeletal Medicine – The Spine* (Lancaster: Kluwer Academic Publishers) (in press)
12. Brügger (1962). Pseudoradikulär syndrome. *Acta. Rheumatol.*, **19**
13. Sutter (1963). Versuch einer Wesensbestimmung pseudoradikulärer Syndrome. *Schweiz. Rundsh. Med. Praxis.*, 842
14. Maigne (1968). Douleur d'origine vertebrale. Expansion scientifique

9
Manual therapy – 1989

Karel LEWIT

This paper is not intended as a historical review or to give the latest 'authoritative' statements about scientific research in manual therapy. Its purpose is to point out some of the most interesting and therefore also most controversial problems in order to stimulate discussion and, if possible, research.

CLINICAL EVALUATION

First, the question of clinical evaluation. This was very adequately dealt with by Arkuszewski[1,2] of the Neurological clinic in Katowice in the following way.

(1)   When mainly muscle energy techniques are used, the patients in the control group cannot distinguish between manual examination (carried out in all patients) and treatment (given only to 50 out of 100 patients).

(2)   Arkuszewski did not rely on pain ratings alone but on clinical examination using a well thought-out three-point system, 1 point standing for slight deviation from the normal, 2 points for medium intensity, and 3 for severe change (Figures 9.1 and 9.2).

(3)   He treated the whole spinal column according to the clinical findings; in fact, patients treated for low back pain including root syndromes in the lower extremities showed greater improvement if upper cervical was found and treated at the same time (Figure 9.3).

(4)   There was also adequate follow-up (Figure 9.4).

Brodin's[3] group of low back pain patients is interesting because he singled out those in whom pain was caused exclusively by segmental movement restriction without root pain, i.e. cases in which manual therapy is assumed to be *the* specific treatment. Evaluation took place after 5 weeks and here the results are as spectacular as could be expected (Figure 9.5). Results were similar in the cervical spine[4] (Figure 9.6).

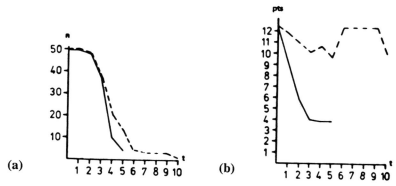

Figure 9.1 Diagram comparing (a) the time of hospital treatment (b) the rate of improvement in the manual treatment group and in controls. Solid curves, manual treatment group; broken curves, control group; *n*, number of patients; pts, symptoms and signs in the points scale, *t*, weeks of treatment

These very encouraging statistical results should not be considered the only criterion for evaluation. Unlike pharmacotherapy, manipulation produces immediate results that can be assessed both subjectively by the patient and by clinical means. If a patient comes with severe pain and impairment of mobility and walks off after treatment with little or no pain and free movement, *his* case does not require statistical evaluation, just as operation for acute appendicitis was accepted by the medical profession long before statistics became a fashion that by now is almost an obsession. The difficulties with statistics in patients with painful conditions of the motor system are that (1) the course is difficult to predict and there is a high rate of recurrence, (2) they are multifactorial, and (3) these factors are interdependent and their relevance changes not only from one patient to the other, but in the course of time even in the same patient[5]. The object of manual therapy, i.e. segmental movement restriction, is only one of many factors of variable relevance. Under such conditions statistics are no easy matter, the more so as, although the final aim of treatment is relief of the patient's suffering, manipulation is no pain killer but can achieve nothing more (or less) than restored mobility, and only if movement restriction is a relevant factor of the painful condition is manipulation profitable.

Joint movement restriction or 'blockage' on the other hand, if correctly diagnosed is always corrected by specific manipulation. This can be assessed by clinical methods: always by palpation, as a rule by measuring the range of movement[6] (Figures 9.7, 9.8), sometimes by X-rays[7] and indirectly by instruments that register reflex effects, e.g. thermography or even EMG (Figures 9.9, 9.10). Again it should be pointed out that reversible movement restriction or blockage in 'somatic dysfunction' if correctly diagnosed and localized, is always corrected by adequate manipulative techniques, as long as there is disturbance of function only, and not of structure.

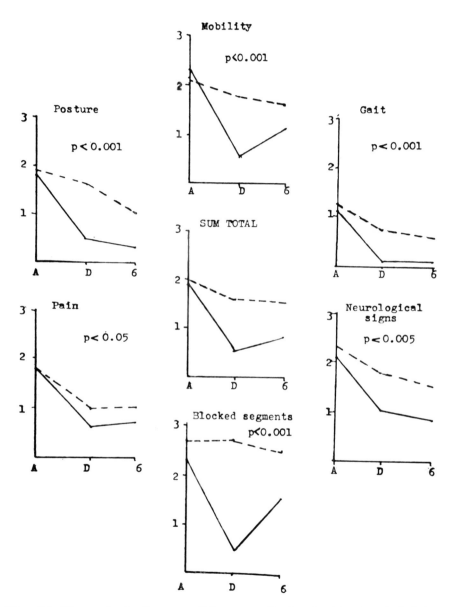

Figure 9.2 Diagram showing the course of disease according to a 3-point system at admission, on discharge and after 6 months

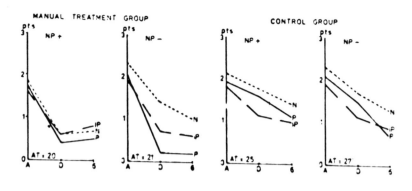

NP+:neck pain present, NP-:neck pain absent
IP-intensity of back pain, N-neurological examination, P-posture
AT-average time of treatment in days
pts-average intensity of a sign on a scale of 0-3 points, A-at
admission, D-at discharge, 6-6 months after discharge

Figure 9.3 Diagram showing that if patients with low back pain have also a cervical problem, their low back pain is likely to improve more if both the cervical and the lumbar area are treated

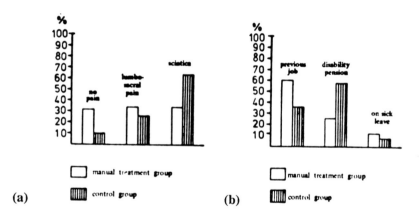

(a)   (b)

Figure 9.4 Diagram comparing (a) pain after 6 months in the treated and control groups and (b) work capacity

Therefore, assessment of the effect of manipulation is part of routine practice for the professional therapist, immediately after treatment; it is made by clinical methods, mainly by palpation.

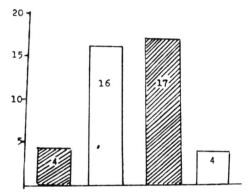

Figure 9.5 Diagram comparing manual treatment group (hatched) and controls in low back pain after 5 weeks. *n* = 41: 21 treatment, 20 control

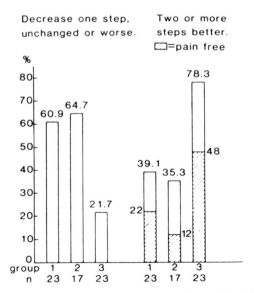

Figure 9.6 Diagram comparing manual treatment group and controls with cervical pain – only group 3 received manual treatment. Hatched: pain free

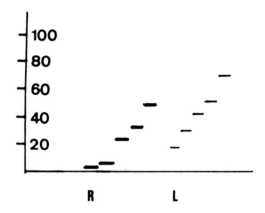

Figure 9.7 Measurement of segmental mobility according to Berger: restriction between C1/2 and C2/3 at right rotation, normal condition at left rotation

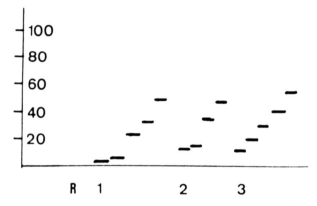

Figure 9.8 1 – Restriction between C1/2 and C2/3 to the right, 2 – After mobilization of C1/2, 3 – after mobilization of C2/3

PALPATION

Palpation is essential in the diagnosis of movement restriction, of tissue changes, even of provoked pain, in assessment of immediate effects and during the process of mobilization as well as while performing soft-tissue techniques. Therefore, an analysis of palpation technique and its implications is of great interest[8,9].

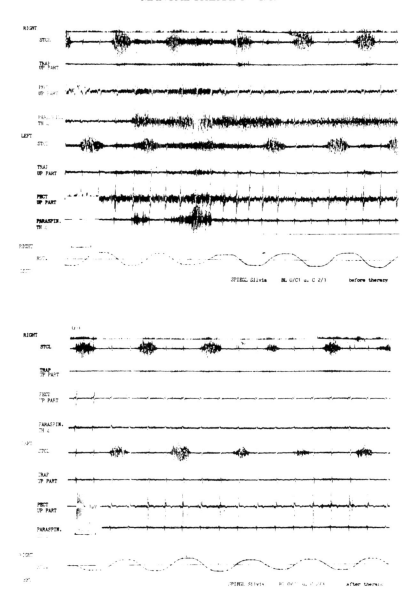

Figures 9.9 (top) and 9.10 (bottom) Compare muscle activity on right and left rotation (undulating line) before and after manual therapy

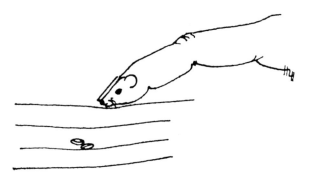

Figure 9.11 Symbolizing the palpating finger

What happens during palpation?

(a) The examiner has to concentrate upon what he intends to study: texture, moisture, temperature, shape, resistance, elasticity, etc. (Figure 9.11).

(b) The main mechanical object that can be measured in palpation is resistance to static pressure.

(c) This, however, is practically never the case. What we do is to try to palpate one layer of tissue after the other, shifting the superficial strata to the side so as to examine in depth; at the same time observing mobility of one layer or structure relative to the next. In order to palpate the shape of a structure – its borders – our fingers again have to move. To palpate muscle bundles we let them slip under our fingers (Figure 9.12), and if there is a trigger point we sense its contractions under our fingers, while the patient experiences pain, i.e. we produce a reaction which we register.

(d) Thus consciously or not, we regularly examine mobility between tissues, e.g. adhesions (movement restriction) in scars, movement restriction during skin rolling or just resistance of the superficial skin layer when examining skin drag. It is only natural if we then learn to palpate joint mobility and its restrictions, in particular the 'endfeel' or the 'barrier'.

(e) The endfeel or the barrier[10] that is so characteristic in joints can also be sensed in the skin, in the connective tissue and in muscles, while stretching skin, stretching connective tissue and muscles, moving one layer (structure) against the other or even when applying pressure.

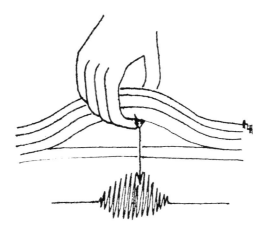

Figure 9.12 Letting a muscle bundle slip between the fingers

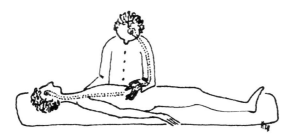

Figure 9.13 Feedback relationship with the patient

(f)   By exerting both pressure and motion, the palpating finger produces a reaction which the examiner registers and on registering it he modifies his own palpation, i.e. an interaction is created between examiner and patient, a feedback relationship between two self-regulating systems of the greatest complexity (Figure 9.13).

(g)   This interaction lends itself most naturally to treatment and is the basis of all massage techniques. Obviously, the secret of the good masseur lies in his ability to make use of this feedback relationship, i.e. to correct the action of his hands so as to achieve the most favourable results.

(h)   The best results if we apply soft tissue techniques can be achieved when engaging the barrier (taking up the slack) and producing 'the release phenomenon'[11]: stretching the skin (Figure 9.14) over a small or large area with very slight force, we reach a barrier. If we then just hold this

83

stretch without increasing our pull, after a latency period of a few seconds, we notice that the skin starts stretching; this will go on for some 10 seconds or longer, until a new barrier is reached. The same will happen if we create a fold of subcutaneous connective tissue, of a scar or of a muscle (Figure 9.15): we first take up the slack, then wait and again a lengthening reaction will ensue which goes on until a new barrier is reached. The same happens when applying pressure ('acupressure') (Figure 9.16). This phenomenon can also be observed in postisometric relaxation[12] and in mobilization using neuromuscular techniques. In the first phase, after taking up the slack the patient applies resistance; then he is told to 'let go' (relax) and after a latency of a few seconds the range of movement increases through muscle decontraction until a new barrier is reached. The same happens by shifting one tissue layer against the other (e.g. fascia).

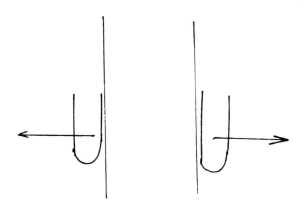

Figure 9.14 Skin stretch

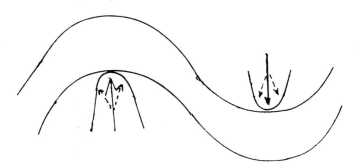

Figure 9.15 Producing the release phenomenon by folding connective tissue

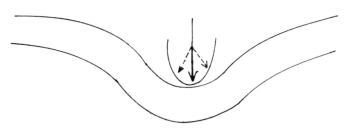

Figure 9.16 Producing release by maintaining pressure

(i)   In all instances the therapy is carried out in tissues or structures where we find increased tension interfering with mobility; in joints or tissues, while release takes place, the therapist feels tension subsiding while lengthening is obtained through stretch or muscle decontraction. Again palpatory skill is decisive: the release phenomenon may last a few seconds or even up to half a minute. If we do not make full use of it, we do not achieve the best results. If we do sense it, we also *know*, that our stretching, mobilization or muscle relaxation has been successful.

The reason why this type of soft tissue technique is much more effective and less time-consuming than the usual massage lies precisely in that it relies on palpation diagnosis of release and we *wait* until it can be fully sensed. In massage, on the other hand, the rhythm is too fast and the tissues are not given the time for full release to take place.

From this analysis palpation is seen to be a clinical procedure providing us with the greatest possible wealth of information. In addition it creates interaction with the patient, resulting in a feedback relationship enabling the therapist to modify his actions to obtain not only diagnostic but also therapeutic results. In this way we can give treatment to any tissue with a degree of control no other instrument can provide, using the techniques of manual medicine (Figure 9.17).

There is, however, a serious snag in this picture, which looks almost too good to be true. This is the difficulty of scientific assessment. From the analysis of palpation it is evident that there is constant change both in direction and in intensity, creating an interaction, a feedback relationship of two such complex systems as the sensing therapist and the patient with his specific changes in his tissue under the control of *his* nervous system. This is so unique that it cannot be reproduced.

Science requires reproducibility – for comparison, verification and further processing of data. What can be seen can be photographed or filmed, what can be heard can be taped, but this does not hold for the wealth of information gained by palpation. It is therefore rejected as 'subjective'. This is true to some extent of other clinical evidence, e.g. extracting information from a patient by personal interview.

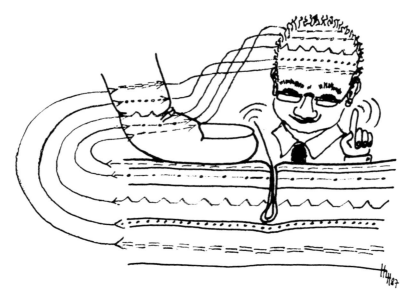

Figure 9.17 The feedback control provided by palpation

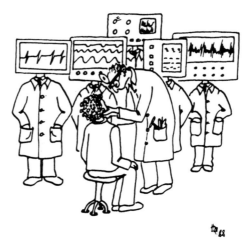

Figure 9.18 The position of the clinician today

This has serious implications. The clinical method, which is our greatest source of information – and which creates a feedback relationship in the spirit of modern cybernetics – is rejected as subjective and non-scientific. To put this dilemma even more pointedly: information obtained from apparatus, including the most sophisticated computers is acceptable, but information from the 'original computer' (our brain) and the most perfect instruments (our hands) is 'unscientific'. This attitude is certainly very detrimental to clinical medicine in which interaction of patient and therapist is an essential element, and carries the threat of dehumanized medicine.

RELIEF OF PAIN BY MANIPULATIVE THERAPY

This is generally considered to be a puzzle. Yet it seems to me that this is so only as long as we ignore clinical evidence that we have literally in our palpating hands. In fact, this section might have been called 'the contribution of manipulative therapy to the puzzle of non-specific pain in the motor system'. Here, non-specific signifies 'without known pathology'. All we can do by manipulation is to restore *function* and it is time we realized that in addition to pathological anatomy, there is also *'functional pathology'*[13]. Just as an engine does not function because a cylinder has burst, it does not function if the ignition is out of order, although the engine may be intact. If we want to understand manual therapy and other methods, in particular in the field of rehabilitation, we ought to understand that they normalize function.

The main and most frequent symptom of disturbed function in the motor system is – pain[14]! The reason is that any dysfunction causes increased *tension*. If we move in the direction of restricted motion, we meet resistance and create tension that is relieved by manipulation. In a muscular trigger point there are muscle bundles that are in contraction and produce tension. By achieving decontraction, tension subsides and so does pain[15]. Dynamic or static overstrain causes discomfort that ends up in pain, which ceases if we rest or change the position that causes strain. This makes sense, for tension is an expression of possible overstrain that may cause damage in the motor system, pain being thus a physiological warning sign of impending danger. It is also in keeping with known facts: pain receptors (high threshold) are found in those structures in which tension manifests itself: the attachment points of ligaments and tendons, joint capsules, root sheaths, muscles, etc. And it is tension we recognize in the tissues with our palpating fingers during manual diagnosis and treatment. We diagnose tension in the skin as well as in muscles and in scars, and if we produce what I have called the release phenomenon we sense tension being released and we *know* that we have relieved pain. Manipulation is effective because by normalizing function it greatly relieves tension. It is particularly effective if we combine it with 'muscle energy'[16] or 'neuromuscular'[17] techniques, because we act on both joint mobility and by muscular relaxation.

Tension in various tissues is coupled with reflex phenomena, as tension in connective tissue and in the skin may disappear after manipulation of joints, and mobility not only of skin layers but also in the spinal column may improve after

87

releasing tension by treating soft tissues. We acquire all this evidence clinically, by our hands.

Although this is done daily by experienced clinicians with similar results, they seem reluctant to draw the logical conclusions on purely clinical grounds – in other words, to stick to their guns. The clinician, who a hundred years ago was the leading figure in medicine, has become something like a humble disciple faced with the physiologist, the biochemist and the anatomist, even if it is he who has the relevant data in his own hands (Figure 9.18).

Manual medicine greatly enhances the ability of the physician to examine by making much better use of his hands than those clinicians who have not been taught these skills. It should therefore make us more confident in drawing theoretical conclusions from the data these skills have provided and allow us to find satisfaction in the fact that we are able to discover things that are hidden even from the most modern apparatus, and should not humbly underrate the human brain and its most precious instrument – our hands. We may also hope that manual medicine will thus help to raise the standing of clinical medicine.

REFERENCES

1. Arkuszewski, Z. (1986). The efficacy of manual treatment in low back pain. *Manual Med.*, **2**, 68–71
2. Arkuszewski, Z. (1986). Involvement of the cervical spine in back pain. *Manual Med.*, **2**, 126–128
3. Brodin, H. (1982). Inhibition–facilitation technique for lumbar pain treatment. *Manuelle Med.*, **20**, 95–98
4. Brodin, H. (1982). Cervical pain and mobilization. *Manuelle Med.*, **20**, 90–94
5. Gutmann, G. (1975). Die pathogenetische Aktualitäts-Diagnostik. In Lewit, K. and Gutmann, G. (eds.) *Functional Pathology of the Motor System. Rehabilitácia*, Suppl.10–11, pp. 15–24. (Bratislavia: Obzor)
6. Berger, M. (1984). Cervikomotographie, ein neues Verfahren zur Funktionsuntersuchung der Halswirbelsäule. In Bergsmann, H., Bischko, J. *et al.* (eds.) *Moderne Schmerzbehandlung. Beiträge zur Anaesthesiologie und Intensivmedizin*, pp. 83–90. (Wien: W. Maudrich)
7. Arlen, A. (1979). Biometrische Röntgen-Funktionsdiagnostik der Halswirbelsäule. *Schriftenenenreihe Manuelle Medizin, Bd.5*. (Heidelberg: Verlag für Medizin, E. Fischer)
8. Greenman, P.E. (1984). Schichtweise Palpation. *Manuelle Med.*, **22**, 46–48
9. Lewit, K. (1987). O vyznamu palpace u bolestivych onemocnení pohybové soustavy (Importance of palpation in painful conditions of the motor system). *Rehabilitácia*, Suppl.34, pp. 23–25. (Bratislava: Obzor)
10. Bourdillon, J.F. and Day, E.A. (1987). *Spinal Manipulation*, pp. 38–40. (London: Heinemann)
11. Lewit, K. (1988). Fenomen uvolnení (Release phenomenon). *Rehabilitácia*, **21**, 152–156
12. Lewit, K. (1986). Postisometric relaxation in combination with other methods of muscular facilitation and inhibition. *Manual Med.*, **2**, 101–104
13. Lewit, K. (1987). The functional pathology of the locomotor system. *J. Orthop. Med.*, **3**, 55–58
14. Lewit, K. (1987). *Manipulative Therapy in Rehabilitation of the Motor System*, pp. 39–43. (London: Butterworths)
15. Travell, J.G. and Simons, D.G. (1983). *Myofascial Pain and Dysfunction. The Trigger Point Manual*. (Baltimore: Williams & Wilkins)
16. Mitchell, F. Jr., Moran, P.S. and Pruzzo, N.A. (1979). *An Evaluation of Muscle Energy Procedures*. (Valey Park: Pruzzo)
17. Schneider, W., Dvorák, J. and Dvorák, V. (1986). *Manuelle Medizin Therapie*, p. 8. (Stuttgart: Thieme)

10
An osteopathic approach to manipulation

Alan STODDARD

Manipulation is only part of the armamentarium of the osteopathic physician. It is important, therefore, to place manipulation into context on the main osteopathic theme, which is that health and disease depend to a large extent on the structural integrity of the body, that when the body has a normal framework it will remain healthy, but if the structure (i.e. the musculo-skeletal components) is faulty then disability and disease ensue. With this in mind, the osteopath's chief concern when treating disability and disease is to restore normal structure whenever possible.

Manipulation of the musculo-skeletal system of the body is in practice an essential component of this osteopathic approach, but other measures to restore structural integrity may be equally important. For example, posture in work and play must be considered in both prevention and treatment. The muscles of the body need to be efficient and strong enough for the tasks of daily life.

Without the body framework and the muscles to move it, none of the other organs of the body could function. The heart and the lungs, the digestive system and emunctory organs are there merely to ensure that the body can move from place to place, so we must if we wish to have our priorities right deal with the most basic of all bodily activity – the musculo-skeletal system. The osteopathic standpoint needs no excuses, therefore, to emphasize the importance of structure.

The title of this chapter restricts any enlargement of the subject and brings it down to the place of manipulation within the global concept of osteopathy. Manipulation is a wide term in itself and it could cover any manual treatment. It is well recognized that manual methods are conveniently divided into three aspects, viz. massage of soft tissue, articulation or mobilization of joints, and specific manipulative techniques to restore normal mobility or to restore normal position of adjacent bones with each other. The treatment of muscles and ligaments is not a prerogative of osteopathy. The principles and methods of those treatments were elaborated long before the osteopathic concept impinged upon mechanical problems, but articulatory techniques and specific manipulations have been developed and improved greatly by osteopaths compared with the earlier ideas of passive joint movements and the old bone setter techniques of putting bones back into position when they have been displaced. The more recent knowledge of the role of disc degeneration in the vertebral complex has modified osteopathic thinking as well as medical thinking in terms of manipulation of the spine, and I will come to this later.

The principle behind articulatory osteopathic techniques is to use gentle, persuasive, repetitive, rhythmic, passive movements that are designed firstly to improve mobility in the joint or joints of the affected area and secondly to increase circulation to the joints and adjacent tissues. Passive movements of the limbs can be shown to increase blood flow to the limb treated. Any healing or repairing process is automatically increased by improvement of circulation.

The details of mobilizing techniques need to be learned by any practitioner who wishes to be effective in treating musculo-skeletal problems, whether using articulation to peripheral joints or to the spine. Normal ranges of movements need to be learned and a tactile sense needs to be acquired by practice, so that joints are not forced beyond their normal ranges. Accessory movements need to be known about and restored when limited. These accessory movements are vital but not always given their due importance. Accessory movements are those ranges that are essentially passive rather than active. The concept has been elaborated by James and John Mennell[1,2]. An example of accessory movements is those found in the interphalangeal joints of fingers. Normal movements exist in flexion and extension, but passively there are small amounts of rotation and side-bending. Without these latter movements even flexion and extension are limited. Another example is the occipito-atlantal joint. There the main movement is flexion and extension, but small amounts of rotation and side-bending are necessary for full flexion and extension.

When it comes to study and practice of specific manipulation, the osteopathic profession has done more to develop and elaborate these techniques than any other school of thought.

The original bone setters developed intuitive techniques handed down from father to son using the 'rule of thumb' methods without much consideration of pathology and the mechanical state of the joint that was being manipulated. The early orthopaedic surgeons used crude techniques on the basis that if a joint was stiff, then it should be simply forcibly stretched in all directions, preferably under an anaesthetic. This method fell into disrepute because no account was taken of the possibility that some of the joints in question were not stiff, but were in fact unstable, and in these earlier days, the knowledge of disc disease was not available. The chiropractors developed techniques that have an application sometimes, but were based on the misconception that bones go out of place and need to be put back. The early osteopaths also evolved techniques of manipulation based on the position of one vertebra relative to the one below. These techniques of the earlier osteopaths and chiropractors have been superseded because of the greater knowledge we all have of mechanical problems in spinal and peripheral joints. The Cyriax school of thought placed excessive emphasis on the role of disc displacements in the management of spinal problems and fails to recognize the earlier mechanical lesions of the spinal column involving reduced mobility, instability and subluxation affecting the apophyseal joints. The physiotherapy schools headed by Maitland have placed emphasis on mobilizing techniques that are modifications of earlier osteopathic articulatory techniques. The terms articulation, mobilization and passive movements cover the same basic procedures and can be collectively grouped together even if there are small differences in practical application.

Each school of thought makes a useful contribution to the whole and to the wider subject of manipulation and each will benefit from the ideas of the others so long as the newer knowledge of mechanical problems is incorporated in the improvements in techniques.

The osteopathic school's main contribution to this wider knowledge has been in the study of spinal mechanics and the application of those studies to the improved techniques of manipulation.

Prior to attempting any form of manipulation the joint or joints in question need to be mechanically assessed and here again the osteopathic methods of mobility tests are vital for this process.

Just as in any peripheral joint problem, before any disease process has taken place and long before degenerative changes have had time to develop, there are painful mechanical problems of sprains and ligamentous damage, leading on to instability when the original trauma was excessive, or to reduced mobility due to tightened capsules and adhesions that form following trauma. In order to diagnose the mechanical problems, mobility has to be checked, not merely in the area in question but at the exact level of damage. There may be other components in the mechanical picture, viz. the position of one vertebra relative to the ones above and below, the state of the muscle tone at the immediate level of the lesion and the relationship of pain and tenderness to these changes.

Of all the tests needed for mechanical diagnosis, the most important one is to test for mobility. Each spinal joint needs to be checked for flexion and extension, side-bending to each side and rotation to each side. These tests require their own study and application. If the tests indicate reduced mobility, then manipulation is probably indicated and may be the only modality that is lastingly effective to relieve pain. If the tests show hypermobility, then manipulation in the sense of specific movements is contraindicated because the joint is already unstable. In such a case, strengthening exercises to reinforce the weak ligaments is indicated and sometimes external support by splintage, corsets and collars is indicated. If weak ligaments persistently cause pain despite the external support and strengthened muscles, then sclerosing injections to reinforce the ligaments are indicated[3].

The mobility tests are not only necessary for detecting which range of movements are limited or excessive, but because such tests lead to the most appropriate form of manipulation. The neck may be stiff from lesions at any level from the occiput to the upper thoracic joints and it is no use manipulating the 2-3C joints if the pain derives from a lesion at 6-7C even though the pain syndrome may be very similar. Manipulating the knee for a painful hip joint is not effective even though both joint lesions may cause pain at the knee.

Having acquired skills in mobility tests and knowledge from study of the anatomy and of the normal ranges and combinations of ranges in spinal joints, we are then in a position to choose which manipulation procedure is most effective in any one case.

Because of the complexity of normal spine movements and because there are always a series of joints involved, the techniques of manipulating one spinal joint to the exclusion of the joints above and below require considerable skill. The skills almost amount to an art form. In painting, anyone can make a daubing representation of a subject, but the great skills are required to paint the subject accurately. Much practice is required. Most people with sufficient practice can play a tune on the piano, but vastly more practice and application is required by a concert painist to interpret a Beethoven or Schubert sonata. The comparisons are applicable to skills in manipulative techniques.

I would like to amplify the contribution that osteopaths have made to the study of normal spinal mechanics with the statement that spinal movements are not purely flexion, extension, side-bending and rotation, but that almost all spinal movements are combinations of all these. What happens when we combine movements? In the cervical spine, rotation is never pure except in the first few degrees of rotation, because when rotating further, a component of side-bending normally occurs by the nature of the shape of the facets comprising the apophyseal joints. Similarly, primary side-bending always involves some degree of rotation. The rule is that when normal movements take place, rotation and side-bending occur to the same side. This applies in the neck even if a component of flexion or extension is the starting point for the other movements. Use is made of this knowledge when manipulating the neck, because if we deliberately rotate and side-bend the neck to opposite sides, we create a jamming of the facets that stops further movements in the opposing directions. This is called facet apposition locking and use is made of this principle to create a firm lever – converting a soft rubber tube into a solid wooden lever so that the forces of manipulation can be directed with precision to the joint that needs manipulating. When we convert a soft, poorly localizing lever into a firm, accurately localizing lever, it enables us to concentrate the forces that culminate precisely at the level of the restricted joint. Furthermore, the joints above and below are protected from undue and haphazard forces.

The application of the principles is not especially difficult, but the accurate localization of the forces requires skill because a sense of tissue tension has to be acquired by the manipulator. A painter needs not only to know which colour is required for the painting, but the precise place to put the colour. This is where the skills also become art. Anyone keen to acquire or adopt these skills must be prepared to study the subject closely and to practise hard to improve his skills.

Continuing the theme of facet apposition locking and applying it to the thoracic and lumbar areas, there is a complication in those areas, because, when combining side-bending and rotation, the normal physiological movements differ according to whether the spine is at first in a position of flexion or of extension. The rule is that when starting from a position of flexion, side-bending to one side promotes rotation to the same side, just as occurs in the neck, but if we start from an erect or extended position the rotation and side-bending quite naturally occur to opposite sides. Why this should be so is not obvious, but it is demonstrable fact radiologically[4].

This rule must be taken into account because it helps us to combine the appropriate functions of flexion, extension, side-bending and rotation to involve the facet apposition component of manipulation in this area. To give an example, if we wish to manipulate the 1-2L level where there is restricted mobility, we can use facet apposition starting either from flexion or from extension. If from flexion, we ought to side-bend and rotate to opposite sides just as in the neck, but if we wish to commence the manipulation from a position of extension, then we must rotate and side-bend to the same side. The choice of commencing in flexion or commencing in extension can depend on other factors. How feasible is it in any one case? A patient with a fat belly cannot be flexed enough because the belly gets in the way, or a patient with an existing lordosis precludes extension because the area is already in an extended state.

The application of these principles could be made clearer by demonstration of such techniques.

The purpose of using combined movements is as I have said to convert a floppy lever into a firm one with the express purpose of localizing the mechanical force with precision to the level where the manipulation is required. Clinically, in many spinal problems there is a combined syndrome of hypo-hyper-mobility. We need to mobilize the stiff joint while protecting the unstable joints above or below. If the patient's symptoms derive predominantly from the unstable levels, then these unstable joints take priority in treatment compared with the restricted ones. The hypermobile joints may need stabilizing with sclerosing injections, with external or internal supports, and increased muscle tone before any attempts are made to manipulate the restricted levels, because more serious consequences ensue from hypermobile spinal joints than do from hypomobile spinal joints.

One of the commonest syndromes in the spine derives from Scheuermann's osteochondrosis, in which the thoraco-lumbar area is kyphosed and rigid. The rigidity places excessive stress on the lower joints. They have to take undue leverage with any spinal movement because of the stiffness above. Eventually, ligaments become over-stretched and such ligaments cause far more symptoms than the hypomobile segments above. The thoraco-lumbar area changes may go unrecognized as a component of the syndrome because pain is usually lower down and because over the years the rigid osteochondrosed joints may have become stabilized.

In passing, I want to emphasize that Scheuermann's osteochondrosis (not osteochondritis as it was previously called) is a common and not a rare condition. My own research (see ref. 5) shows that even in the normal population of people not specially complaining about back pain there is an incidence of 13% of Scheuermann's osteochondrosis, whereas in the patients coming primarily for advice about back pain the figures show a 42% incidence of osteochondrosis even if the affected area is not causing the precipitating symptoms.

As I have said, the principle of accurate manipulation should be the accurate localization of forces, and one of the techniques of achieving this is facet apposition locking. Another way is to use ligamentous-tension locking. In these techniques, the ligaments of the area are stretched fully and then extra force is applied at the limit of such leverage. Instead of an elastic band remaining loose, we put it to a maximum stretch whereby it cannot go any further without giving way. This sounds as if damage could occur to the elastic band, but here the analogy is inappropriate because in human ligaments there is an 'end feel' to ligamentous stretch beyond which there is discomfort yet a few more degrees are possible before tearing takes place. It is these few degrees that are used effectively for this technique of manipulation. We sense the ligamentous tension, feeling for it all the time, during the manipulation and at the 'end feel' point, we exert an extra force at the exact site of the manipulation.

Again, skills are needed and practice is required to obtain this sense of tissue tension to avoid damage to the ligaments. The sense of restriction by adhesions again is different from the physiological stretch limit and this sense has to be acquired by the operator.

The mobilizing techniques of Maitland and articulatory techniques of osteopathy are a great safeguard against excessive force, because the principle behind such techniques is only to stretch the ligaments or capsules to their pain limit. The passive stretching is stopped when pain occurs and this makes it a safe procedure. By using the stretching short of pain in a repetitive persuasive manner, we find that joints begin to yield slowly and safely. In experienced hands this compares favourably with specific manipulations, which are often applied beyond the pain range. Such specific manipulations should only be used by practitioners of wide knowledge and experience.

Coming to the question of manipulation in the presence of disc degeneration, another concept is required. As we know, the process of degeneration can be entirely silent for years and then, owing to some trivial leverage, the structure gives way and the disc either swells or protrudes or prolapses. Such changes are often the result of several years of degeneration following major trauma or repeated minor stresses. Impaired mobility is often a sequel to spinal injury and is frequently overlooked or the signs and symptoms are misinterpreted; and this leads slowly to the degenerative changes of the cartilage. When degeneration has occurred as a result of previous injury or when osteochondrosis is present, then such sites are vulnerable and they react adversely to relatively minor new stresses. Then an acute episode demands attention. There is little hope in such situations of restoring normality. We may be able to restore comfort at the site, but we cannot regenerate the cartilage. A swollen disc may resolve itself in a matter of days even without treatment. A herniated disc without prolapse may be resolved more quickly by appropriate manipulative techniques, but inappropriate manipulations can easily convert the hernia into a prolapse. Without knowledge and clinical experience, it is wiser not to use manipulation at all in those cases and to allow time and support to solve the immediate symptoms. The most effective and safest manipulative technique in a herniated disc is traction. Adjustive manual traction can often shorten the duration of the acute episode by many days. Sustained traction has very little place in these cases except when nerve root pressure is present and when the traction affords relief.

Once disc degeneration has become painfully manifest, then we need to change the policy of trying to manipulate to restore mobility to the avoidance of specific manipulation. We must only apply articulatory techniques and keep these within the pain limit.

Can manipulation be of any value if a disc protrusion occurs, giving rise to nerve root irritation or compression? I say yes to this, in certain specific circumstances. These circumstances are reached after an acute episode has largely subsided but then gives rise to a persisting chronic pain. We know that one of the sequels to inflammation, whether from trauma or infections, is the formation of fibrous tissue. In the capsule of joints we refer to this fibrous tissue as adhesions. Such adhesions are inelastic and painful. Strong stretching of these adhesions is appropriate in some cases, but again skill and clinical judgement are required.

If nerve roots are tethered by adhesions and the protruding disc has become slowly smaller, often a quick response to relieve the root irritation can be achieved by stretching those adhesions. Manipulation in such circumstances is best given under anaesthesia to minimize the forces that are required for it to be effective, and to minimize any reactive swelling following the manipulation. There are appropriate techniques for brachial nerve root pressure, femoral nerve root pressure and sciatic nerve pressure. These techniques, which are designed specifically to release adhesions and not to make any attempt at 'replacing an offending disc', are safe when the correct techniques are used and correct indications are present for such a manoeuvre.

More recent changes in some osteopathic thinking have been called functional techniques, muscle energy techniques, kinesiology and cranial techniques, and other chapters will deal with these.

REFERENCES

1. Mennell, J.B. (1945). *Physical Treatment by Movement, Manipulation and Massage.* (London: Churchill)
2. Mennell, M. McM. (1964). *Joint Pain.* (London: Churchill)
3. Ongley, M.T. *et al.* (1987). A new approach to the treatment of chronic low back pain. *Lancet,* 2, 143–146
4. Stoddard, A. (1983). *Manual of Osteopathic Practice,* p.299. (London: Hutchinson)
5. Stoddard, A. (1979). Scheuerman's disease or spinal osteochondrosis. *J. Bone Jt. Surg.,* **61B**, 56

11

Low back pain of thoracolumbar origin

Robert MAIGNE

Pain in the lumbosacroiliac or gluteal regions is usually attributed to disorders of the lower lumbar or lumbosacral spine. The author's clinical experience indicates that this pain is commonly derived from irritation of the posterior branches of the lower thoracic and/or the first lumbar spinal nerves. This irritation takes place at the corresponding zygoapophyseal joints of the same segments with which these nerves are anatomically related.

An entrapment of the posterior ramus at the level of the iliac chest may also be present.

Diagnosis of this form of low back pain is purely clinical. Findings on X-ray examination and computerized tomography of the lower thoracic and upper lumbar spine are usually normal. The clinical picture may frequently be confused by the findings of radiological abnormalities at the lumbosacral region to which the cause of the low back pain is erroneously attributed.

ANATOMIC CONSIDERATIONS

In 1974 it was realized that the thoracolumbar junction frequently played a role in the causation of low back pain[2].

Posterior primary rami of the thoracolumbar spinal nerves

These rami innervate the skin and the intrinsic muscles of the back, the apophyseal joints and the supra- and interspinous ligament. Each posterior ramus separates at right angles from a merging spinal nerve. The ramus passes about the apophyseal joint along the superior articular apophysis of the underlying vertebra. Each ramus divides immediately into two branches: a lateral branch that carries motor and sensory fibres and becomes subcutaneous several vertebral levels below its origin, and a medial branch that is almost exclusively motor and is distributed to the multifidus, rotatory muscles and interspinous muscles. The cutaneous branches penetrate the lumbar fascia, descend in the

96

subcutaneous tissue and end in the skin of the lower lumbar area. Anastomoses between these branches are frequent.

Classically the cutaneous innervation of the lower lumbar and gluteal regions has been attributed to the lateral branches of L1-L2 and L3. The author has, however observed more frequent other cutaneous innervation of the gluteal region derived from higher levels of the thoracolumbar region: 37 dissections have been performed (J.Y. Maigne). The result is shown Figure 11.1. Anastomoses between these nerves are also common, so lateral branches of posterior rami contain nerve fibres from two or three spinal segments[4].

The most medial cutaneous ramus crossing the iliac crest is L1 (65%), L2 (25%) and L2 anastomosed with L3 (10%). It crosses the iliac crest at 7–8 cm from the middle line through an osteofibrous canal, in which it may be entrapped as observed in some of our dissections.

Apophyseal joints of the thoracolumbar junction

The direction and extent of motion in the vertebral column are determined at each vertebral segment by the orientation and form of the posterior articulations. In the cervical spine, the articular plane exhibits an inclination of 45° from the horizontal plane.

In the thoracic spine the inclination reaches 60° and is 90° in the lumbar region. In the cervical and thoracic spine the posterior articulations are approximately in the frontal plane, while in the lumbar spine they are in the sagittal plane. As a result of this organization, forward flexion and extension are essentially all that is permitted in the lumbar spine. The thoracic spine, by virtue of the orientation of the facets, should have a high degree of mobility, especially of rotation. The ribs, however, prevent much of this rotatory movement. No rotation is possible in the lumbar spine because of the facet orientation and form. Therefore, the greatest degree of rotation and lateral flexion must take place at the level of the thoracolumbar junction.

T12 (sometimes T11) is considered to be an intermediate vertebra with its superior joints acting as those of the dorsal spine and its inferior joints as those of the lumbar spine.

MATERIAL AND METHODS

In 500 patients having common back pain the origin of pain was found to be thoracolumbar in 30% and to be combined with lumbosacral in 25%.

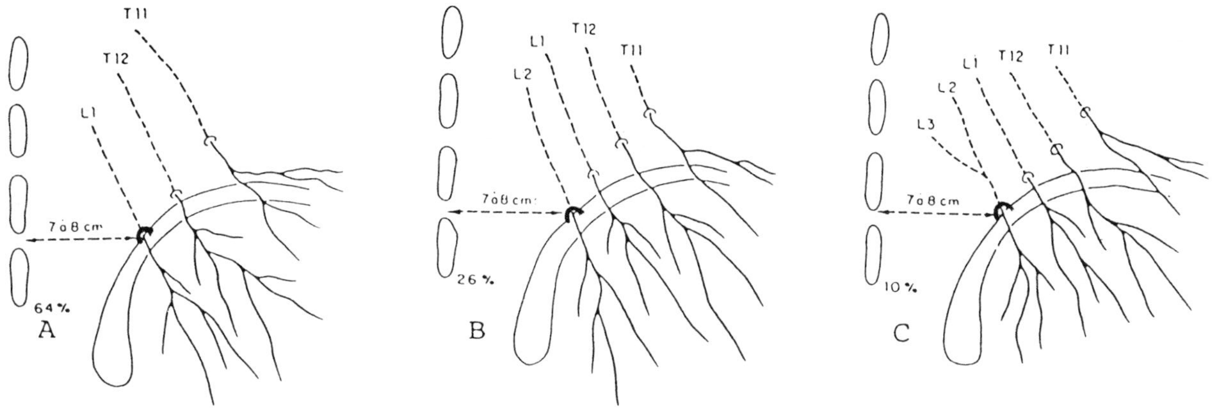

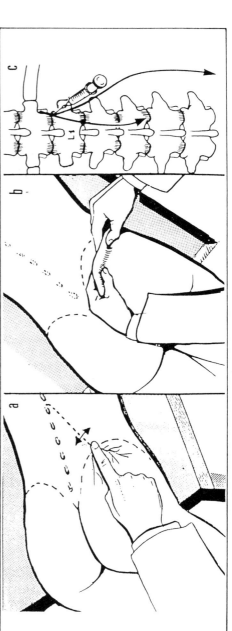

Figure 11.1 Cutaneous innervation of the lower lumbar and gluteal region

Figure 11.2 (a) How to look for the 'iliac crest point'.
(b) The skin-rolling test.
(c) Procaine injection of the painful joint should suppress the pain and discomfort of the patient, eliminate the tenderness over the 'iliac

To confirm that the back pain originated in the thoracolumbar junction, five factors were found to be essential: (1) the 'iliac crest point' sign; (2) positive skin-rolling test; (3) clinical evidence of specific level involvement in the thoracolumbar region; (4) tenderness to deep palpation over the involved apophysial joints; and (5) specific responses to diagnostic block with procaine.

1. The 'iliac crest point' sign. Pain and deep tenderness are located at the level of the iliac crest at a point that corresponds to the cutaneous emergence of the posterior branches of the affected spinal nerves (anastomoses are frequent). Pressure at this point causes a sharp pain similar to the patient's complaint. This sign requires careful, precise localization. The patient is placed across the examining table, lying on a pillow placed under the abdomen to flex the back and cause him to be in a relaxed position. The examiner places his finger along the iliac crest with moderate pressure being exerted every half-centimetre in an attempt to isolate the exquisite tender point. The examiner moves his finger slightly laterally, medially and vertically in a probing manner (Figure 11.2(a)). Once the irritated nerve is located, deep pressure and gentle movement arouse marked hypersensitivity that is clearly demonstrated by the patient's reaction. The opposite iliac crest is usually examined in a similar manner and is commonly not affected.

2. Skin-rolling test. Thickening and hypersensitivity of the skin and subcutaneous tissues of the gluteal and iliac crest region are noted when a fold of the skin and subcutaneous tissues is taken gently between the thumb and forefinger of the examining hand and rolled (Figure 11.2(b)). The area of painful, thickened skin found on the involved side differs from the contralateral region, where the skin is normal in texture and sensitivity. This sign is difficult to elicit in an obese patient or if the examination is hurried.

3. Clinical evidence of specific level involvement in the thoracolumbar region. The thoracolumbar spine segments from T10 to L5 are examined with the patient prone. Pressure is applied by the thumb upon the spinous processes one by one tangentially in a slower unhurried manner (Figure 11.3(a)). At each spinal segment pressure is applied both to the left and to the right. Upon reaching the involved segment, tenderness is unequivocally elicited. This manoeuvre exerts a rotatory force upon the vertebra. At the segment that is the source of pain, the patient feels unilateral pain. Rarely (20%) is pain noted upon movement of the same vertebra in the opposite direction.

4. Palpation of the apophyseal joints. To confirm the diagnosis, tenderness to deep, palpation over the corresponding apophyseal joint can be elicited. Pressure is applied in a direct, deep, vertical manner, approximately 1 cm lateral to the spinous processes, and is followed by a slow, gentle rubbing movement of the fingers (Figure 11.3(b)). In this manner, the pressure is

exerted over the facet joint of the specific vertebral segment. It may be controlled under radiography.

5. Diagnostic block with procaine. That the pain is referred from the thoraco-lumbar region to the iliac-gluteal region can be confirmed by infiltration of a local anaesthetic around the painful apophyseal joint. The anaesthetic (2 ml) is injected 1 cm lateral to the spinous process (Figure 11.2(c)) directly into the joint region. The injection should, within minutes, suppress the pain and discomfort previously initiated by the patient's rotatory movement, eliminate the tenderness over the 'iliac crest point', and diminish or relieve the cutaneous tenderness and thickening of the subcutaneous tissue and skin previously detected by the skin-rolling test.

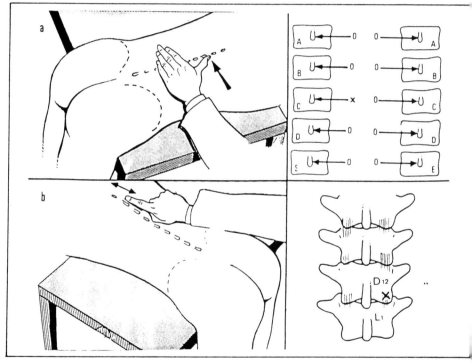

Figure 11.3 Examination of the thoracolumbar junction.
(a) Lateral pressure on the side of the spinous process. This manoeuvre usually provokes a painful response on one side.
(b) The involved zygoapophyseal joint is painful to deep palpation.

DISCUSSION

The role of the posterior facet joint and of the posterior dorsal ramus is clearly demonstrated by tests of anaesthetic injection and by therapeutic results. Another factor that needs to be considered since our first description of this lumbalgia[1] emerged from our recent clinical observations and anatomical research.

In most cases the iliac crest point is located 7–8 cm from the middle line and does not depend on the involved dorsolumbar vertebral segment. This iliac crest point corresponds, as our discussions have shown, either to the posterior ramus of L1 (65%) or L2 (25%) or to anastomosis of L2 and L3 (10%). Furthermore, this posterior ramus goes through a fibro-osseous canal where it may be entrapped. We have often observed this condition.

As many others have shown, there are frequent anastomoses between the different posterior rami as the ramus crossing at the medial level of iliac crest point contains fibres that can come from a different segment of the thoracolumbar junction. Thus, the lumbalgia often seems to be the result of two factors: one – the most important – of vertebral origin, the other of local origin. In some cases suppression of one factor may give relief to the patient. In other cases both factors must be suppressed.

TREATMENT

The treatment includes manipulations and/or infiltrations of the involved facet joint with corticosteroids and in some cases percutaneous radiofrequency facet denervation.

REFERENCES

1. Maigne, R. (1980). Low back pain of thoracolumbar origin. *Arch. Phys. Med. Rehabil.*, **61**, 389–395
2. Maigne, R. (1974). Origine dorso-lombaire de certaines lombalgies basses. Rôles des articulations interapophysaires et des branches postérieures des nerfs rachidiens. *Rev. Rhum.*, **41**, 781–789
3. Lazorthes, G. (1972). Les branches postérieures des nerfs rachidiens et le plan articulaire vertébral postérieur. *Ann. Med. Phys.*, 1, 192–203
4. Maigne, J.Y., Lazareth, J.P. and Maigne, R. (1988). Etude anatomique de l'innervation cutanée lombosacrée. *Rev. Rhum.*, 55, 107–111

12

The Cyriax contribution to manipulation

M.A. HUTSON

It is appropriate in such a volume to identify the contribution of James Cyriax (1904–1985), the more so as he became an Honorary member and the first Fellow of the British Association of Manipulative Medicine in 1975. That James Cyriax, truly the father of orthopaedic medicine, was a genius and became a legend in his own lifetime might tend to be forgotten on a stage such as this when a spectrum of learned opinion (by the very essence of the subject) often holds diametrically opposite views. It is of some significance perhaps that, of all the principles, concepts and doctrines emblazoned by Cyriax across the field of orthopaedic medicine, the topic I have been asked to address is his contribution to manipulation. Meantime we have digested and accepted into common usage his other radical concepts, such as:

(1)   The differentiation between inert and contractile tissues in soft tissue lesions;
(2)   The establishment of exact localization of tissue injury in the majority of cases of 'fibrositis';
(3)   The capsular pattern of joint injury;
(4)   The nature of referred pain: segmental and extrasegmental.

What appears to be particularly contentious (although considered sacrosanct by his disciples) is his conclusion, first published in 1945 in the *Lancet*, that the majority of spinal problems responsible for the diverse aches and pains labelled previously as fibrositis by Gower are due to lesions of the intervertebral disc. They give rise to intra-articular derangement – thus the concept of the partial articular pattern of restriction of joint movement, due to a displaced fragment within a joint, was born. Cyriax visualized the existence of two types of disc lesion: the annular cartilaginous fragment that he felt was the manipulative lesion, and the nucleus pulposus herniation or 'soft disc' prolapse, which is unlikely to be reduced by manipulation – responding, however, to traction or epidural injections. Thus he was at odds with, and very outspoken against, the osteopathic concepts of spinal dysfunction and the osteopathic examination techniques of segmental localization. He was particularly critical of palpatory techniques, which he felt yielded only misleading information.

Cyriax considered that intra-articular derangements occurred at the peripheral joints (when they were due to loose bodies or meniscus detachments), and also at spinal joints owing to annular detachments. The correct treatment was manipulative reduction. Usually this was a combination of manual traction, a passive movement (e.g. rotation, side-flexion or extension, depending upon the site of injury) and then over-pressure. Often the combination of a stamp of the foot and Cyriax's imposing physical presence made for an impressive performance. Assistance from trained physiotherapists was necessary.

From 1949, when he was appointed Honorary Consultant in Orthopaedic Medicine at St Thomas' Hospital, he transmitted his ideas to his physiotherapists and detailed his treatment techniques in the second part of his *Textbook of Orthopaedic Medicine*. His conclusion that manipulation without anaesthesia should be available to all patients within the medical sphere was an attempt to introduce a management strategy that had hitherto been confined to bone setters, chiropractors and those 'despicable' osteopaths, to a medical profession that forty years ago (and nowadays too for that matter) was trenchantly conservative. No doubt he was influenced by his father, Edgar Cyriax, who treated painful musculoskeletal disorders by exercise and manipulation using manual vibration techniques. Additionally, the elder Mennell (J.B.) must have been influential: Mennell inaugurated the teaching of orthopaedic and manipulative medicine for graduate and undergraduate students, and for graduate physiotherapists and physiotherapists in training, in his department at St. Thomas' Hospital from 1916. Within his department, the School of Physiotherapy started, and James Cyriax worked there in the 1940s.

Whilst both Mennell Senior and Mennell Junior believed in the use of mobilization for joint derangement, and the concept of restriction in the involuntary range of joint movement (giving rise to joint dysfunction), Cyriax decided that hard disc fragments were the manipulable lesions. His decision that the physiotherapist was the proper person to carry out manipulative treatment was hardly original. Of greater impact, however, was his doctrine that therapists should assess patients clinically, thereby (on adopting the Cyriax examination routine) assuming greater responsibility for the patient. The result was the release over twenty years of a considerable number of highly trained physiotherapists into the community. Some of these therapists assisted Cyriax in teaching the principles and practice of Orthopaedic Medicine to both doctors and therapists on Cyriax courses of instruction. Cyriax believed that physiotherapists should manipulate at doctors' requests, despite the fact that a Cyriax-trained therapist was often considerably better placed to assess a patient's musculoskeletal problem than the majority of trained doctors!

Of his techniques, he argued in favour of manual traction:

1. Separation of the facet joint surfaces occurred, thereby facilitating the procedure and making it safer.
2. Pain was abolished, therefore the patient relaxed.

3. The production of a suction effect caused the cartilaginous fragment to move towards the centre of the joint.
4. A tautening effect on the posterior longitudinal ligament also created a centripetal force.

Re-examination of the patient after each procedure was imperative. Cyriax was sensitive to the criticism that the techniques were to some degree 'non-specific', although he countered this argument by stating that 'the strain is borne by the blocked joint', which must, I think, be true. With regard to the criticism concerning specificity, and to the techniques involved, he considered that 'what matters is effectiveness not elegance'. I believe this to be a most profound dictum and one that may not generally be recognized as attributable to Cyriax. I take it to argue in favour of empiricism, i.e. that the techniques are acceptable if they are successful even if the reasons are unknown or disputed.

Some manipulations were performed without manual traction, e.g. in the lumbar spine when manual traction proved to be ineffective. In the cervical spine, gliding movements without traction are considered to be useful to 'fine tune' the spine, for instance to abolish slight residual restriction of extension when an otherwise normal range of movements has been restored.

Cyriax was influential in the formation of the British Association of Manipulative Medicine and was responsible for the establishment of the Society of Orthopaedic Medicine, the Institute of Orthopaedic Medicine and of course the Cyriax Foundation. Amongst the many honorary appointments and honours bestowed upon him, he was made an Honorary Fellow of the Chartered Society of Physiotherapy, London, in 1983. Within his attitude towards and teaching of physiotherapists lies a doctrine that has significant political ramifications. On this and other matters I consider that he was often politically naive, although he may have given medical politics little thought. In respect of this contribution to manipulative practice, a number of factors were responsible for the love–hate relationship that he had with the medical profession in general, or to be more exact that the medical profession had with him. The teaching and resulting competence of physiotherapists who were willing to learn, compared to the intransigence of large sectors of the medical profession, led to a feeling of unease in many quarters. The teaching of doctors by Cyriax-trained physiotherapists, some of whom have been given 'internal' examiner status for accreditation of those doctors who follow certain courses of tuition, creates a potential 'Achilles' heel in the progress of orthopaedic medicine, particularly in respect of the establishment of its rightful place amongst other medical disciplines. The speciality of orthopaedic surgery, for instance, has reacted in a seemingly critical, cynical and threatened manner in the face of those Cyriax doctrines that I have discussed. It is regrettable that, despite major advances in the academic status of orthopaedic (or 'musculoskeletal') medicine, both osteopathic techniques and Cyriax's concepts continue to stimulate such antagonism within groups of the medical profession that have the intellectual capacity for a more tolerant and learned view.

13
Manipulation of the sacroiliac joint

A. STEVENS

The function of the sacroiliac joints remains a mystery. They constitute two components in the pelvic joint complex. Because of the strong ligamentous fixation of the joints and their complex irregular topography, the suggestion is made that they produce minimal amount of motion. Rotations in a paramedian plane, anterior-posterior and cranial caudal translation have been identified. Even rotation in the frontal plane has been shown. Little is known concerning rotation in the transversal plane. In the Congress of Manual Medicine in Madrid one paper was dedicated to this item[3]. The mean axial rotation of the sacrum in the horizontal plane inside the pelvic ring was estimated at 3.3° (SD 1.3) on side-bending. Biomechanical research *in vitro* carried out by Miller and associates has demonstrated this rotatory movement on axial torsion and anteroposterior strain.

OBJECTIVES AND METHODS

This study is the continuation of our investigations concerning the evidence of rotatory movement of the sacrum against the superior iliacal spines in the transversal plane by means of sacroiliac goniometry[4].

Measuring technique with goniometers

Applying this measuring method, the rotation of the pelvic girdle is determined by the angle constructed between the parallel line to the superior posterior iliacal spines and the reference line in the transversal plane (Figure 13.3). In the same way, the rotation of the sacrum is measured by the parallel to two points at the same distance from the sacral crest. The subtraction of these angles gives the amount of rotation of the sacrum against the superior posterior iliacal spines in the horizontal plane.

Two different measuring instruments were used:

(1)   A mechanical goniometer with optical reading (accuracy 1°);

(2)   A three-dimensional electrogoniometer with computer system.

As these measurements are carried out in sequence, change in the position of the pelvic girdle may falsify the results. In order to avoid these postural changes, subjects are allowed to lean with the thighs against a support.

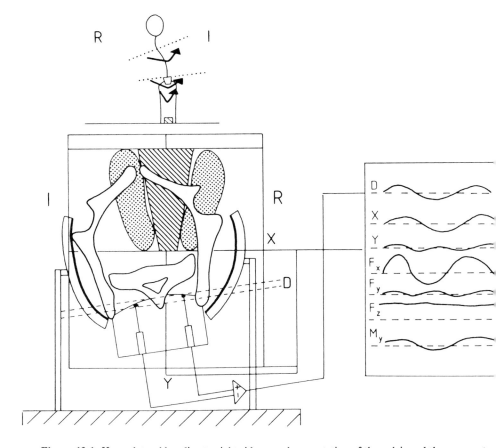

Figure 13.1 *Upper:* lateral bending to right side provokes a rotation of the pelvis and the sacrum to the left.

Lower: seen from above, the pelvis is stabilized between both fixators. The pelvis and the sacrum are rotated in different degree to the left. The measurement of this rotatory movement occurred by means of linear displacement transducers, which are mounted in a bridge over both iliac spines. The moveable beams inside the cylinders show a difference in length D, revealing the displacement. This displacement is a measure of the tangent of the rotation angle (as the distance between both cylinders if fixed). The amount of displacement and the coordinates of the centre of vertical pressure are recorded on the polygraph. This is also the case for the forces (F_x, F_y) in the horizontal plane and in the vertical plane (F_z) as well as the moment (M_z) provoked around the centre of vertical pressure.

Measuring techniques with linear displacement transducers

The difference between the length of both transducers gives the value of the tangent of the angle formed by the rotation of the sacrum in the transversal plane against the superior posterior sacroiliac spines (Figure 13.1). The changes of this tangent are displayed continuously and synchronously by the analogue signal on the 8-channel polygraph. On the other channels are displayed the coordinates of the centre of the vertical pressure and the three components of this force as well as its moment, measured on the force plate (Kistler).

Tested movements

Three different samples are examined by means of different measuring instruments:

(1)   Linear displacement transducers in subjects of sample A ($n=31$) invest-
      igated by the author;
(2)   Mechanical goniometer in sample B ($n=32$) examined by two physio-
      therapists instructed in the use of this measuring instrument;
(3)   Electrogoniometer in sample C ($n=28$) investigated by the author.

Experimental conditions

The test settings are different in the three samples. In sample A the pelvis was stabilized by means of shell-like fixators round the pelvis. In sample B the subjects were facing ahead while side-bending in a sitting or standing position. In sample C they were watching the computer screen located on their right side during the whole experiment.

Complementary experiments

The subjects of sample B were examined by two physiotherapists independently of each other. These subjects underwent test and retest with one week interval.

In a small sample ($n=7$) of subjects with dysfunction discovered by the usual examination techniques, the amount of rotation was recorded before and after treatment by means of linear displacement transducers.

In the same way another sample ($n=14$) was examined by means of the electrogoniometer.

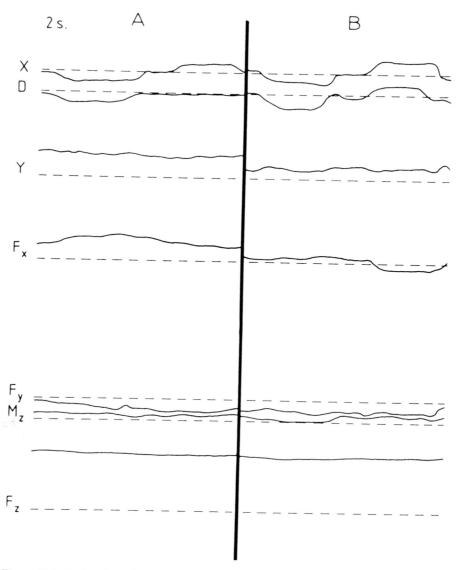

Figure 13.2 Registration of the coordinates of the centre of vertical pressure on the X and the Y axis on lateral bending (X) and ante- retroflexion (Y). One centimetre on the record equals 10 cm on the force plate. A positive deflection indicates a lateral bending to the right.
D is amount of displacement as a measure of the tangent of the rotatory angle (0.1 cm = 0.5°). A negative deflection indicates a rotatory movement of the sacrum to the right in this set-up.
F_x is force in lateral direction in the horizontal plane (1 cm = 40 N)
F_y is force in the anterior-posterior direction (1 cm = 40 N)
M_z is moment around the centre of vertical pressure (1 cm = 4 NM)
F_z is vertical force (1 cm = 400 N)
A No rotatory movement to the left is recorded on side-bending to the right before manipulation.
B Restored rotatory motion to the left after treatment.

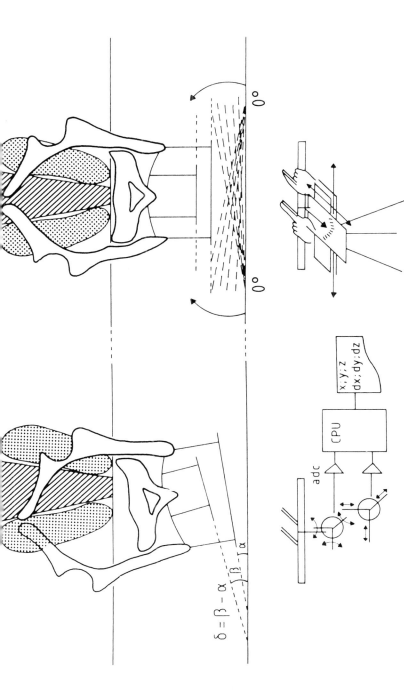

Figure 13.3 *Left.* measurement of the rotatory movement of the sacrum inside the pelvic ring by means of the three-dimensional goniometer. The rotation of the pelvis (angle α) and of the sacrum (angle β) are measured in sequence. The translation and rotatory movements in the three planes are recorded and printed out by the computer. The program calculates also the difference between both measurements in sequence (angle δ). *Right.* measurement of both components (angles α and β) in the neutral position by means of the adaptable mechanical goniometer; only rotatory movements are recorded

The change in the amount of vertical pressure on each foot on standing and side-bending is investigated through two force plates. The changes were recorded in three different conditions: (1) the set-up with stabilized pelvis, (2) looking ahead, and (3) keeping eyes fixed on the screen at the right side.

While measuring with goniometers the results may be falsified in consequence of differences in pressure force acting on the soft tissues by the cross-beams of the goniometer. The margin of error is estimated by using soft materials in a controlled test setting.

In prone postion with drooping leg and with one half of the pelvis outside the table, the position of the sacrum is determined against the posterior sacroiliac spines through the electrogoniometer (Figure 13.4).

Objectives

(1)   What is the position of the sacrum inside the pelvic ring before lateral bending from different postures?

(2)   Does side bending provoke a significant rotatory motion of the sacrum against the posterior superior sacroiliac spines?

(3)   What is the movement pattern while side-bending?

(4)   Does the amount of motion differ significantly between the different postures?

(5)   What effect do the following conditions have on the amount of rotation such as stabilization of the pelvis, looking ahead or to the right?

(6)   Are the results reproducible and independent from the observer?

(7)   What is the behaviour of the sacrum inside the pelvic ring when the function in these joints is disturbed?

(8)   Does manual treatment change the behaviour of the sacrum while side-bending?

(9)   What kind of decisions concerning the treatment may be deduced from these results?

(10)   Does sacroiliac goniometry improve the examination and treatment techniques?

RESULTS

Different postures and the position of the sacrum

Keeping the eyes fixed on the right side is accompanied with a significant rotation of the sacrum of about 1° in the following conditions:

(1)   In the upright posture in a standing position;

(2)   In the anteflexed posture in a standing and sitting position;

(3)   In the extended posture in a sitting position (one-sample statistic, significance level ⩽ 0.01).

This rotation inside the pelvic ring is directed:

(1)   To the right side with regard to the erect posture in a standing position and with respect to the anteflexed posture in a sitting position;
(2)   To the left side for the anteflexion in a standing position.

Looking straight ahead does not coincide with any rotation that is significantly different from zero (one-sample analysis).

Side-bending and rotational motion of the sacrum

Lateral bending from different postures in a standing position is associated with a significant rotatory movement of the sacrum inside the pelvic girdle. The amount of this motion is much more pronounced in a standing than in a sitting position. The excess value ranges from 1.5° to 3.5° (paired comparisons test significance level ⩽0.01).
    Side-bending from the different postures in a sitting position while looking straight ahead is not combined with any rotation.

Side-bending and movement pattern

Lateral bending from different postures in a standing position provokes a rotational motion of the sacrum according to certain movement patterns in a constant way (sign test for location, significance level ⩽0.001).
    In upright and extended posture the direction of rotation is opposite to that of side-bending. But in the anteflexed posture the rotatory movement and the side-bending are oriented in the same direction. The amount of rotation of the sacrum is in accordance with the degree of lateral bending.
    In a very small number of observations a unidirectional movement pattern is seen on lateral bending to either side. Further analysis of these cases revealed a lumbosacral scoliosis with asymmetries on the X-rays ($n=3$) and one case of sacroiliitis (confidence limits for occurence between 1% and 10%).

Pelvic stabilization and the amount of sacral rotation

The use of shell-like fixators round the lateral sides of the pelvis increases the amount of rotation significantly in comparison with the values measured without the use of stabilizers. This enhanced motion of the sacrum is found on side-bending to either side from different postures (Kolmogorov–Smirnov two-sample test, significance level ≤0.05).

Steady fixed look and the amount of sacral rotation

Side-bending while keeping the eyes fixed on the screen on the right side is correlated with an increase of rotatory motion of the sacrum to the right in comparison with the amount of rotation to the left. On average this increase amounts to 1.4° with confidence limits ranging from 0.1° to 2.7° (paired comparisons test, significance level ≤0.05).

This observation is valid for side-bending to the left from the upright posture and for lateral bending to the right from the anteflexed one. Making the latter movement while gazing to the right is also associated with an enhanced motion to the right when we compare these measurements with those while looking ahead (Kolmogorov–Smirnov, significance level ≤0.001). Further comparison between both experimental conditions shows that the amount of rotation to the left is significantly decreased under the influence of the fixed look to the right (Kolmogorov–Smirnov, significance level ≤0.001). This is the case on side-bending to the right from the erect posture and also to the left from the anteflexed posture in a standing position.

Keeping the eyes fixed on the right affects the amount of rotation not only upon side-bending but also upon standing. The two-sample analysis shows a significant difference in means ranging from 0.5° to 2° (95% confidence interval).

This observation is valid for the following attitudes and movements:

(1)   Upright and the anteflexed posture in a standing position with predominance of rotation to the right and to the left side respectively (significance level ≤0.001 and ≤0.01);

(b)   Ante- or retroflexed posture in a sitting position (significance level ≤0.01);

(c)   Lateral bending to the left from the extended posture in a sitting position (significance level ≤0.01).

Hypofunction and the motion of the sacrum

The investigation of patients with an established sacroiliacal dysfunction ($n = 7$) shows a mean difference of about 1° in rotatory motion to either side. This mean value; measured by means of linear displacement transducers, is not significantly different from zero (paired comparisons ≤0.05). The 95% confidence interval in this condition ranges from 0.5° towards the left to 2.3° towards the right (Figure

13.1). After treatment the mean value of differences is estimated at about 5° with a 95% confidence interval ranging between 3° and 6.6° (significance level ≤0.001).

In a second sample of patients ($n = 14$) investigated by means of the electrogoniometer, no movement in the expected direction is observed in 44 recordings gathered upon lateral bending to either side. After treatment the direction of movement improves with a high level of significance (sign test for paired samples $p \leq 0.005$).

Inter- and intra-examiner reliability

The data collected by both physiotherapists were expressed on an ordinal scale; hypofunction, normal function, hyperfunction. This was done because an ordinal scale is more suited for making decisions in clinical practice than a metric one.

The paired sign test is applied to the ratings obtained on examining 10 subjects. The null hypothesis supposing that the observers measure differently is rejected at a high level of significance ($p = \leq 0.005$) for all the postures and lateral bendings.

There is a concordance between the ratings in this sample with a confidence of 99.5%.

This sign test is also applied to the ratings belonging to test and retest ($n = 32$). The null hypothesis assuming that the ratings are not reproducible is rejected at a significant level for all postures and lateral bendings ($p \leq 0.025$). Consequently, test and retest with an interval of one week give the same ratings with a confidence of 97.5%.

Possible measuring errors

Difference in compression forces acting on the soft tissues by means of cross-beams may be the source of measuring errors.

Using soft materials in a controlled test setting, these errors are estimated at the maximum of 1° while measuring with the mechanical and the electro-goniometer. Measuring with the linear displacement transducers, bulging and folding of the soft tissues may provoke the same error. This is the reason why only lean subjects are asked to undergo this test.

The vertical forces acting on each foot on side-bending

The ground reaction force or the vertical pressure on each foot is measured by means of two force plates while side-bending to either side. The amount of this pressure is expressed as a percentage of the body weight.

BACK PAIN – AN INTERNATIONAL REVIEW

In normal standing the load on the right foot amounts to about 57% of the body weight. Only when using pelvis stabilizers is the vertical force equally distributed on each foot.

Table 13.1 Distribution of the values in the different samples

Upright					
Left bending	Stabilized pelvis	=	Looking to the right	>	Facing ahead
Difference in ground reaction in % body weight	82%		45%		77%
Type of movement	Coupled motion		Coupled motion + torsion		Coupled motion
Right bending	Stabilized pelvis	>	Facing ahead	>	Looking to the right
Difference in ground reaction in % body weight	90%		72%		55%
Type of movement	Coupled motion		Coupled motion		Coupled motion
Anteflexed					
Left bending	Stabilized pelvis	>	Facing ahead	>	Looking to the right
Difference in ground reaction in % body weight	90%		72%		59%
Type of movement	Coupled motion		Coupled motion		Coupled motion
Right bending	Stabilized pelvis	=	Looking to the right	>	Facing ahead
Difference in ground reaction in % body weight	90%		86%		73%
Type of movement	Coupled motion		Coupled motion		Coupled motion
Extended					
Left bending	Stabilized pelvis	>	Facing ahead	=	Looking to the right
Difference in ground reaction in % body weight	76%		46%		40%
Type of movement	Coupled motion		Coupled motion		Coupled motion
Right bending	Stabilized pelvis	>	Facing ahead	>	Looking to the right
Difference in ground reaction in % body weight	90%		32%		37%
Type of movement	Coupled motion		Coupled motion		Coupled motion-tors

On side-bending from different postures with stabilized pelvis, the difference in vertical pressure between both feet rises to approximately 90% of the body weight (Table 13.1). This difference in load on both feet decreases to about 75% while looking ahead and diminishes further to some 57% while looking to the right. This is true for side-bending from erect and flexed postures.

Lateral bending to the right from the flexed posture in comparison with that to the left is associated with a stronger ground reaction force, amounting to about 75% of the body weight.

On side-bending from the extended posture, the difference between these ground reaction forces reaches 40% of the body weight while looking ahead or to the right.

114

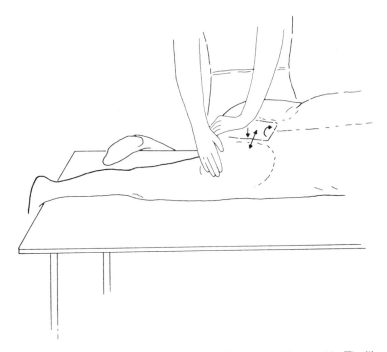

Figure 13.4 The patient is in prone position with drooping leg outside the table. The ilium on the table is fixed by the weight of the patient and the compression force exerted on the ischial tuber by the physician. The weight of the drooping leg provides a distraction force in the sacroiliacal joint on the side of the fixed ilium. This distraction force is augmented by the distraction component of the compression force. The other hand of the physician pushes in a ventral direction on the sacrum. In this way a shear force in the sacroiliac joint is provoked.

Rotation of the sacrum in prone position with drooping leg

Lying in prone position with one half of the pelvis on the table and the other half outside the table, the leg upon the table is extended, the other is drooping and bent at the hip and knee (Figure 13.4).

In this position an average rotation of the sacrum of about 3.8° (SD 1.3°) is observed towards the ilium located on the table ($n=9$).

DISCUSSION

Only the measurements carried out in a standing position are outside the margin of error. This applies to the three samples investigated by different measuring instruments.

On side-bending from different postures in a standing position, the sacrum rotates in the horizontal plane inside the pelvic girdle according to well-defined movement patterns.

The direction of rotation is opposite to that of side-bending in upright and extended posture, but in the anteflexed posture lateral bending and rotatory movement of the sacrum occur in the same direction. Side-bending alternately to the left and to the right provokes rotational motion in alternating direction (Figure 13.2). In this way movement patterns in mirror image are created. When both elements of motion and movement patterns in mirror image are present, the function of the sacroiliacal joint may be considered as normal. In some cases of lumbosacral scoliosis unidirectional motion may be observed on lateral bending to either side. This uniform, unidirectional pattern replaces the motion in mirror image in these cases without dysfunction.

Alternating or uniform motion is absent on bending to either side when the function of the sacroiliacal joint is disturbed. No movement at all may be measured in either direction. This is the case when impaired function is due to distortion of the sacrum inside the pelvic ring. In our sample the sacrum was often distorted to the left. In this situation the sacrum was rotated 3° or 4° to the left against the superior posterior iliac spines. This position remained fixed on bending to either side.

In sacroiliacal dysfunction without distortion, rotatory movement in only one direction may be present. After treatment the amount of motion and the movement pattern are restored in the restrained direction. Consequently, in a standing position and in normal circumstances the rotatory movement of the spine in the frontal plane is combined with a rotatory movement of the sacrum in the horizontal plane. This combination implies that the rotational motion of the sacrum is a coupled one. The movement pattern of the sacrum is similar to that of the lumbar vertebral bodies on side-bending. This coupled motion is obvious in a standing position, but it is insignificant when the subjects are seated.

Our findings are in agreement with the load-displacement behaviour of the sacroiliac joints investigated on cadaver specimens by Miller and associates[1]. These authors also found coupled rotation of about 3° while applying antero-posterior shear of 294 N to the centre of the sacrum. This motion was detected when the specimens were gripped by one ilium only. On torsion the amount of rotatory motion rises to 6° (SD 3.3°).

When both ilia were fixed, motion in the two joints tended to be small. The authors also found that the sacroiliac joints were much less stiff in torsion than the lumbar motion segments. In their experiments shear in the posterior direction provoked coupled rotation of the sacrum turning away from the fixed ilium. But shear in the anterior direction produced coupled rotation towards the fixed ilium. These findings are in accordance with the motion patterns observed in our experiments. In consequence, the load–displacement behaviour may offer an explanation:

(1) For the predominance of the standing position in provoking coupled rotatory motion of the sacrum on side-bending;

(2) For the different motion patterns belonging to different postures.

Lateral bending in a standing position results in a firmer fixation of the ilium on the bending side. The stronger the fixation is applied the better the conditions are for provoking coupled rotational motion inside the pelvic girdle. This is shown in Table 13.1.

On using stabilizers round the pelvis the difference in vertical pressure between both feet reaches or exceeds 80% of the body weight in favour of the foot on the bending side. This considerable ground reaction at the foot reveals that the subjects are practically standing on one leg. In consequence, the mathematical model described by Goel and Svensson[2] in order to evaluate the forces in muscles and ligaments acting on the hipbone while standing on one leg could be applied in this case. The magnitude of the reaction force at the sacroiliac joint ranges from 85% to 110% of the body weight. This range is calculated as a function of the angle that the reaction force at the sacroiliac joint forms with the horizontal.

Stabilization of the pelvis during lateral bending is realized by avoiding compensatory translation movement in the opposite direction of the bending. In this way the highest values of vertical pressure upon the foot are created on the bending side. Without stabilization by means of the fixators a similar ground reaction force is observed only on lateral bending towards the right side starting from the flexed posture. During this movement the subjects keep the eyes fixed to the right. In these circumstances it is not surprising that the distribution of the range of coupled rotation of the sacrum provoked by this bending movement does not differ from that recorded while the pelvis is stabilized. In consequence, lateral bending to the right from the anteflexed posture together with fixing the attention to the right produces coupled rotation of the same magnitude as in the test setting where stabilizers are used.

Table 13.1 reveals some parallelism between the differences in distribution of the coupled rotations and the differential changes in vertical pressure upon the foot on the bending side. The smaller the difference in the ground reaction force on both feet, the less the unilateral fixation of the ilium on the bending side. Decreasing difference in vertical load implies increasing fixation of both ilia. This results in a diminishing magnitude of rotatory movement in the following sequence: (1) on side-bending while the pelvis is stabilized, (2) on lateral bending while looking straight ahead, (3) on performing lateral flexion while focusing attention on the right side.

Only lateral bending to the left from the erect posture and bending to the right from the flexed posture while keeping the eyes fixed on the right side are an exception to this sequence (Table 13.1). The difference in vertical pressure in the former movement is out of order. In the latter, the difference in ground reaction force equals the values recorded in the testing while the pelvis is stabilized as already mentioned.

Continuously looking at the screen at the right seems to induce torsion of the sacrum to the right. In consequence, a supplement of primary rotation may be added to the amount of coupled rotatory movement provoked on lateral bending to the left from the upright position (Table 13.1). This induced torsion to the right may also brake the coupled rotation to the left from the extended posture.

Lateral bending from the extended posture without using stabilizers is associated with the smallest differences in vertical pressure between both feet. The average difference is estimated at about 40% of the body weight. It is not surprising that, on side-bending to the left from the extended posture, the rotational motion does not differ between samples that vary only in the direction of the gaze or attention.

CONCLUSIONS

On side-bending in a standing position, a significant coupled motion is observed. This coupled rotation of the sacrum in the horizontal plane occurs according to well-defined movement patterns. The direction of the rotatory movement is determined by mechanical factors. This coupled rotation on side-bending is only observed when one ilium is fixed and when motion in the sacroiliac joints is free. The amount of this coupled rotation is determined by the degree of unilateral fixation of the ilium on the bending side and the direction of the fixed look.

A disturbed function in the sacroiliac joints is characterized by the absence of this coupled rotation in one or both directions (Figure 13.2). The treatment consists in the restoration of the coupled rotatory movement. This can be achieved by exerting a shear force in anterior direction on the sacrum. While applying this force, the ilium into which the sacrum does not move is kept fixed on the table (Figure 13.4).

REFERENCES

1. Miller, J.A.A., Schultz, A.B. and Andersson, G.B.J. (1987). Load-displacement behaviour of sacroiliac joints. *J. Orthop. Res.*, **5**, 92–101
2. Goel, V.K. and Svensson, N.L. (1977). Forces on the pelvis. *J. Biomech.*, **10**, 195–200
3. Stevens, A. and Vyncke, G. (1986). Sacrum rotation in the horizontal plane on lateral bending. *8th Congress of the International Federation for Manual Medicine, Madrid, 24 – 28 June*
4. Stevens, A. and Vyncke, G. (1988). Die Bewegungsfähigkeit des Sakrums in der Transversalebene. *Manual Med.*, **26**, 85–88

14

The diagnosis and therapy of sacroiliac joint dysfunction utilizing manual medicine techniques, in particular the muscle energy technique by Mitchell

H.-D. NEUMANN

Somatic dysfunctions of the sacroiliac joint (SIJ) are among the most frequent causes of acute and chronic disability of the lower spine. There is no active movement in the SIJ. It moves passively with lumbar flexion and the walking cycle. Any of these movements can be restricted. Additionally, there are dysfunctions that do not follow these physiological motion directions. The following possibilities exist:

(a)   The entire innominate has slipped superiorly, e.g. missing a step (upslip).
(b)   The entire innominate has slipped inferiorly, e.g. in a skiing accident when the straps did not open or falling off a horse while being caught in the stirrups (downslip).
(c)   The innominate is flared out (outflare).
(d)   The innominate is flared medially (inflare), e.g. after falling on the side of the pelvis; such lesions have been reported after vaginal delivery, for instance.

As in the remaining portion of the spine, one should never be content with diagnosing the existence, but rather investigate as to the nature and direction of the somatic dysfunction.

DIAGNOSIS

The diagnosis of somatic dysfunction of the SIJ is made by examining the relationship of certain landmarks (static diagnosis) and by functional motion testing (functional diagnosis).

Static diagnosis of the pelvis

Specific landmarks are used when examining the pelvic girdle for the presence of somatic dysfunction and include the following:

(1)   The ASIS, anterior superior iliac spine;
(2)   The PSIS, posterior superior iliac spine;
(3)   The pubic tubercle;
(4)   The sulcus;
(5)   Spinous and transverse processes of the fifth lumbar vertebra;
(6)   Inferior lateral sacral angle;
(7)   Ischial tuberosities.

The following positional changes can be observed:

(1)   Pubic bone is either inferior or superior.
(2)   (a)   The sacrum is unilaterally flexed to either side (left or right).
        (b)   The sacrum is unilaterally extended to either side (left or right)
(3)   Combination of abnormal positions (see Table 14.1):
        (a)   Sacral base is anterior: rotated about the left diagonal axis, or the right diagonal axis;
        (b)   Sacral base is posterior: rotated about the left diagonal axis, or the right diagonal axis.
(4)   The ileum is rotated either anteriorly or posteriorly.
(5)   The ileum is slipped either up or down.
(6)   The ileum is flared in or out.

The type and direction of somatic dysfunction are diagnosed by landmark palpation, the side of the dysfunction by functional motion testing.

Functional motion testing of the sacroiliac joints

The most reliable indicator for a somatic dysfunction involving the SIJ is the standing or seated flexion test.

Additional tests have been utilized aiding in the differential diagnosis, and they include the spine test, variable leg length assessment and springing test. The description of these individual tests would be beyond the frame of this presentation, and would probably cloud rather than elucidate the salient points to be made (Table 14.1).

Table 14.1 Sacrum dysfunctions

Type	Flexion/extension lesions				Torsions			
	LSF	LSE	RSF	RSE	L/L	L/R	R/R	R/L
	sacral base (sb) left ventral	sb left dorsal	sb right ventral	sb right dorsal	sb ventral right LCSA dorsal left	sb ventral right LCSA dorsal left	sb ventral left LCSA dorsal right	sb ventral left LCSA dorsal right
Findings								
Side of dysfunction	L	L	R	R	R	L	L	R
Rotation of L5	L	R	R	L	R	R	L	L
Sulcus deeper	L	L	R	R	R	R	L	L
LCSA	L dorsal caudal	L ventral cranial	R dorsal caudal	R ventral cranial	L dorsal caudal	L dorsal caudal	R dorsal caudal	R dorsal caudal
Positive spine test	L	L	R	R	R	L	L	R
Sitting flexion test	L	L	R	R	R	L	L	R
Backward bending test	–	–	–	–	Decreased	Increased	Decreased	Increased
Lumbar lordosis	Supple	Rigid	Supple	Rigid	Supple	Rigid	Supple	Rigid
Functional leg length difference	L longer	L shorter	R longer	L shorter	L shorter	R shorter	R shorter	R shorter

LCSA: lateral caudal sacral angle. LSF: left sacral flexion. LSE: left sacral extension
RSF: right sacral flexion. RSE: right sacral extension
L/L: The sacral base is rotated left over the left diagonal axis
L/R: The sacral base is rotated left over the right diagonal axis
R/R: The sacral base is rotated right over the right diagonal axis
R/L: The sacral base is rotated right over the left diagonal axis

121

By *combining* the results from the *static* positional examination and the *functional* motion testing, not only is one then able to deduce the correct *diagnosis*, i.e. the type, direction and side of the dysfunction, but one has a set of diagnostic indicators for the appropriate *treatment* procedure.

THERAPY

Once the diagnosis of a somatic dysfunction of the SIJ has been established, various treatment procedures are available. I shall describe and apply the so-called muscle energy technique (MET), which was originally developed in the early 1960s by the American osteopathic physician Fred Mitchell, Senior.

The treatment of the different types of somatic dysfunction is demonstrated by means of the following examples.

EXAMPLES OF TREATMENT

Example 1

- Diagnosis: the pubic bone is superior on the left.
- Clinical findings: the pubic bone is superior on the left, inferior on the right.
- Seated flexion test: positive on the left.

(1)   The patient is supine.
(2)   The operator stands on the side where the lesion is.
(3)   While one hand reaches over to support the ASIS (anterior superior iliac spine), the other hand is placed over the patient's knee, pressing the thigh downward to the barrier. The patient's leg rests on the lower leg of the operator.
(4)   The patient is then requested to bend the leg at the hip against the counter-force provided by the operator. The patient, after contracting his muscles for 5–6 seconds, is instructed to relax as much as possible.
(5)   Engage the new barrier and repeat above process about 3 times.
(6)   The situation is then reassessed and the technique may be repeated if the expected treatment success has not occurred. This reassessment is crucial and must be done after each treatment as control of the success of therapy (Figure 14.1).

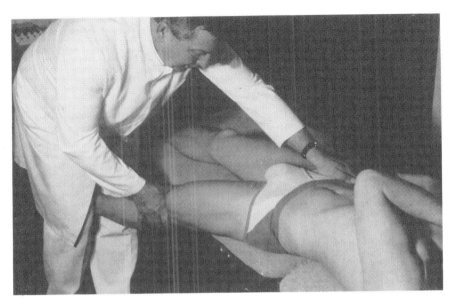

Figure 14.1

Example 2

- Diagnosis: the pubic bone is inferior on the right.
- Clinical findings: the pubic bone is superior left, inferior on the right.
- Seated flexion test: positive on the right.

(1) The patient is supine.
(2) The operator stands on the side opposite to the diagnosed lesion and introduces flexion to the hip by moving the flexed knee. Flexion is introduced until the palpating hand starts to feel the ischial tuberositiy to move.
(3) With the third and fourth finger of the other hand, the operator then palpates the PSIS (posterior superior iliac spine) in such a way that the thenar and hypothenar eminences come to rest on either side of the ischial tuberosity. Slight pressure from a medial direction is exerted. It is important that the SIJ should not be pushed together or pulled apart.
(4) The patient is requested first to extend his hip isometrically for 5–6 seconds against equal but opposite resistance, and then to relax.
(5) During the relaxation phase, the hip can then be flexed further, while at the same time the ipsilateral side of the pelvis is carried to the barrier through pressure applied to the ischial tuberosity (Figure 14.2).

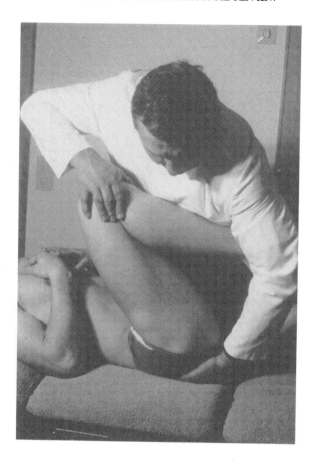

Figure 14.2

Example 3

- Diagnosis: sacrum flexed on the left.
- Clinical findings: left sulcus deep, left inferior sacral angle inferior and posterior.
- Seated flexion test: positive on left.

(1) The patient is prone.
(2) The operator stands on the same side as the dysfunction.
(3) The palpating finger rests over the sulcus on the ipsilateral side.
(4) Abducting and rotating the hip internally by about 15° will 'engage' the hip, that is take up the 'slack'. The SIJ is then carried to its neutral or so-called loose-packed position.

(5) The opposite hand provides a constant pressure to the inferior lateral sacral angle on the same side as the restriction. It is important that the heel of the hand be used while the arm is held straight.

(6) The patient is requested to take a deep breath and hold it. Assure maximal inhalation by having him attempt to take in more air if possible.

(7) After the patient has held his breath he is requested to exhale slowly while the operator simultaneously exerts pressure upon the inferior lateral sacral angle (Figure 14.3).

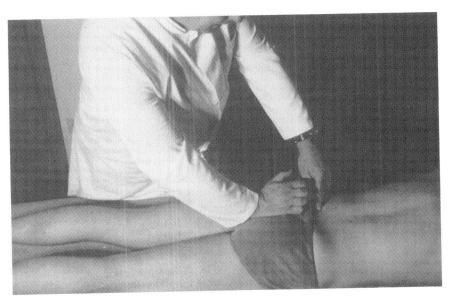

Figure 14.3

This technique takes into account that, as a consequence of the physiological motion associated with the respiratory cycle, the sacrum extends along with the flattening of the spinal curves during maximal inhalation. The opposite is true during maximal exhalation when the sacrum flexes and the spinal curves are more pronounced.

Example 4

– Diagnosis: sacrum flexed on the right.
– Clinical findings: right sulcus is shallow, the right inferior sacral angle is not posterior.
– Seated flexion test: positive on the right.

125

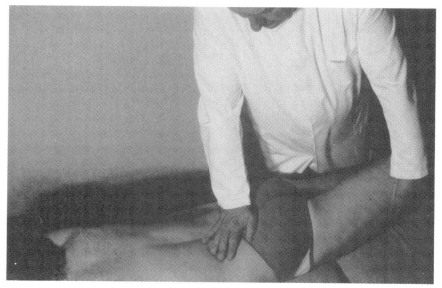

Figure 14.4

(1)   The patient is prone. Sometimes the patient may need to be positioned on his elbows and knees. Again, it is important that the SIJ is in its neutral, the loose-packed, position.

(2)   The hip on the same side as the restriction is extended to the point at which the sacral base is perceived to start to move.

(3)   The patient is requested to take a deep breath and exhale to maximum. The operator exerts continued pressure to the sacral base during the entire procedure (Figure 14.4).

Example 5

− Diagnosis: sacrum rotated left on the diagonal axis (forward lesion).
− Clinical findings: the right sulcus is deeper, the left inferior sacral angle is posterior and inferior.
− Seated flexion test: positive on the right.
− Springing test: lumbar lordosis is supple.

(1)   The patient lies in the lateral recumbent position, with the same side of the body on the table as the side of the axis involved. Thus, if the patient has a lesion on the left axis, he or she lies on the left side.

(2)   The operator faces the patient.

126

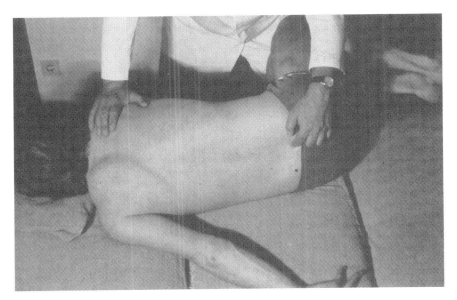

Figure 14.5

(3)   The lateral recumbent position, also known as the Sims position, is assumed from a prone position. With the patient draping his right arm over the examination table, the operator introduces flexion to both the knee and the hip joint and then rotates the pelvis such that the sacrum is perpendicular to the table, which is very important. The patient is to be as close to the table's edge as possible.

(4)   One hand, the monitoring hand, always stays at the sulcus.

(5)   The other hand flexes the hip passively until one perceives the ileum to move while the sacrum remains stationary. One of the most frequently observed mistakes at this point is that this movement is carried up too far, even up to the lumbar spine.

(6)   The monitoring hand is now moved to the patient's shoulder, while the other hand comes to rest over the sulcus.

(7)   The patient is requested to take a deep breath and then, while exhaling, he moves the right hand towards the floor. The operator assists this movement by pushing carefully onto the patient's shoulder. This is repeated several times (Figure 14.5).

(8)   With the patient remaining in this position, the operator again switches hands; that is, the hand moves from the shoulder to the sulcus, and the hand over the sulcus is placed around the patient's malleoli.

(9)   Through the malleoli the operator guides the patient's legs towards the floor, until the movement is just transferred to the ileum. From this

position the patient is requested to push his legs in direction of the ceiling for about 5–6 seconds against equal but opposite resistance. The patient can then relax and the procedure may be repeated from this newly engaged barrier in a similar fashion (Figure 14.6).

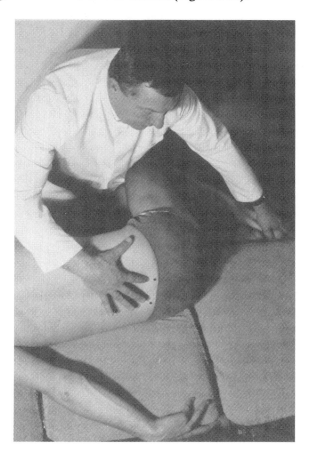

Figure 14.6

Example 6

- Diagnosis: sacrum rotated left on the right diagonal axis (backward lesion).
- Clinical findings: sulcus deep on the right, the left inferior sacral angle is posterior and inferior.
- Seated flexion test: positive on the left.
- Springing test: lumbar spine rigid.

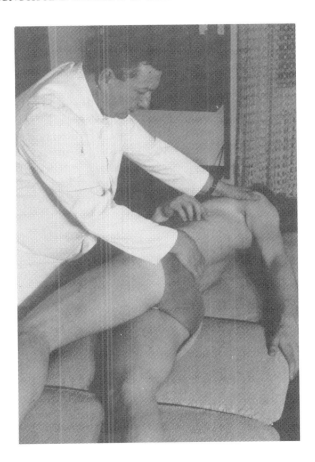

Figure 14.7a

(1)   The patient is lying on his right side, which is the incriminated side of the axis (right axis, position lying on the right side, etc.).

(2)   The operator stands on the opposite side, facing the patient.

(3)   The patient's pelvis is as close to the edge of the table as possible. The patient's trunk is then rotated so as to bring the back closer to the table's surface, which is also enhanced by bringing the shoulder that is making contact with the table more towards the edge of the table. The leg on which the patient rests should be as straight as possible (including at the hip). The upper leg is placed downward on the table in front of the other leg.

(4)   The monitoring hand palpates the depth of the sulcus while also stabilizing the pelvis. Together with the lower leg the extended spine should form a wide arch.

(5)   The other hand grasps the patient's shoulder. The patient is then requested to inhale deeply. While the patient exhales, his shoulder is further rotated. This procedure is repeated several times. One should always make sure that the posterior surface of the sacrum is perpendicular to the treatment table.

(6)   The operator switches hands; that is, the movement hand is now placed over the sacral sulcus, while the other hand now cradles the upper leg at the knee, guiding it over the table's edge in the direction of the floor, until he perceives the ileum starting to move. The lumbar spine should not move.

(7)   The patient is then requested to push the upper leg in the direction of the ceiling and hold it up for 5–6 seconds, whereupon he can relax (Figures 14.7a and b).

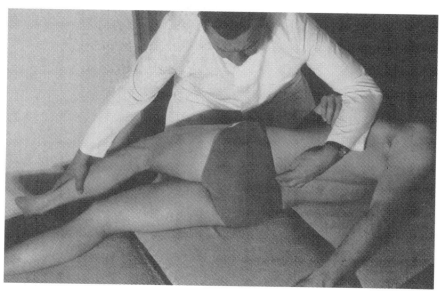

Figure 14.7b

Example 7

- Diagnosis: ileum anterior on the right.
- Clinical findings: the right anterior superior iliac spine is inferior, the left anterior superior iliac spine is superior.
- Seated flexion test: positive on the right.

(1)   The patient lies on the non-involved side.
(2)   The operator faces the patient.
(3)   Starting position: the hip and knee are bent until movement is perceived in the ileum, but not yet in the sacrum. The patient's upper foot is pressed against the operator's thigh. The operator places one hand over the sulcus, while the other grasps the patient's knee, guiding the leg to the barrier (bringing it into the loose-packed position).
(4)   From this position the patient attempts to extend his hip, with the operator providing an equal but resistive force for 5–6 seconds. Then, the patient relaxes at which time the new barrier is engaged (Figures 14.8a and b).

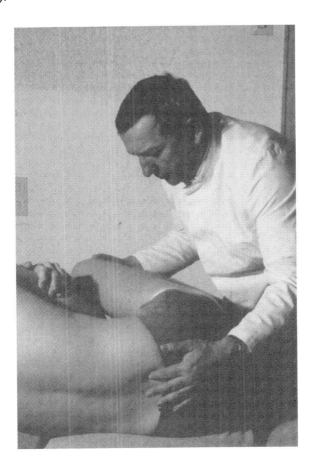

Figure 14.8a

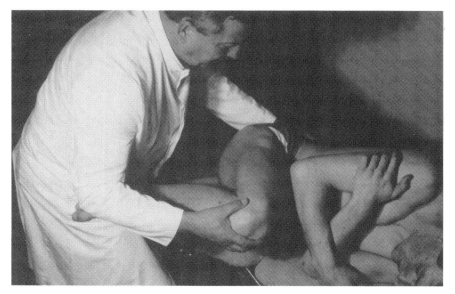

Figure 14.8b

Example 8

- Diagnosis: ileum posterior on the left.
- Clinical findings: the right anterior superior iliac is inferior. The left anterior superior iliac spine is superior.
- Seated flexion test: positive on the left.

(1)   The patient is supine.

(2)   The operator stands on the same side as the incriminated joint.

(3)   With one hand the operator takes hold of the opposite superior anterior iliac spine while the   other hand grasps the patient's distal thigh. The patient's leg rests on the crossed lower legs of the operator.

(4)   Slack is taken up in the hip joint. With the SIJ in the neutral position the thigh is somewhat internally rotated. Now one guides the leg that is draped over the table's edge towards the floor until the movement is transmitted to the ileum. The patient then attempts to flex the hip against the resistive force of the operator for 5–6 seconds (Figure 14.9).

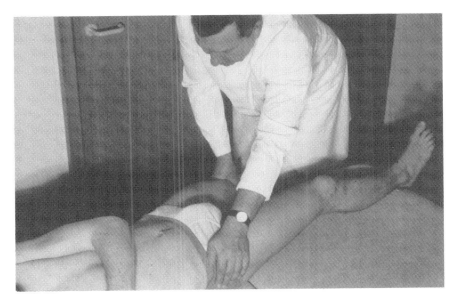

Figure 14.9

Example 9

- Diagnosis: left ileum superior (upslip).
- Clinical findings: both the anterior and superior iliac spines on the left are superior to the same landmarks on the opposite side. The ischial tuberosity is also superior on the left.
- Seated flexion test: positive on the left.

(1)   The patient is prone.
(2)   The operator stands at the foot of the table.
(3)   The patient's foot on the non-incriminated side is placed against the operator's thigh.
(4)   The operator cradles the patient's malleoli with both hands. The leg is slightly abducted, internally rotated and hyperextended at the hip.
(5)   The operator then slowly but steadily pulls on the leg so as to take up any slack.
(6)   A sudden quick tug on the leg is then introduced; that is, an impulse force is utilized, making this a 'thrust' technique rather than a muscle energy technique (Figure 14.10).

133

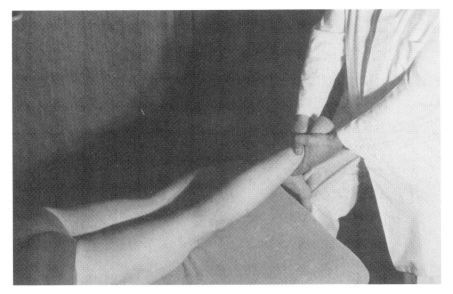

Figure 14.10

Example 10

- Diagnosis: ileum inferior on the right (downslip).
- Clinical findings: the ischial tuberosity, ASIS, PSIS, are inferior on the right, in contrast to the left, where these landmarks are superior.
- Seated flexion test: positive on the right.

(1)   The patient rests in the lateral recumbent position, on the non-incriminated side.
(2)   The operator palpates with both hands the patient's ischial tuberosity and the pubic bone. So as to have the SIJ in as neutral, that is loose-packed, a position as possible. The patient's leg rests on the operator's shoulder.
(3)   The operator pushes the ileum in a superior position in synchronization with the breathing cycle (Figure 14.11). *Slip lesion should always be treated before the flare lesion!*

134

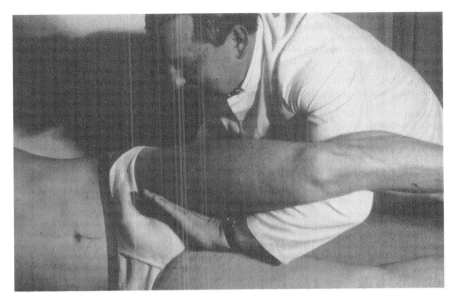

Figure 14.11

Example 11

- Diagnosis: iliac inflare, left.
- Clinical findings: the ASIS-to-umbilicus distance is shorter on the left than on the right.
- Seated flexion test: positive on the left.

If, in addition to a flare lesion there is an iliac rotation lesion, the former may impede proper treatment of the latter. *In such a case one should treat the flare lesion first.*

(1)   The patient is supine.
(2)   The operator stands on the same side as the dysfunction.
(3)   With one hand the operator palpates the ASIS of the non-incriminated side and provides stabilizing support.
(4)   With the other hand he grasps the patient's ankle on the ipsilateral side to the dysfunction. The hip on the incriminated side is slightly flexed, abducted and externally rotated to its present barrier.
(5)   The operator's forearm rests with the elbow against the patient's poplitea.
(6)   Against equal but opposite resistance provided to the patient's knee, the patient is requested to adduct his hip.
(7)   While the patient relaxes, the hip is abducted and externally rotated so as

to engage the newly established barrier.

(8)   While abduction and external rotation of the hip joint are maintained, the leg is extended and returned to its neutral position (Figure 14.12).

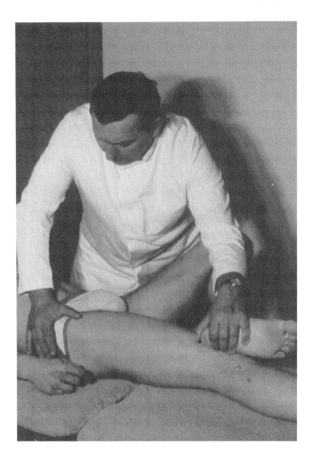

Figure 14.12

Example 12

–   Diagnosis: iliac out-flare, right.
–   Clinical findings: the ASIS–umbilicus distance is shorter on the left than on the right.
–   Seated flexion test: positive on the right.

(1)   The patient is supine.
(2)   The operator stands on the same side as the lesion.

(3)   With one hand in its supinated position, the operator reaches under the patient's buttocks so as to palpate the sulcus on the restricted side. This will also introduce lateral traction on the PSIS.

(4)   The hip and knee are flexed only until the ileum is perceived to begin to move. The patient's foot rests flat on the examination table. The hip is adducted to a point where one can feel the ileum begin to move. Then the patient is requested to isometrically abduct his hip against equal but opposite resistance.

(5)   The patient is allowed to relax. The hip is then adducted and externally rotated further, guiding it to its new barrier (Figure 14.13).

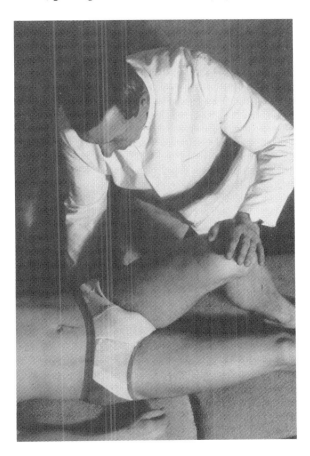

Figure 14.13

Again, if there are both flare and rotation lesion of the ileum, *one is to treat the flare lesion before the rotation lesion.*

Having mastered the biomechanical and theoretical concepts of dysfunctions affecting the pelvic girdle, one can apply them in practice by paying particular attention to diagnostic findings. Once a diagnosis has been made, one can utilize various manual treatment techniques, in particular the MET.

As with many other treatment modalities, much practice is required to become proficient in treating these dysfunctions.

SUMMARY

The anatomical structure of the pelvic girdle and its physiological movement are described. The diagnosis 'blockage (somatic dysfunction) of the sacroiliac joint' is differentiated by the bone primarily involved (os pubis, os ilium (innominate), os sacrum) and the exact description of the direction of motion restriction by means of combined palpatory and functional examination. A sequence of examples describes the manual therapy for different types of blockage using the muscle energy technique.

FURTHER READING

Mitchel, F. Jr., Moran, P. and Pruzzo, N. (1979). An evaluation and treatment manual of osteopathic muscle energy procedures. PO Box 371, Valley Park, MO 63088, USA

Neumann, H.D. (1989). *An Introduction to Manual Medicine*. (Berlin: Springer)

15
Injections in the lumbar area

G. MARX

We hear quite a lot about manual techniques to achieve good results in the treatment of vertebral and peripheral joint dysfunction. I believe that in some cases we can achieve better results with certain injection techniques. There is a very important difference between these two kinds of therapy. For manual techniques we need an exact diagnosis of joint or vertebral dysfunction, including the amount and quality of mobility. For the special kinds of injections to be discussed we need special findings of tissue texture change in the following tissues:

(1)   cutis and subcutis
(2)   fascia
(3)   muscle
(4)   neural structures
(5)   ligaments
(6)   cartilage

Each one of these may show abnormal tissue textures. Often we will find a combination of texture changes in various tissues. For this reason, in one case we will need only one type of injection, in other cases we will need a combination of different injections. This depends on good palpatory skills and a lot of experience.

Another problem is determining what kind of drug we are going to inject. We have to consider:
−   Is it an acute or chronic disease?
−   What kind of tissue texture have we found?
−   What quality of drug for one injection?
−   What is the dose limit for all injections for this patient (toxic dose)?
−   Is there any problem of allergy?
−   Last but not least, what kind of human being is our patient?

Now, let us see what type of injection and which technical procedure will be successful for different types of tissue texture changes.

1. Cutaneous tissue

Ramus dorsalis; local superficial infiltration and ramus ventralis; peripheral superficial infiltration with mepivacaine 0.5% about 5–10 ml. Do not overlook the scars of operations, for example disc prolapse at the back and appendix at the front.

2. Fascial tissue

Consider the penetration points of the nerves, for instance the narrow passage of nervus ilioinguinalis through the abdominal wall or the rami dorsales in the back. Inject mepivacaine 1% 2ml around the painful nerve near the narrowness. With a special technique of infiltration if may be possible to get adherent tissue to glide.

3. Muscular tissue

Pay attention to the well-known trigger points. This is a small point within the muscle with a local and radiating pain when we apply a local pressure. The typical localization of these trigger points is related to the clinical symptoms. For pains in the lumbar and pelvic area, trigger points of gluteus medius and maximus muscle, erector trunci and quadratus lumborum are important. At the front, look at the rectus abdominis muscle near the symphysis and the pectineus muscle near by. Mepivacaine 1% 0.5 or 1 ml to each trigger point is adequate.

Another speciality of muscle tissue is the myogelosis. We can treat it in the same way. The muscle should be massaged and stretched afterwards.

4. Nervous tissue

The symptoms of nerve compressions often are imposing. There may be severe pain and the muscles activated by this nerve can be paretic or even paralysed. The reason can be constriction around this nerve, perhaps a compression by a disc or an inflammation with oedema.

After analysing the exact localization or segment of this painful nerve, one may give an injection of mepivacaine 1% 5 or 10 ml. If signs of inflammation are found, add about 20 mg of soluble dexamethasone. This injection may be repeated two or three times a week. If there is no lasting effect it will be necessary to proceed with diagnostic procedures such as CAT-scan.

The epidural sacral injection is a very successful method for treatment of painful dysfunctions of the lumbar area. Inject about 10 ml of mepivacaine 1% into the aperture of the sacral channel.

If there is also a narrow spinal channel, it is better to add 20 or 40 mg of soluble dexamethasone.

If there is irritation of the sympathetic nervous system in this area, the lumbar truncus sympathicus should be infiltrated. The patient will report cold legs and crawling pain increasing during the night and there will be cold skin on one or both legs, perhaps with dysaesthesia.

It is adequate to give bupivacaine 0.5% 10 ml in such a case. Better blood circulation will result for at least eight hours. Repetition of this injection three to five times within a month is recommended.

In every case the patient should remain lying for at least one hour, because the legs may be paralysed after these injections.

If the patient is without pain after the injection it will be better to use soft methods of manual therapy. In this painless phase it can be dangerous to manipulate with high velocity, because the warning mechanisms of the segment are switched off and it is possible to produce injury of anatomical structures. Our first rule always must be: *nil nocere*.

5. Ligamentous tissues

Special kinds of injections are a well-known therapy for achieving a sclerosis of the lumbar and pelvic ligaments. One of the famous names in this field is that of R. Barbor, who gives an effective composition for a solution for injection by various routes.

From my own experience, sclerosing injections of iliolumbar, iliosacral and interspinal ligaments, deep and superficial, are important.

It can be dangerous to give this type of injection into the deep spinal ligaments because of the vicinity of the spinal channel.

Important points are the addition of stabilization of segmental and regional muscles, the re-establishment of normal muscular patterns and elimination of disturbing foci.

6. Chondral tissue

Very often we will find microlesions of the cartilage of lumbar vertebral joints if we pay attention to dysfunction of the articulation, painfulness and reduced range of motion. There will be more pain in compression, less pain in traction of the vertebral joint. These typical findings of manual diagnosis primarily demand manipulative therapy.

However, after a short time and without any new accident, we may once again find the same vertebral dysfunction, perhaps more painful and more irritated. Investigating the middle-aged or older patient we may discover that a sports, traffic or occupational accident occurred several years previously.

Unfortunately, it is difficult to demonstrate this chondral microlesion objectively, even with the help of the different radiological methods. In this case, it is recommended to give about three to five injections of a chondroprotective remedy, like Ney-Chondrin or Ney-Arthros, precisely into this facet joint. The tissue texture will normalize and another manipulation will be lastingly successful. This treatment is well known and widely used at the knee joint.

It is always important to consider muscular stabilization, to correct the muscular patterns and to instruct the patient exactly how to conduct and perform his or her daily activities.

By the application of a combination of manipulation, local and/or peripheral injection and proper instructions to the patient as to behaviour, successful therapy for the vertebral as well as for the peripheral joint dysfunction is possible.

FURTHER READING

Auberger, M. (1969). *Praktische Lokalanaesthesie* (Stuttgart: Thieme)
Barbor, R. (1966). Sklerosierende Behandlung von Ileo-Sakral-Schmerzen *FAC-Information 4*, 1, 16–17
Dosch, P. (1977). *Lehrbuch der Neuraltherapie*. (Heidelburg: Haug)
Eder, M. and Tilscher, H. (1982). *Schmerzsyndrome der Wirbelsäule*. (Stuttgart: Hippokrates)
Eder, M. and Tilscher, H. (1986). *Lehrbuch der Reflextherapie*. (Stuttgart: Hippokrates)
Eder, M. and Tilscher, H. (1987). *Chirotherapie*. (Stuttgart: Hippokrates)
Lewit, K. (1977). *Manuelle Medizin im Rahmen der ärztlichen Rehabilitation*. (Wien: Urban & Schwarzenberg)
Travell, J.G. and Simons, D.G. (1983). *Myofascial Pain and Dysfunction*. (Baltimore: Williams & Wilkins)
Zimmermann, M. (1981). *Physiologische Mechanismen von Schmerz und Schmerztherapie*, 20, 1–2

16
Drug therapy

R. PASTRANA

Musculoskeletal pain is due to different aetiologies.

Physicians must therefore make as accurate a diagnostic approach as possible. We can sometimes find that pain is caused by serious pathological processes like infections, tumours, inflammatory rheumatisms, etc. However, the great majority of patients are suffering minor pathology (microtraumata, static and postural problems, degenerative osteoarthritis), which occasionally will benefit from manipulative therapy, though sometimes we have to consider alternative procedures such as physical therapy or drug therapy.

The most important medication is analgesic. We prefer drugs with analgesic action and non-steroid anti-inflammatory drugs (NSAIDs), mainly propionics and those with long-lasting activity and good digestive tolerance in order to allow a simple treatment (one pill per day).

A second group we utilize are myorelaxants. They increase the effectiveness of analgesics and we recommend them when a patient is suffering muscle contracture, anxiety and stress. In this group we use mostly diazepam.

Group B vitamins as neurotrophics and cartilage regenerators, apart their 'placebo' effect, are indicated in some radiculitis and osteoarthritis. In symptomatic osteoporosis and algodistrophies we use a combination of calcitonin and calcium for several months.

In ankylosing spondylitis we prefer oral indomethacin schemes of drug therapy for different problems, and different evolutive periods are shown.

17

The causes of poor results of surgery in low back pain

H. TILSCHER and M. HANNA

INTRODUCTION

According to Krämer[1,2], of 100 radicular lumbar syndromes in the Federal Republic of Germany, about 98% receive conservative treatment and just 2% require an invasive intervention in the form of conventional or percutaneous discotomy or chemonucleolysis. Owing to the high number of intervertebral disc disorders, in the FRG some 40,000 disc operations are performed per year and in the USA about 200,000.

Kane ascertained a frequency of disc operation in various countries ranging from 15 per 100,000 inhabitants in the UK to 80 per 100,000 inhabitants in some regions of the western parts of the USA[3]. According to the operational results of 2000 disc-operated patients by Thomalske and his colleagues, 54.15% are considered to be cured, but 39% as only improved, and 6.85% as not improved[4].

In our own study[11] of a comparison between 33 low back pain patients without surgical treatment and 33 patients with surgical treatment 10 years afterwards, 2 patients in the surgical group had no pain, no reliable information was given from 2 patients, 16 had much less pain, 12 had less pain, and 3 had the same amount of pain.

In the department for conservative orthopaedics and rehabilitation, patients with symptoms following a disc operation demand special consideration. Of 4123 patients with lumbar syndrome, 1828 patients had neurological lesions, 631 (34.51%) of whom had already been disc-operated.

Fifty-three disc-operated patients with lumbar complaints from 1988 were chosen corresponding to the admission figures. The group consisted of: 21 patients L4/5 operated, 14 patients L5/S1 operated, 18 patients repeatedly operated on at one or both of the above mentioned levels. The computerized pain topic showed interesting results, namely, the L4/5 operated had pains in the lumbar and sacral regions, the L5/S1 operated had pains in the lumbar and sacral regions with referred pain in the lower extremities, and the repeatedly operated had lumbar, sacral, and gluteal pains with intensive referred pain in the L5/S1 area, right more than left (Figure 17.1).

When considering the possible reasons for the poor results, five groups of faults can be listed, each of which can be subdivided further as in Table 17.1.

Table 17.1 Possible causes of failure

---

1. **Faults in the operational indication**

    1.1 Wrong interpretation of clinical findings
    1.2 Wrong interpretation of auxiliary findings

2. **Faults in operational technique**

    2.1 Wrongly indicated techniques
    2.2 Lesions of vessels, dura and nerves
    2.3 The wrong level
    2.4 Infection
    2.5 Unattached sequestra overlooked

3. **Faults despite optimal indication and technique**

    3.1 Persistent anulus formation
    3.2 Recurring prolapse
    3.3 Segment instability
    3.4 Epidural fibrosis
    3.5 Post-discectomy syndrome

4. **Faults that are not eliminated by operation**

    Ligamentous insufficiency
    Blockages
    Hip participation with pseudoradicular symptoms
    Psychological factors (depressive symptoms)
    Pension request with aggravation tendency
    Polyneuropathy (diabetic and alcoholic)
    Focal systematic
    Serious pathomorphologies (spondylolisthesis, Baastrup's syndrome, nearthrosis, and osteoporosis)
    Postischialgic circulatory disturbances

5. **Faults in rehabilitation**

FAULTS IN THE OPERATIONAL INDICATION

Wrong interpretation of clinical findings

Apart from the rare lesions of cauda equina, one of the most important reasons for an intervertebral disc operation is doubtless primarily the pain. The referred pain in the leg is more positively affected by an operation than the back pain itself.

145

L4/5 operated

21

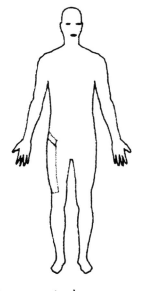 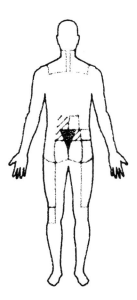

repeatedly operated

18

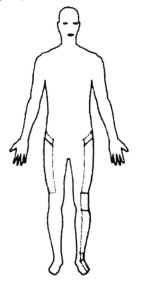 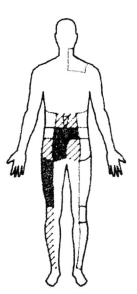

L5/S1 operated

14

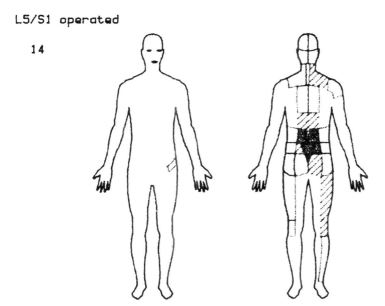

Figure 17.1 Comparison of the pain topography
■ more than 60%
☑ more than 40%
☐ more than 20%

Therefore, it would seem that backache alone, apart from the infrequent intervertebral disc protrusion in the form of a sliding disc, is not an ideal indication for a disc operation. Indications are rather given by referred pains in the leg with paresis. Whereas once signs of dorsiflexion weakness of the foot presented a definite indication to operate, and although a dorsiflexion weakness of the foot has a worse prognosis than plantar flexion weakness, non-surgical treatment can be effected for 2–3 weeks.

An ideal indication seems to be the free sequestrum of a young intervertebral disc patient.

Anamnesis period

Our experience was that our once-operated patients had a short-lived pre-operative anamnesis. On the average it was 6 months for the L4/5 operated and 8 months for the L5/S1 operated, but up to 45 months preceding the first surgical event for the repeatedly operated (Table 17.2).

This might indicate that one should show careful restraint in treating patients with long-lasting anamnesis of pure sciatica pain.

Table 17.2 The length of complaints before surgery

L5/S1	(*n* = 14)	8 months
L4/L5	(*n* = 21)	6 months
Repeatedly operated	(*n* = 18)	45 months

Wrong interpretation of auxiliary findings

Objectification of the luxation of an intervertebral disc is a special problem. An exact neurological examination is of particular importance, which means searching for motor and sensory deficits. Computerized tomography continues to be superior to nuclear spin tomography, although the latter can better detect a free sequestrum. Computerized tomography is of particular importance in determining morphological changes in the spinal canal in the analysis of extreme lateral disc herniation and of spinal stenosis, but cannot differentiate fibrosis from relapse of disc herniation.

Myelography, as an invasive method, should remain a reserve procedure for unclear cases, and it is of interest for patients with poor results after surgery. Electrical tests generally serve to objectify clinical findings.

Often one can observe trivial objective results in combination with clinically serious symptoms: on the other hand, one may see impressive radiographic results with negligible clinical symptoms. Imperative indications are so-called root death and caudal lesion.

FAULTS IN OPERATIONAL TECHNIQUE

Wrongly indicated techniques

Discotomy

The operation most frequently performed is discotomy. It appears to be inadequate from morphological changes in the spinal canal by spinal stenosis, and by intermittent claudication of the spine. Spinal stenosis is, after recurring prolapse, one of the most frequent causes of poor results[6,7]. Either the stenosis was the cause of complaints before the operation or it was decompensated by the surgery and developed problems afterwards. Another form of operation – hemilaminectomy – comes into consideration here.

Hemilaminectomy

Hemilaminectomy is a chance to provide space for the lumbar epidural cavity and the roots. It has, however, the disadvantage of an increasing instability and of ligamentary insufficiency as well as destruction of muscular and nervous structures.

Microsurgery

The advantage of microsurgery is the atraumatic procedure of the operation; the disadvantage is that if a revision is at the wrong level the whole operation procedure must be repeated.

Chemonucleolysis

This is only indicated by an intervertebral disc protrusion with intact spinal ligaments.

Percutaneous discotomy

The long-term results of this operation are still outstanding, and as with chemonucleolysis of disc L5/S1, anatomically caused difficulties must be reckoned with.

Lesions of vessels, dura and nerves

The lesions of vessels, particularly the large abdominal ones, represents a periculum vitae and is not considered as a cause of postoperative pain.

On the other hand nerve root lesions, particularly by powerful attacking retracting hooks during the operation, might be the cause of neurological deficit syndromes, pain and the feeling of pins and needles as the result of so-called de-afferentation complaints.

Dural injuries belong to the most common operation complications, particularly by a severe adhesive prolapse on the nerve roots and epidural cavity, and by re-discotomy. Dural injuries are more often found in poor results (8.8%) than in good results (3.1%)[8].

The wrong level

Pain radiation into the dermatome and neurological findings are important in finding the correct segment. The comparison of the pain topic and the operated level shows distinct differences in our group of repeatedly operated patients (28%).

The L4/5 operated patients had 24% differences, the L5/S1 no differences.

Negative findings during the operation are often the result of surgical treatment of the wrong level, and particularly by the microsurgical technique. The radiological identification of the level is an important aid here.

Infection

According to Nelson[9] discitis developed in 2.5%. Personal experience shows that so-called postoperative irritation is of particular importance. It is characterized by the reappearance of symptoms on the average 14 days after the operation, with clearly increased sedimentation and subfebrile temperatures. Neither the common X-ray nor other laboratory reports show typical findings.

However, in similar cases of complaints arising after the 22nd day, radiological changes, such as increased sclerosing and alterations in the bone structures near the disc, corresponding to spondylodiscitis, can be seen[5]. It still has to be clarified to what extent the occurrence of discitis is connected with the intrathecal application of corticoids in order to prevent dura cementation or arachnoiditis.

Unattached sequestra overlooked

Displaced sequestra behind the vertebral arch can easily be overlooked, as well as extremely laterally positioned prolapses.

FAULTS DESPITE OPTIMAL INDICATION AND TECHNIQUE

Persistent annulus formation

When retrospondylogical changes with distinctly diminished distance of the disc space are to be seen on the plain film, more or less fixed annulus deformities are sometimes found. A local excision of the annulus results in a cauliflower-type protrusion again and again.

Recurring prolapse

Weir and Jakobs found in 11% of all operations a so-called recurring prolapse within the first 2 years, of which 60% were on the same side and in the same segment.

Clinically, the pain-free interval between the first operation and the time when the same pain reappears, must be mentioned.

Essential for the prevention of a recurring prolapse is the extensive scraping out of the disc space; however, with present instruments only 30% of the material can be obtained. To objectivize a recurring prolapse, its differential diagnosis from scar formation is often very difficult in computer-assisted tomography.

Segment instability

Particularly by discotomy and hemilaminectomy, there is extensive removal of ligaments, whereby the so-called 'discoligamentary tension balance' is disturbed. The instability is characterized by a limited mobility with increased joint play; this is in contrast to hypermobility, which shows increased mobility *and* increased joint play. This increased mobility in the sense of the translatoric slide is recognized by receptors, especially by those in the vertebral joints, but also in the muscular insertion, which induces local and referred pain. Of our 53 patients with pain, instability was shown by repeatedly operated patients (22%), 3 of those operated on L5/S1 (14%) and 7 of those operated on L4/5 (24%).

Epidural fibrosis

Scar formation in the epidural space occurs after every disc operation and is also asymptomatic. On the average, the pain begins a year after the operation and never in the first two months. In unfavourable cases, particularly when simultaneous instabilities are present, scars can pull on the nerve roots[1,2] and thus cause radicular lesion. A sure clinical sign of fusions and scarring is painful restricted movement as measured by the finger–floor distance and by the straight leg rising test, the 'Lasegue's sign', but particularly by bilateral Lasegue.

Six of those repeatedly operated on had positive Lasegue's signs (33%), 4 of them bilaterally (22%), 6 of the L5/S1 operated had Lasegue's sign (29%), 3 of them bilaterally (14%), 5 of the L4/5 operated had a positive Lasegue's (19%), but not bilaterally (Figure 17.2). Accordingly, the finger–floor distance of 10 of the 18 repeatedly operated on was extremely limited (56%) (Figure 17.3).

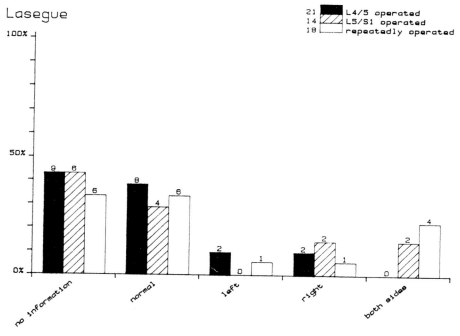

Figure 17.2 Comparison of Lasegue's signs

Post-discectomy syndrome

Included in this generic term are combinations of epidural fibrosis, segmental instability, etc. There are persistent, or also newly appeared radicular, often polysegmental symptoms with usually bilateral pseudoradicular and referred pain irradiation.

FAULTS THAT ARE NOT ELIMINATED BY THE OPERATION

The symptoms of a sciatica syndrome are usually a combination of radicular complaints with muscular tension, referred pain from painful ligaments, blockages, dysfunction of the sacroiliac joint, hip complaints, polyneuropathy, etc. It is one of the most important duties of the clinical examination to diagnose whether one of the above-mentioned reversible dysfunctions dominates the symptoms. The so-called 'test treatment' is of particular importance here.

Blockages of the atlanto-occipital joint in L5/S1 operated and in the area of the cervical vertebral column, but particularly blockages between L4/5 and to

152

some extent also L5/S1 and L3/4 as well as the sacroiliac joint, D12/L1, could be seen in our 53 disc-operated patients. In a study made in 1979 of 105 other patients who had had disc operations and had symptoms, the following factors, which had certainly not been eliminated by the operation, were established[5].

Ligamentous insufficiency	22 patients
Blockages	21 patients
Hip participation with pseudoradicular symptoms	18 patients
Psychological factors (depressive symptoms, pension request with aggravation tendency)	14 patients
Polyneuropathy (diabetic and alcoholic)	13 patients
Focal systematic	7 patients
Serious pathomorphologies (spondylolisthesis, Baastrup's syndrome, nearthrosis and osteoporosis)	6 patients
Postischialgic circulatory disturbances	4 patients

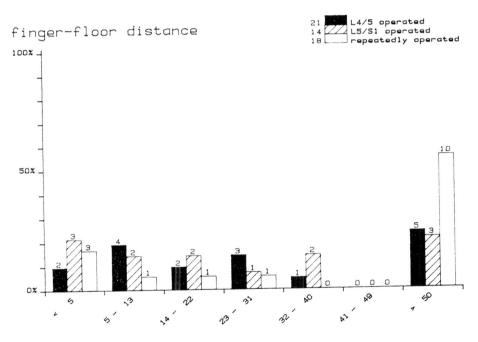

Figure 17.3 Comparison of finger–floor distance

For these faults, which were not and will not be eliminated by the operation, but where the pain syndrome dominate, as shown by these patients, an exact clinical diagnosis and the corresponding anamnesis must be obtained.

Ligamentous insufficiency must be ruled out by definite tests before an operation. Coxarthrosis with its L3, L4 and often even S1 imitative pain syndromes (tension of the ischiocrurale muscles – ham strings) is also a diagnostic trap.

The psychological factor is often expressed by a panalgesia, i.e. widespread expansive pain, of which the sciatica is only a partial symptom.

Polyneuropathy with its definite neurological symptoms once more demands a neurological examination, whereas serious pathomorphologies such as spondylolisthesis, Baastrup's syndrome, nearthrosis and osteoporosis should be demonstrable by a normal standard X-ray of the lumbar–pelvic–hip areas.

Postischialgic circulatory disturbance, which may exist even before operation, is a very common but seldom-diagnosed condition. The principal clinical sign, namely cramp and pain in the calf, which might occur particularly at night and also after walking for any length of time, and which can imitate real circulatory disorder, shows as a definite clinical phenomenon, a side-to-side difference in the skin temperature. Just above the ankle joint, the calf of the affected side is cooler than the other and the objectivizing methods of angiology do not help here. These symptoms, which are improved by sympathetic blocking, will also not be influenced by operation. Some of these problems must be tackled during postoperative rehabilitation.

FAULTS IN REHABILITATION

The rehabilitation of a disc-operated patient has two main aims. On the one hand it should take care of existing dysfunctions or pathological findings that cause pain or could cause pain at a later date, by reflex therapy, physical therapy or physiotherapy. On the other hand it is also necessary to advise the patient in ergotherapeutics so that circumstances that could lead to a new outbreak of the illness can be avoided. This includes regular physiotherapeutic exercises, sanatorium treatment, restrictions in professional life and in sport, just as much as considering certain positions and movements in everyday life.

It is clear that unsatisfactory rehabilitation – that is, medical failure in this case, can influence the future fate of the patient, and the failure to comply can do so equally. Both factors can be seen as reasons for an unsatisfactory operational result.

DISCUSSION

From the problems mentioned above follow a multitude of factors that lead to unsatisfactory results after a disc operation. Many can be avoided by exact diagnostic clarification, by strict adherence to the positive indications for surgery, by clear-cut operating methods, and by specific rehabilitation.

It is, however, quite conceivable that postoperative care, ergotherapeutic advice, physiotherapeutic exercises, sanatorium treatment, as well as restrictions in professional life and sport, all influence the fate of the intervertebral disc-operated patient to a very great degree.

Summing up, given that the potential sources of error are so vast, and also taking the human error factor into account, one might say that mistakes must happen, and that the optimism of the surgeon should be somewhat guarded. For the future, with the exception of caudal paralysis and so-called root death, the conservative treatment of patients with an intervertebral disc prolapse should be given priority. It is interesting that this is exactly what many patients wish for, and personally affected surgeons are no exception.

REFERENCES

1. Krämer, J. (1986). *Bandscheibenbedingte Erkrankungen*, 2nd edn. (Stuttgart: Thieme)
2. Krämer, J. (1987). Das Postdiskotomiesyndrom – PDS. *Z. Orthop.*, **125**, 622
3. Kane, W.J. (1983). World-wide incidence of surgery for lumbar disc herniation. Vortrag, 10. *Society for the Study of the Lumbar Spine*
4. Thomalske, G., Galow, W. and Plake, G. (1977). Operationsergebnisse bei 2000 Fällen lumbaler Bandscheibenläsionen. *Munch. Med. Wochens.*, **36**, 119
5. Tilscher, H., Friedrich, M., Bogner, G. and Landsiedl, F. (1980). In Schöllner, D. (ed.) *Ursachen für rezidivierende Schmerzzustände nach Bandscheibenoperationen*, pp. 22–27. (Uelzen: Medizinisch-literarische Verlagsges)
6. Fitting, P.L., Fankhauser, M. and De Tribelet, N. (1989). Erkenntnisse über 137 Reoperationen nach Behandlung lumbaler Diskushernien: die Bedeutung der Ossälen Stenose. In ref. 7
7. Benini, A. (ed.) (1989). *Komplikationen und Misserfolge der lumbalen Diskus-Chirurgie*. (Bern: Huber) (*Aktuelle Probleme in Chirurgie und Orthopädie*, Vol. 35)
8. Schmitt, O., Fritsch, E., Massinger, M. and Schmitt, E. (1984). Epikritische Langzeitergebnisse nach lumbalen Bandscheibenoperationen. In Hohmann, D., Kügelgen, B., Liebig, K. and Schirmer, M. (eds.) *Neuroorthopädie 2*, (Berlin: Springer)
9. Nelson, M.A. (1982). Survey of surgical management of lumbar disc prolapse in UK and N. Eire 1981. *Congress of the International Society for the Study of the Lumbar Spine, Toronto 1982*
10. Weir, B.K.A. and Jacobs, G.A. (1980). Reoperation rate following lumbar discectomy; an analysis of 662 lumbar discectomies. *Spine*, **5**, 175
11. Lörincz, St., Tilscher, H. and Hanna, M. (1988). Lumboischialige – 10 Jahre danach. Vergleichende Untersuchung von operierten und nichtoperierten Patienten. *Manuelle Med.*, **26**, 55–60
12. Schöllner, D. (ed.) (1980). Rezidive nach lumbalen Bandscheibenoperationen. (Uelzen: Medizinisch-literarische Verlagsges) (*Buchreihe für Orthopädie und orthopädische Grenzgebiete*, Vol.1)

18
Treatment of pain with electrical stimulation (TENS) and acupuncture

M. MEHTA

TRANSCUTANEOUS ELECTRICAL NERVE STIMULATION (TENS, TNS)

Basic mechanisms

Electrical stimulation for pain relief has been known as far back as Socrates' era, but its current use and understanding followed the publication in 1965 of Melzack and Wall's gate control theory for the modulation of sensory transmission in the dorsal horn of the spinal cord. It was envisaged that stimulation of large myelinated 'A' sensory fibres exerted an inhibitory influence on sensory input into the spinal cord. From a practical point of view it is important to realize that high levels of excitation, exceeding the thresholds of the usual pain-conducting 'C' afferents, only result in pain. At lower levels the mechanoreceptors of A-β fibres are brought into play, producing the non-painful paraesthesiae that are useful for our purpose. Pain relief is also centrally mediated by descending tracts from the mid-brain to the dorsal horn. Neurotransmitters at this level are being identified[1], such as enkephalin and dynorphin, and they may be significant in the development of analgesic and psychothopic drugs to reinforce the effects of TNS[2].

Technique

There are a whole range of machines available for TNS, details of which will be found elsewhere[3]. The emphasis in this paper will be on practical aspects. Output from the power source, mainly with a spike or square wave form and repetitive firing rate, is transmitted to sponges or malleable carbon electrodes that are applied to the skin surface. These must be flat and maintain good skin contact with moisture or special gels. Recently introduced gels with adhesive properties are a useful advance, in that stimulation can be maintained for long periods without the need to use sticking plaster or manually hold the electrodes in position, which is tedious and not entirely satisfactory. Optimum siting is

156

achieved by trial and error in the area of maximum discomfort, although it should be noted that treatment is totally ineffective when applied to skin that is completely insensitive. Intensity of stimulation for conventional TNS should be the highest tolerable by the patient and is usually 2 or 3 times the sensory threshold. On the other hand, for acupuncture-like TNS, a higher intensity is required, which is tolerated at a low repetition rate. Muscle twitches should occur and enhanced effects are said to be due to activation of deep receptors. Pulse width 0.1–0.5 ms is not an important parameter. Frequency, with the conventional method is 80–100, but for the acupuncture mode it is 1–2 in bursts of at least 8 pulses at a time and the electrodes are placed over the nerves innervating related myotomes. Duration of stimulation is variable, depending on the resultant analgesia, which varies from patient to patient and is difficult to predict. Usually 30 minutes 2 or 3 times daily is sufficient, but some patients need much longer and occasionally almost continuous stimulation. Close supervision is recommended for better results but this may be only a placebo effect. Conventional TENS consist of continuous stimulation at 50–100 Hz and this is effective in 30–40% of patients. However, Sjolund and his co-workers[4,5] developed the use of a pulsed stimulator giving low-frequency, high-threshold stimulation, which they call acupuncture TENS. Results were improved by approximately a further 20%. Since these developments, other forms of TNS stimulation listed below have been described[6] that may be useful in difficult cases.

(1)   *Conventional TENS*
        Output: high (up to 50 mA), continuous stimulation
        Pulse width: low (75 ms), output raised to limit of patient tolerance
        Rate: high (85–100 Hz pps)

(2)   *Acupuncture TENS*
        Output: high (up to 50 mA), muscle contraction
        Pulse width: high (200 ms) – stimulation of deep afferents
        Rate: low (1–2 Hz), better for chronic pain

(3)   *Brief intense mode TENS*
        Output: high, sudden bursts
        Pulse width: high – joint pains
        Rate: high – useful for mobilization techniques

(4)   *Bursts and train mode*
        Output: high, low-frequency, high bursts
        Pulse width: high – analgesia maintained for long periods
        Rate: low

(5)   *Modulation*
      Parameters: reduces likelihood of accommodation but not the effectivness
      of analgesia

Patient selection and indication for TNS

Careful investigation, preliminary diagnosis and assessment of individual patients
for suitability of treatment in this way is essential in every case[7]. TNS is relatively
simple to apply, non-invasive and free of complications, so it is very tempting to
use it when the cause is not immediately apparent or the painful condition is not
responding to a particular form of treatment. Temporary relief acheived in this
way may be dangerous if it delays recognition of serious underlying pathology,
for example an early malignant tumour. Some patients are unsuitable for other
reasons.   There are those with high expectations that are unfulfilled by a
technique that often does not provide immediate or complete analgesia as with a
nerve block. Others accept the benefits grudgingly but focus entirely on what is
left. Many of these problems are resolved by brief explanation of the basic
mechanisms and the way treatment should should be conducted. Paraesthesia
after electrostimulation is then not unexpected and rarely discourages
continuation of the technique. Elderly or anxious patients need to be reassured
that this level of electrical stimulation is perfectly safe and of the need to persist
before improvement is noticed. Some are sufficiently intelligent to anticipate the
onset of pain and start treatment before the symptoms are intense. This is
particularly necessary for amputation stump and phantom limb syndromes. For
this reason, in the author's practice, a trial is started in the out-patients clinic
and, if necessary, continued in the patient's home with a loaned machine. A
relative or the district nurse can assist if the patient is unable to manage the
technique on his own.
  In general, pain emanating from parietal structures is particularly suitable for
treatment by TENS and many practitioners will find it a useful adjunct in their
practice. Stimulation techniques not only increase the effectiveness of other
pain-relieving methods but facilitate the reduction of analgesic drugs required,
with consequent lessening of complications.
  TENS has been used uncritically in a whole host of acute and chronic pain
conditions, but those who are selective and have considerable experience[1]
suggest the following conditions for which TENS is recommended or
contraindicated.

Conditions for which TENS is recommended

(1)   *Musculo-skeletal disorders* – post-traumatic soft tissue injuries, low back muscle strain, torticollis

(2)   *Joint pain* – as an adjunct to mobilization and analgesic drugs in rheumatoid and osteoarthritis; ? 'frozen' shoulder, tennis elbow

(3)   *Peripheral nerve disorders* – peripheral nerve compression, post operation scar pain, neuromas, amputation stump, phantom limb

(4)   *Neuralgias* – trigeminal and facial pain, intercostal neuritis, post-hepatic neuralgia

(5)   *Deafferentation pain* – causalgia and peripheral nerve injuries, branchial plexus avulsion, post-cordotomy and post-rhizotomy dysaesthesia

(6)   *Central* – migraine, intractable headache, spinal cord injury

(7)   *Neoplastic* – particularly if associated with nerve compression or neuralgia

Unlikely to respond to TENS

(1)   *Peripheral nerves* – neuropathy

(2)   *Central pain* – e.g. severe brain or spinal cord damage, thalamic pain, cerebro-vascular incident (e.g. 'strokes')

(3)   *Others* – e.g. visceral pain, coccydynia

Relative contraindications

(1)   *Emotional instability* – psychiatric disorders, narcotic dependence

(2)   *Industrial injury* – compensation claims

(3)   *Cardiac pacemaker* or other implanted electrical devices

Complications

Complications are unusual and are mainly at the electrode site. Electric burns may be due to inadequate insulation with the gel or faulty connections. Allergy may be the reason for skin irritation, which will respond to a steroid cream. The affected area should be cleaned daily if treatment is continued for any length of time. Sudden increase in electrical activity over a hypersensitive area, notably in the face and neck, may cause a surge in blood pressure. It may also cause intense bradycardia if stimulation takes place over the carotid sinus.

The use of TENS over a pregnant uterus is prohibited, also in a patient with a pacemaker, because it may interfere with the action of this vital apparatus.

Very occasionally the pain is temporarily improved by electric stimulation.

159

On the other hand, improvement gradually declines as tolerance develops. In this situation it may be better to stop treatment, resort to analgesics and resume the TENS at a later date.

ACUPUNCTURE

Acupuncture is an ancient Chinese art that is steeped in tradition and oriental mysticism with overtones of national and traditional fervour. It is a subject of much controversy, even between the barefoot doctors and their more traditional counterparts. Cynicism is heightened by extravagant, anedoctal claims unsupported by proper scientific criteria. However this is a cheap and relatively non-invasive technique that undoubtedly produces analgesia[8]. After a recent visit to China, I believe that a great deal of misunderstanding arises from our failure to appreciate the entirely different philosophy, culture and life-style of the Chinese people. They are brought up to believe that life is a compromise between extremes, for example sorrow and happiness or love and hate; sickness and pain are a reflection of the imbalance between essential life forces and acupuncture an important means of restoring equilibrium. Strong belief is an essential ingredient for success in all branches of medicine and this is especially so for acupuncture as a cheap remedy in the health care of a vast population with extremely limited medical and economic resources. However, the purpose of this article is to assess the worth of this treatment in the context of our more sophisticated medical practice, where acceptance is guided by more basic realities.

Mechanism of action

Acupuncture is essentially a means of stimulating subcutaneous nerve plexuses with hollow needles and applied heat, electricity, manual or digital pressure and even a laser beam. Details of the technique for practitioners in the Western world are well described elsewhere[9,10]. In many ways acupuncture and TENS are very similar, in that both are relatively simple, non-invasive methods of diminishing pain by utilization of inhibitory pathways. Melzack[11], the distinguished Canadian scientist, calls this hyperstimulation analgesia where initial discomfort from stimulation is used to achieve prolonged pain relief. However, there are also essential differences between the two techniques. While acupuncture is being induced there is often a dull ache locally with pain referred on occasion to a more distal site. Characteristically, there is also a sense of heaviness or tingling away from the source of stimulation. Analgesia, which is immediate after TENS, is often delayed after acupuncture. More general effects are lethargy, weakness, vertigo and sometimes dizziness. Experienced observers believe these are evidence of a neuro-hormonal basis for acupuncture and

160

popularly this is ascribed to endorphin release. On the other hand, TENS is more dependent on integration of central inhibitory pathways. Where the two come together is when muscle excitation is produced, as it is with both acupuncture and acupuncture-type TENS. In both methods there is stimulation of deep afferent pathways[11].

Practical aspects

Most clinicians in Western countries agree that the mode of stimulation, whether by manual rotation or electricity, is less important than the site and depth of needle penetration. It is a common practice to locate subcutaneous nerve plexuses with instruments that detect areas of lowered electrical resistance. In most cases these acupuncture points are found in the affected dermatome and correspond with trigger points and motor areas well known in electro-myography[12]. Stimulation results in muscle excitation, suggestive of activity in deep sensory nerve afferents, although some acupuncturists prefer to introduce needles to a much greater depth, for example to the periosteum, and others rely on acupuncture charts from traditional Chinese medicine. This is not a generally accepted view. Whatever technique is used, it is important to elicit a dull ache locally with heaviness or paraesthesia referred to a distal site, a phenomenon known as 'Te-Chi', before proceeding to more prolonged stimulation. Another unusual aspect of acupuncture is the different sensations elicited by needle puncture at the same site. For example, a needle introduced perpendicularly might result in a sensation of warmth or dysaesthesia referred to another more remote part of the body. It is difficult to explain why the same needle introduced more tangentially in exactly the same place may elicit a totally different response, such as diffuse tingling in another dermatome or even temporary pain relief. Presumably this is some sort of neurohormonal effect.

Elderly, nervous or unduly sensitive individuals are alarmed at the sight of long needles, which they immediately associate with painful injections in other treatments, as for example the repeated administration of antibiotics or prophylactic tetanus toxoid. This is most unusual, but some physicians favour concomitant use of an antidepressant like amitriptyline in a small dose of 10–25 mg. The drug both allays anxiety and reinforces analgesia but I have seldom felt it necessary to adopt this routine.

Great care is needed when using acupuncture in sensitive areas of the face, head and neck. Reflex slowing of the pulse (bradycardia) and a temporary fall of blood pressure is not unknown in elderly patients and cardiac invalids. It is essential to have oxygen and drugs immediately available for resuscitation to avoid a disaster, even if this is a highly unlikely eventuality. Deep needle insertion in the face, neck and chest and in the vicinity of major blood vessels is not only unnecessary but potentially dangerous. Haemorrhage or a pneumo-thorax are rare complications that can occur in this way.

Low-intensity, high-frequency stimulation is mediated by serotonin and is more effective for acute pain, whereas the high-intensity low-frequency mode is said to be due to endorphin release and may be more suitable for chronic pain. For this reason some clinicians start with the former stimulation and proceed to the latter for more prolonged effect.

Complications

Repeated needling is a potential source of infection unless strict standards of asepsis are observed. Most workers in this country scrub their hands with soap and water, followed by application of a disinfectant, as they would prior to surgery. The wearing of gloves is probably unnecessary. The patient's skin is also cleansed with a suitable antiseptic, while acupuncture needles are better autocleaned and stored in small, sterile pockets. Some acupuncturists keep their needles in a spirit or alcohol container but this is not, in the author's opinion, necessarily entirely safe. It is not unknown for infective hepatitis to be transmitted by repeated injection and, although not reported so far, the risk of transmitting the AIDS virus cannot be dismissed unless the recommended precautions are observed.

Manual rotation or electric stimulation often causes intense muscle spasm, which will gradually subside and facilitate gradual withdrawal of needle. Accidents have occurred after forcible attempts to remove the needle. If it is inadvertently broken, the retained fragment is secured with a pair of forceps and removed later, under local anaesthesia if necessary.

With any pain-relieving technique, and acupuncture is no exception, complications may occur that are entirely unrelated to the procedure. It is therefore important to know the patient's history and concurrent medication. Following pain relief by acupuncture in arthritis, for example, a patient may ill-advisedly discontinue not only analgesic drugs but also those that are essential to health, such as antihypertensives, steroids and cardiac glucosides. Subsequent deterioration is then unfairly attributed to the acupuncture. Another dilemma is the patient on anticoagulant therapy for cardiac or peripheral vascular ischaemia. There is no need to stop these drugs, because there is very little risk of bleeding from acupuncture, although the patient should be warned of possible bruising, which can be controlled with a pressure bandage or ice pack.

Indications for acupuncture

These are very similar to those already listed for transcutaneous stimulation. Indiscriminate use of either method without proper evaluation is strongly deprecated. Temporary relief in an undiagnosed patient may critically delay recognition of serious underlying pathology, such as a brain tumour or aneurysm in a person with intractable headache or migraine. As for TNS, there are impressive lists of indications for acupuncture in the literature. In my view, pain emanating from a musculo-skeletal disorder or various neuralgias are the ones that should be carefully scrutinized for TENS or acupuncture. It is only by trial and error that the clinician will find which of the two modes is suitable for each individual. More debateable is the choice of these non-invasive methods for severe intractable pain of unknown origin that is unresponsive to conventional analgesic drugs. Occasionally, their use is justified by their preventing the need for complicated and potentially dangerous invasive procedures.

Summary

Pain management can be a very difficult problem on some occasions. Acupuncture and TENS are particularly useful in this situation because they are safe, relatively uncomplicated and inexpensive methods, and are often the means whereby potent analgesic or psychotropic drugs can be reduced or withdrawn altogether. Although either technique can be used as the main therapeutic option, experience has shown that these non-invasive methods are ideally suited as an adjunct to some other form, such as medical manipulation. It is essential to understand the basic mechanisms of acupuncture and TNS before the principles can be applied intelligently in each case. It is also necessary to know of current medication and perform an examination, if necessary with investigations, to reach a provisional diagnosis in the first instance. This has been stressed repeatedly. Patient selection is also important, to see whether the individual understands what is involved, does not expect immediate or complete analgesia and is willing to persevere until significant benefits are achieved. Nevertheless, even within these constraints, 50–70% of those with pain that is difficult to resolve in any way are improved and the effort is rewarding for both the individual and his medical adviser.

REFERENCES

1. Woolf, C.J. (1984). Transcutaneous and implanted nerve stimulation. In Wall, P.D. and Melzack, R. (eds.) *Textbook of Pain*, Vol. 3; Chap. 1; 679–689. (Edinburgh: Churchill Livingstone)
2. Thompson, J.W. (1987). The role of transcutaneous electric nerve stimulation (TENS) for the control of pain. In Doyle, D. (ed.) *International Symposium on Pain Control* pp. 28–47. (London: Royal Society of Medicine)
3. Stamp, J.M. and Wood, D.A. (1981). *A Comparative Evaluation of Transcutaneous Nerve Stimulators (TENS)*. (Sheffield UK: Sheffield University and Area Health Authority)
4. Sjolund, B. (1988). Clinical aspects of TENS. *Intractable Pain Soc.*, 6(2), 35–38
5. Sjolund, B. and Eriksson, M. (1985). *Relief of Pain by TENS*. (Chichester: Wiley)
6. Yeh, C., Gonyea, M., Lemke, J. and Volpe, M. (1985). Physical therapy: evaluation and treatment of chronic pain. In Aronoff, G.N. (ed.) *Evaluation and Treatment of Chronic Pain*, pp. 251–266. (Baltimore: Urban and Schwarsenberg)

7. Mehta, M. (1987). Simple ways of treating pain. In Andersson, A., Bond, M., Mehta, M. and Swerdlow, M. (eds.) *Chronic Non-Cancer Pain*, pp. 133–145. (Lancaster: MTP Press)
8. Pomeranz, B., Cheng, R. and Law, P. (1977). Acupuncture reduces electrophysiological and behavioural responses to noxious stimuli. *Exp. Neurol.*, **54**, 172–178
9. Chu, L.S.W., Yey, S.D.J. and Wood, D.D. (1979). *Acupuncture Manual – A Western Approach.* (New York: Dekker)
10. Wensel, L.O. (1980). *Acupuncture in Medical Practice.* (Resor, Va.: Reston)
11. Melzack, R. (1984). Acupuncture and related forms of folk medicine. In Wall, P.D. and Melzack, R. (eds.) *Textbook of Pain*, (Edinburgh: Churchill Livingstone)
12. Melzack, R., Stilwell, D. and Fox, E. (1977). Trigger points and acupuncture points for pain. Correlation and implications. *Pain*, **3**, 3

19
Hypnosis in musculoskeletal medicine

H.B. GIBSON

It is important to realize that hypnosis is not a form of alternative therapy. Hypnosis in itself has no therapeutic value and, contrary to popular belief, the various physical and mental ills to which we are subject cannot simply be hypnotized away. The term 'hypnotherapy' has led to a great deal of misunderstanding, and there are now many quite unqualified people calling themselves 'hypnotherapists' who offer their services for hire and capitalize on the numerous misconceptions about the power of hypnosis.

Any procedure or any neutral preparation that is applied with a therapeutic intent will generally have some initial success owing to the psychological mechanism of the placebo reaction[1]. Therefore, when hypnosis is used even by ignorant and unprofessional quacks, there may be some initial improvement in the patient's condition, just as there would be if a bottle of coloured water were prescribed with due solemnity. But so-called 'hypnotherapy' in the hands of inadequately qualified people may do a great deal of harm, since it may conceal serious conditions that need to be adequately diagnosed in their early stages and given appropriate treatment.

What then is the value of hypnosis in therapy? It has a value as an adjunctive procedure: that is, it can be very useful to various sorts of professional people in the exercise of their different therapeutic skills, provided that they are prepared to work within the strict limits of their own professional training and expertise. Hypnosis is being used fruitfully by various medical specialists, clinical and educational psychologists, speech therapists, physiotherapists, dentists, and a number of other professional people, all working within their own specialisms and often contributing to interdisciplinary units.

The techniques of inducing hypnosis are very easy to learn, and hence there is a certain danger of some professional people, once they have had some succes in the legitimate enhancement of their own professional skill, coming to regard themselves as 'hypnotherapists' and trying to treat conditions that are quite outside their relevant range of competence. Thus, there have been cases of physiotherapists and dentists who have made good use of hypnosis in treating conditions that are within their proper province going on to try to treat cases of emotional and psychosomatic disorder with very unfortunate results[2]. It is for this reason that the British Society of Experimental and Clinical Hypnosis (BSECH) stipulates that all members give an undertaking that they will use hypnosis only in areas in which they are qualified.

It has been necessary to give this rather lengthy caveat because there is so much misunderstanding about the nature of hypnotic techniques and how and for whom they should be employed before we get on to the question of their usefulness in musculoskeletal medicine.

I shall not attempt to define too closely just what hypnosis is. At best is must be defined ostensively rather than operationally. The nature of hypnosis has always been the subject of lively controversy, and in his recent book David Rowley outlines seven separate theories of hypnosis. Such theoretical points need not concern us here. I am content to accept the rough and ready description of hypnosis that is given in an educational pamphlet issued to the public by BSECH. 'Hypnosis can be described as a state in which your mind pays attention to things in a different way. In hypnosis you are more open to acceptable suggestions and more likely to follow them whether the suggestion is to achieve something, to think of something, or to imagine something vividly which you may find difficult in your normal state of waking consciousness.' Hypnosis alters how we perceive and experience our environment, both temporarily, and also by effecting long-term changes in properly planned therapeutic programmes.

Because hypnosis can produce an alteration in perception, it can be used to screen out from consciousness the perception of pain. Here I must counter a misconception that is very common even in the medical and allied professions. Hypnosis does not confer analgesia automatically[3]. You have to work quite hard with a hypnotized patient to build up what is in fact a negative hallucination for pain, and the means by which this is achieved fits in quite well with the gate control theory of pain first proposed by Melzack and Wall. Many of you will have had the difficult task of treating chronic pain patients who used to have some organic condition that has remitted long ago, but who still continue to suffer pain chronically and because of that painful experience continue to move in an odd manner or inhibit movements so that a maladaptive habit develops and secondary disorders ensue. According to Loeser[4], 60–78% of patients suffering from low back pain have no apparent physical signs. It used to be thought until quite recently that while hypnosis had some power to overcome or attenuate acute pain, it was of little use in programmes designed to help chronic pain patients. Such a view was put forward in Melzack's 1973 book *The Puzzle of Pain*. However, by 1982, when he came to revise and enlarge that book in collaboration with Patrick Wall[5], Melzack had modified his views on hypnosis, partly, I think, owing to his collaboration with Campbell Perry, a noted expert on hypnosis. They carried out a most interesting study that merits a brief description[6]. Melzack and Perry studied a group of chronic pain patients who suffered from low back pain, arthritic pain, cancer pain and other disorders. Patients were treated in different groups using placebo, biofeedback and hypnosis, either as separate treatments or in combination. I will quote Melzack and Wall's brief description of the part of the results relevant to hypnotic training[7].

> Melzack and Perry (1975) found that EEG biofeedback alone had no demonstrable effect on chronic pain compared to the level of pain relief obtained in 'placebo' baseline sessions. In contrast they found that hypnotic training instructions produced substantial relief of pain – significantly greater than the effect of biofeedback. The subjects reported on average 22% pain reduction, and 50% achieved pain decreases of 33% or more. Despite the magnitude of the effect, it was not statistically greater than that of the 'placebo' baseline sessions. However, when the hypnotic training instructions were presented together with biofeedback the pain relief was significantly greater than that produced by baseline placebo sessions.

This study shows us that hypnosis is a technique that is especially effective when it is carefully combined with other techniques, and has a place in therapeutic programmes of rehabilitation. We should get out of the habit of thinking in terms of 'hypnotherapy' and study how best hypnosis can be used in conjunction with other techniques to enhance our existing therapeutic skills.

I would point out that it is only comparatively recently that hypnosis has been taken seriously by responsible clincians and has ceased to be regarded as the exclusive province of some rather eccentric doctors and others. The eccentrics still continue to flourish, of course, and do a roaring trade in various brands of cult alternative therapy. But the serious use of hypnosis in the treatment of both acute and chronic pain has resulted in the publication of a number of excellent books and chapters in books in the 1980s relating to the use of hypnosis in the treatment of painful conditions. I would mention Burrows and Dennerstein[8], De Piano and Salzberg[9], Elton, Stanley and Burrows[10], Gibson[11], and Hilgard and LeBaron[12]. The increased interest in the use of hypnosis in therapy for painful conditions is manifest if we study the presentations at the successive International World Congresses on pain. At the First World Congress in 1975, of the 148 published papers only two referred to the treatment of pain in humans by means of hypnosis. At the 4th World Congress in 1984 there was more time devoted to hypnosis in clinical pain control, one of the eight workshops being entirely devoted to hypnosis. There was also an extended video programme, and a presentation concerned with experimental pain and hypnosis. At the 5th World Congress in 1987 there were no fewer than seven presentations relating to the utilization of hypnosis in treating various pain conditions. At last responsible scientists and clinicians are taking hypnosis seriously.

So far I have referred only to the role of hypnosis in the management of painful conditions. This has the double function of contributing to the patient's comfort and wellbeing, and of permitting forms of treatment that would otherwise be too painful to be endured. But hypnosis has a wider role to play in therapy for musculoskeletal disorders. By the use of hypnotic techniques a degree of deep muscular relaxation can be obtained that is very difficult to obtain in the normal waking state. In Japan, Kimura and his colleagues[13] use hypnosis in treating patients with spastic paralysis where remedial therapy involves their executing movements that would be impossible for them in the normal waking state because of their muscular tension. This practice is common in Japan where their own tradition of Zen has merged with the system of Autogenic Training of Luthe, and has been influential in both sports training and clinical physiotherapy. Japan is a country where hypnosis is generally accepted in medical and psychological treatment by both lay persons and professionals, and it is not regarded with the suspicion that has been generally accorded to it in the West.

Similarly, Pajntar, Roskar and Voldovnick[14] in Yugoslavia use hypnosis extensively in the rehabilitation of patients suffering from various forms of musculoskeletal disorders. In other countries too there is a growing use of hypnosis both for diagnosis and treatment. Various therapists in the USA make such use of hypnosis. William Kroger[15] devotes a chapter of his book to it. Finkelstein[16] reports the successful treatment involving hypnosis of a woman with disrupted flexor function after an injury to the hand, and Spiegel and Chase[17] report the successful use of self-hypnosis and daily flexing exercises in a patient with severe post-traumatic contractures of the hand. Schneiderman and his colleagues[18] report a case of spasmodic torticollis treated by general relaxation and specific hypnotic suggestions for control of the neck muscles. I could go on mentioning single case studies but unfortunately we are still too dependent on such reports, and more controlled trials are needed to establish more precisely just what the role of hypnosis is in rehabilitative programmes of behaviour therapy.

Finally I shall mention a rather unusual paper by Van Strien[19] who reports the treatment of 31 patients suffering from hernia nuclei pulposi in which hypnosis was involved. Seventeen of these patients are described as 'completely cured' and the rest either dropped out of treatment, or were suspended from treatment because of unsatisfactory progress. Dr Van Strien has a somewhat individual explanation of the aetiology of the prolapse of intervertebral discs and the methods by which such patients should be treated, but his claims seem worth investigation.

The diagnostic value of hypnosis lies in the fact that if a partially disabled patient can perform certain movements quite easily when hypnotized but finds them impossible to execute in the normal waking state, that is evidence that the disability is largely functional rather than organic. Many disabilities have a large psychological component, torticollis being the classical example. I shall not call this component hysterical; I think it is more useful to regard it as the result of a conditioning process that has taken place over a long period of time following a neuromuscular or similar lesion that has cleared up but has left the patient with a maladaptive habit that cannot be broken by conscious intention. Hypnotic treatment is ideally suited to re-educating the patient whose physical disabilities have a large psychological component.

Many patients do not like to admit to themselves that their physical disabilities are maintained partly by psychological factors, and in my opinion it is a mistake to introduce too large a component of what is generally regarded as 'psychotherapy' into the treatment of people with musculoskeletal disorders. I think that some psychiatrists and others who have been over-influenced by psychoanalytic thinking have been far too prone to attribute psychodynamic motivation in people with physical disorders. If we fail to alleviate the distress and disability of patients who suffer from such disorders, it is a rather easy let-out for the unsuccessful therapist to claim that it is really the patients' fault because they 'want' to cling on to their disability because of the supposed secondary gains that incapacity may bring. I do not dispute the fact that secondary gains may exist, but I think that this aspect of the treatment of musculoskeletal disorder has been grossly exaggerated in some quarters. Some therapists using hypnosis seem to have convinced themselves that if they spend enough time in hypnotic sessions, age-regressing their patients to early childhood and allegedly probing the murky depth of the Freudian unconscious, they will somehow clear up the existing disorder. Although I have read a great number of case studies where this approach has been adopted, they are of an anecdotal nature and I have found no real evidence for the success of such methods. In my opinion, while we should recognize the role that psychological factors may play in the maintenance of physical disorders, we should be very cautious in venturing psychological explanations for physical disability. And when we use hypnosis it should be directed to the remedy of the presenting disorder rather than trying to remodel a patient's personality. Hypnosis is a useful tool, but it is a dangerous tool when therapists become too involved in psychodynamic speculation.

It will be apparent that I am a psychologist broadly of the behaviourist persuasion, and because of my rather pragmatic orientation some people wonder why I have taken such an interest in the clinical and experimental aspects of hypnosis over the past thirty years. There is still a strong reluctance among some behavioural scientists to interest themselves in the practical possibilities of hypnosis in therapy. Fortunately this has been breaking down over the past two decades, and controlled clinical trials have convinced more enlightened therapists that hypnosis may play a very valuable part in well-designed programmes of behaviour therapy directed to both psychological and physical disorders.

In the UK there is little employment of hypnosis by one profession that could well make more use of it. I refer to the chartered physiotherapists. BSECH has had applications for membership from a few of them, and should be glad to offer them help and training, and to extend their general knowledge of hypnosis and its application, for they get no formal training in hypnosis under the NHS. Some physiotherapists are using hypnosis in the course of their work, but the society is reluctant to admit them as a body because it seems that some individuals are setting up as part-time 'hypnotherapists' and trying to treat emotional disorders although they lack the proper professional education and training in this area of therapy. I commented on this general problem earlier, and it is one that will be with us for some time.

What then do I advocate for those who are seriously interested in the possibilities of using hypnosis in their professional work? There are national societies for professional people concerned with hypnosis and they run training programmes, conferences, etc. Most of them are affiliated to the International Society of Hypnosis, which has some 15,000 members. Most societies publish their own professional journals. Despite the great proliferation of commercial trash that is published about the alleged wonders of hypnosis, there are some good modern books and I have already referred to some. Last year a book edited by Michael Heap[20], was published; it is contributed to by numerous British authors on a great range of aspects of hypnosis, and it runs to 40 chapters. Finally, like most proud authors, I must mention my own book written jointly with Dr Heap[21], which deals in detail with many of the questions I have not space to cover here.

REFERENCES

1. Gibson, H.B. (1987). Is hypnosis a placebo? *Br. J. Exp. Clin. Hypnosis*, **4**, 149–155
2. Kleinhaus, M. and Eli, I. (1986). Potential deleterious effects of hypnosis in the clinical setting. *Am. J. Clin. Hypnosis*, **29**, 155–159
3. Hilgard, E.R. and Hilgard, J.R. (eds.) (1985). *Hypnosis in the Relief of Pain*, Chap. 4. (Los Altos, Calif.: W. Kaufmann)
4. Loeser, J.D. (1980). Low back pain. In Bonica, J.J. (ed.) *Pain*. (New York: Raven Press)
5. Melzack, R. and Wall, P. (1982). *The Challenge of Pain*. (Harmondsworth: Penguin)
6. Melzack, R. and Perry, C. (1975). Selfregulation of pain: the use of alpha-biofeedback and hypnotic training for the control of chronic pain. *Exp. Neurol.*, **46**, 452–469
7. Melzack, R. and Wall, P. *op. cit.*, p.349
8. Burrows, G.D. and Dennerstein, L. (eds.) (1981). *Handbook of Hypnosis and Psychosomatic Medicine*. (New York: Elsevier Press)
9. DePiano, F.A. and Salzberg, H.C. (eds.) (1986). *Clinical Applications of Hypnosis*. (Norwood, N.J.: Ablex)
10. Elton, D., Stanley, G. and Burrows, G. (1983). *Psychological Control of Pain*. (Sydney: Grune & Stratton)
11. Gibson, H.B. (1982). *Pain and Its Conquest*. (London: Peter Owen)
12. Hilgard, J.R. and LeBaron, S. (1984). *Hypnotherapy of Pain in Children with Cancer*. (Los Altos, Calif.: W. Kaufmann)
13. Kimura, S. (1975). Behaviour therapy for cerebral palsy by hypnotic methods. *Bull. Br. Psychol. Soc.*, **28**, 240
14. Pajntar, M., Roskar, E. and Voldovnick, L. (1985). Some neuromuscular phenomena in hypnosis. In Waxman, D., Misra, P.C., Gibson, M. and Basker, M.A. (eds.) *Modern Trends in Hypnosis*. (New York: Plenum Press)
15. Kroger, W.S. (1977). *Clinical and Experimental Hypnosis in Medicine, Dentistry and Psychology*. (Philadelphia: J.B. Lippencott)
16. Finkelstein, S. (1982). Re-establishment of traumatically disrupted finger flexion: a brief communication. *Int. J. Clin. Exp. Hypnosis*, **30**, 1
17. Spiegel, D. and Chase, R.A. (1980). The treatment of contractures of the hand using self-hypnosis. *J. Hand Surg.*, **5**, 428

18. Schneiderman, M.J., Leu, R.H. and Glazeski, R.C. (1987). Use of hypnosis in spasmodic torticollis: a case report. *Am. J. Clin. Hypnosis*, **29**, 260–263
19. Van Strien, J.J.A. (1987). The role of hypnosis is the understanding and treatment of hernia nuclei pulposi. Paper presented at the *Fourth European Congress of Hypnosis in Psychotherapy and Psychosomatic Medicine*, Oxford, UK
20. Heap, M. (ed.) (1988). *Hypnosis: Current Clinical, Experimental and Forensic Practices.* (London: Croom Helm)
21. Gibson, H.B. and Heap, M. (1989). *Hypnosis in Therapy.* (London: Lawrence Erlbaum Associates) (in press)

Section II
DIRECTED PAPERS

20
Comments on the evolution of the sacroiliac joint

H.-D. WOLFF

INTRODUCTION

The sacroiliac joint plays the role of an 'outsider', both in arthrology and in human medicine. It has even been doubted repeatedly whether it is a joint at all. It lacks active mobility because there is no autochthonous musculature. Its mechanics are not clearly defined and are variable. What appears certain, at least to a practitioner of manual medicine, is that joint play exists there and that loss of this joint play is clinically relevant.

This chapter is devoted to the conclusions that can be drawn from the phylogenesis of the articulation, and the changes in the connection between the pelvis and the sacrum. It is particularly interesting to trace how and under what conditions the sacroiliac joint (SIJ) has evolved in *Homo sapiens*.

THE DEVELOPMENT OF THE PELVIS AND SACRUM IN GENERAL

The earliest vertebrates living in water needed neither a pelvic nor a shoulder girdle, as they were not exposed to the forces of gravity during locomotion.

When the change from life in the water to life on land took place, at the end of the Devonian period about 380 million years ago, the static and dynamic forces of gravity posed great problems. The fins had to be transformed into weight-bearing and moving extremities. A connection had to be formed between the longitudinal structure of the endoskeleton and the extremities. Two models evolved to meet this need:

(1) The forward extremities were attached to the spine mainly by muscles;
(2) The hind legs were connected to the pelvic girdle either by ligaments or by bones and joints.

FISH

Although fish need no pelvic girdle, species exist that have a bony structure in the anterior abdominal wall, stabilizing the abdominal fins. This part of the trunk can also be found in the Crossopterygia, the fossils which are of greatest interest for dating the transformation from aquatic to terrestial life. (Figures 20.1 and 20.2).

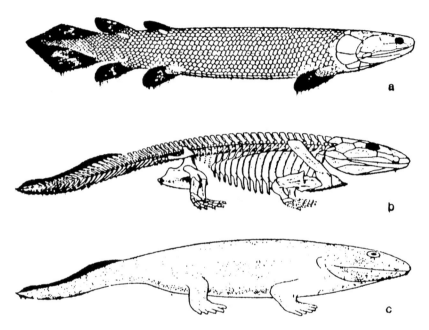

Figure 20.1 (a) A *Crossopterygia* (Upper Devonian) (b) *Icytyostega* from Grönland. The oldest known quadruped with a fishtail (Upper Devonian). (From Ref. 2)

AMPHIBIA

In the early amphibia (380–250 million years ago), for the first time a ventral bony structure, the 'pelvic plate', shows three characteristic parts: the ilium, the pubic and the ischial bones. At the junction of these three pelvic bones there is the acetabulum, the joint cavity for the femoral head.

The ilium lengthened and came into contact with the spinal column. It met with a vertebra having an enlarged costal process as a point of contact. The other pelvic bones grew quickly, too, and provided the necessary attachments for a powerful musculature. It is at this early stage that the original model of the pelvic girdle with the sacrum was firmly established (Figure 20.3).

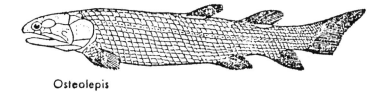

Osteolepis

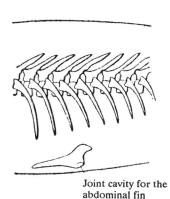

Joint cavity for the
abdominal fin

Figure 20.2 Osteolepis (*Crossopterygii*) and pelvis plate. (From Ref. 4)

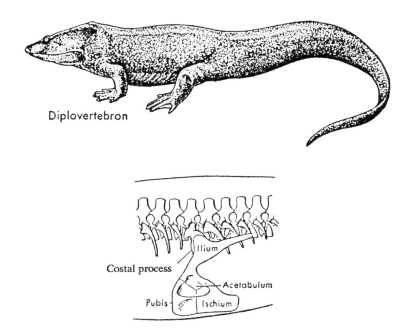

Diplovertebron

Ilium

Costal process

Acetabulum

Pubis

Ischium

Figure 20.3 Diplovertebron (early Amphibia) and pelvic girdle. (From Ref. 4)

177

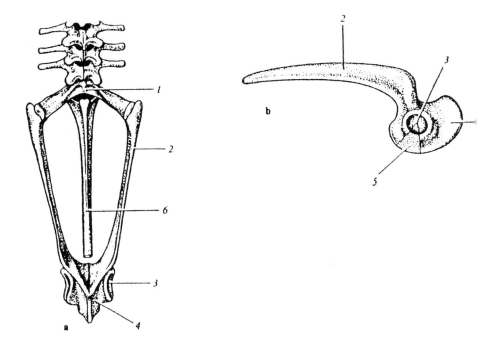

Figure 20.4 Frog (*Rana esculenta*) pelvis: (a) from dorsal, (b) from the left.
1, Sacral vertebra; 2, ilium; 3, acetabulum; 4, ischium; 5, pars pubica; 6, urostyl (os cossygis). (From Ref. 5)

This model was adhered to consistently during later periods no matter how much the shape and function of the individual elements changed during adaptation to new demands.

As early as in the amphibian stage there is great variability in the course of phylogenesis. The developmental history of the frog is particularly interesting. Here the centre of gravity had to shift to accomodate forward leaping. For this purpose the spinal column was reduced and the single sacral vertebra situated almost at the centre of the body. The ilium therefore became very long. It remained in contact with the transverse process of the sacral vertebra by a very mobile articulation (Figure 20.4). On the other hand, in other living amphibia (salamanders, newts) the ilium lies in a dorsal and caudal direction; they have kept to the ancient form of forward motion. The pelvic girdle is closed in front by cartilage between the pubic bones.

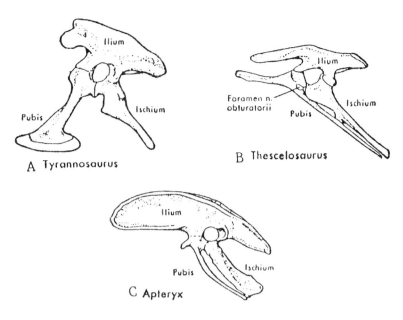

Figure 20.5 Reptilia: (A) pelvis of a saurischia (*Tyrannosaurus*); (B) pelvis of an ornithischia (*Thescelosaurus*); (C) pelvis of a bird (*Apteryx*). (From Ref. 4)

REPTILES

The trunks of reptiles are shaped very much like those of the amphibia. The most ancient reptile was recently found in Scotland, in geological strata about 340 million years old. It shows a caudal ilium in contact with 1–2 sacral vertebrae. The pubic and ischial bones are still plate shaped.

In the course of 150 million years during which reptiles predominated, considerable modifications of this basic pattern took place during specialization. In particular, the giant species of dinosaurs showed some significant variations. Scientifically, two types of saurian pelvis have been distinguished: in the Saurischia and the Ornithischia. The Saurischia were very large and fleet predators that were able to stand on their hind legs. A powerful tail played an important static as well as a dynamic role. A large pubic bone turned forward closed the pelvic girdle. The latter carried the weight of the abdominal viscera, exerting pressure in a caudal direction (Figure 20.5 (A)).

On the other hand, in the bird-like type of pelvis, what remains of the pubic bone is thin, and like a rod turned in a dorso-caudal direction; it lies in front of the very large ischial bone. This development is connected with erect posture and bipedal locomotion. The differences between these two types of pelvis can

179

be explained by a different type of locomotion, a smaller tail, and a different position of the centre of gravity (Figure 20.5 (B)). The Ornithischia pelvis was the starting point for all later changes during this evolution of birds, which are phylogenetically related to the reptiles.

BIRDS

The reptiles were the first vertebrates to conquer the air. This new change again caused far-reaching reshaping of the skeleton and of the motor system. Flying required a greatly enlarged sternal bone and massive ossification of the spinal column and the pelvis. In the course of this process, up to 22 somites were fused to form the sacrum. The very large ilia are joined on the back, behind the spinal column. There is no pelvic girdle or pubic symphysis. Here we see the most extensive ossification in the pelvic and sacral regions.

MARITIME REPTILES

Unlike those reptile forms that developed into birds, there were species that went back to aquatic from reptilian life, just as some mammals did later. Theoretically, the return to aquatic life (e.g. in Ichthyosauri, whales, Cetacea and others) meant that acquisition of the pelvis and the extremities were superfluous. In reality, however, there was no return to the original condition as in fish, rather those structures and functions already acquired were subjected to restructuring. The pelvic bones frequently atrophied until they were hardly recognizable. The connection between the ilium and the sacrum disappeared and the symphysis opened.

MAMMALS

The expansion and differentiation of the numerous species of mammals began about 65 million years ago, after the previously dominant dinosaurs became extinct. Early forms of mammals, however, appeared as early as the primitive forms of reptiles and even of amphibia. Consequently, the pelvis in early mammals closely resembled the pelvis of early reptiles and amphibia.

Characteristic differences arose later, when the laterally turned acetabula and horizontal thighs that made sliding and creeping propulsion possible gave way to vertical extremities placed laterally and allowing mammals to run and trot. This made faster and more differentiated motion possible. The tail became less heavy and lost its importance for body statics. Consequently the SIJ moved in a cranial direction, in front of the hip joint. The ilium not only lengthened in a cranial direction, but became broader, so as to provide attachment for the longer and more powerful pelvic musculature. Those mammals that learned to fly or that returned to the water developed the same characteristics as we have found in the corresponding species of reptiles:

- Flying species (bats) developed wider ossifications between the sacrum and the ilium;
- Aquatic forms (seals, sea lions, etc.) show reduction and atrophy of the connection between the sacrum and the ilium.

PRIMATES, HOMINIDS AND MAN

Not unlike the change from water to land, the change from quadruped to erect posture caused unmistakable changes.

The primate evolved from insectivorous mammals living in trees. The anthropoid ape is believed to stem from the Tupaia. The extinct Proconsul is thought to be the lost common ancestor from whose family tree the orang-utan was the first to branch off, followed later by the gorilla and the chimpanzee, and finally by man. About 10 million years ago the first signs of bipedal habit appeared. The first certain proof of erect posture was found in the anthropithecus Lucy, that is to say, more than 3 million years ago. The famous footprints of Laetoli date from the same period.

Erect posture was accompanied by a shortening of the trunk and the forelimbs. The centre of gravity of the body was shifted to the surface of the sacrum. The formerly flat and thin ilium turned from a directly frontal to a more lateral direction and became much larger (Figures 20.6 and 20.7), stabilizing the labile body.

The motor system had the urgent task of maintaining balance. For this purpose the entire pelvic musculature had to be reorganized: stabilization in the sagittal plane led to enormous growth of the gluteus maximus; stabilization in the frontal plane became the task of the abductors (especially of the gluteus medius) and of the adductors. The femoral neck and the pelvic ligaments were included in this reshaping. At the same time the differentiation of the sacroiliac joint took place. As long as the horizontal SIJ in the quadrupeds is not subject to much pressure, it remains thin and lies parallel to the sacrum. With erect posture the SIJ becomes broader (in the gorilla and chimpanzee) (Figures 20.7 and 20.8). The shape of the joint becomes angular. The wide section at S_1 lies in the direction of the plumb-line; the part at S_2 and S_3, however, is horizontal and at right angles to the first. The articular surface of S_1 is open in a ventral direction and that of S_3 in a dorsal direction, with ligamentous fixation. This points to a specific mechanical joint function: 'nutation'. The iliosacral connection possesses all the characteristics of a true joint.

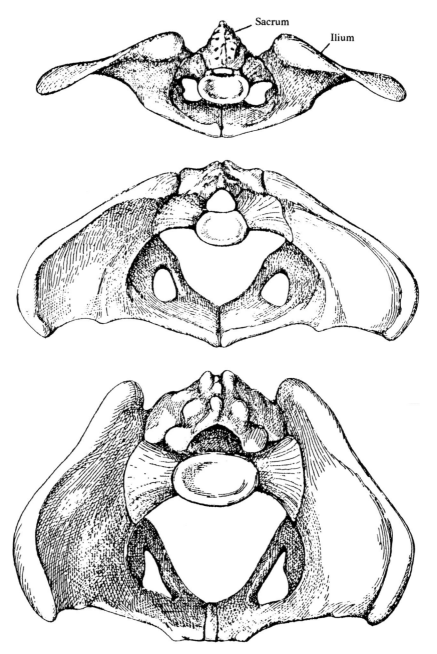

Figure 20.6 Primate pelvic girdle in topview: (a) chimpanzee; (b) Lucy (*Australopithecus*); (c) Human pelvis (woman). (From Ref. 3)

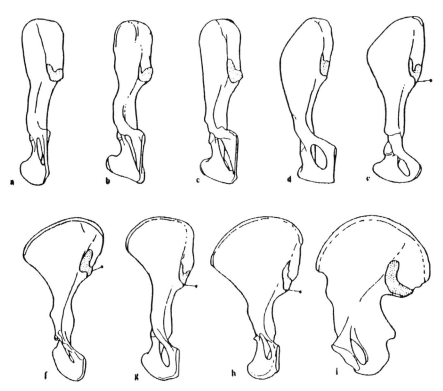

Figure 20.7 Change in pelvic bone and SIJ of primates: (a) *Macuca*; (b) *Papio*; (c) *Presbytis*; (d) *Hylobates*; (e) *Symphalangus*; (f) *Pongo* (urang-utang); (g) *Pan* (chimpanzee); (h) *Gorilla*; (i) *Homo*. (From Ref. 5)

The greatly increased pressure on the sacrum requires a pelvis that is both elastic and firm. The firmness is guaranteed by the linea terminalis, the elasticity by the spring in the SIJ and (with a different mechanism) by the symphysis. From the point of view of phylogenesis, it can be concluded that the SIJ is not an archaic relic but that the existing structures are the result of adaptation to the specific requirements of erect posture.

CONCLUSIONS

Phylogenesis offers further confirmation that the SIJ plays a very subtle though passive role in pelvic statics so as to make erect posture and movement possible in man. As always happens, sophisticated construction implies increased vulnerability. The diagnosis of disturbed function by the practitioners of manual medicine is a practical response to this liability to disturbance.

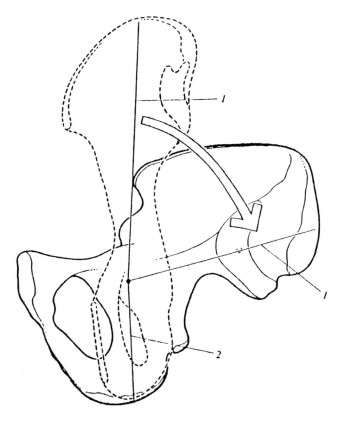

Figure 20.8 Comparison between chimpanzee pelvis (quadruped) and human pelvis (biped). (From Ref. 5)

SUMMARY

The following conclusions can be drawn from the phylogenesis of the sacroiliac joint (SIJ).

(1)　The change from water to land necessitated the evolution of limbs from fins. The forelimbs are connected to the spinal column by means of muscles via the shoulder girdle. The caudal extremities are connected to a transformed spinal column by means of the pelvis.

(2)　The ventral structure, i.e. the pelvic plate of early fishes, became the three pelvic bones. They are in contact with the costal processes of the first sacral vertebra via the budding ilium.

(3)   In all original species of amphibia, reptiles and mammals, there is a similar original model.

(4)   The actual adaptation to various functional demands caused differentiation and great variability from the original structure. In keeping with the shape of the pelvic girdle, the iliosacral junction may be diarthrotic, syndesmotic or even osseous. The sacral part may be one vertebra or the product of 20 somites. In birds the pelvic girdle is formed by considerable sections of the spinal column and constitutes an osseous block.

(5)   Only in primates has erect posture been established during the last 10 million years. This development has not yet been documented by fossil remains. It took place 3 million years ago and brought about a transformation of the pelvic girdle, producing the specific and unique shape and function of the human SIJ.

(6)   From the point of view of phylogenesis, it follows that the SIJ is not an accidental or superfluous developmental relic but a particularly subtly functioning solution to the specific problem of effective erect posture.

REFERENCES AND FURTHER READING

1.   Herm, D. (1987). Unweltveränderungen und Evolution in der Erdgeschichte. In Wilhelm, F. (ed.) *Der Gang der Evolution*, pp. 177–192. (München: Ch. Beck)
2.   Kuhn-Schnyder, E. and Rieber, H. (1984). Paläozoologie. (Stuttgart: G. Thieme)
3.   Lovejoy, C. Owen (1989). Die Evolution des aufrechten Ganges. *Spektrum Wiss.*, 1, 92
4.   Romer, A.S. (1976). *Vergleichende Anatomie der Wirbeltiere.* (Berlin: Paul Parey)
5.   Starck, D. (1979). *Vergleichende Anatomie der Wirbeltiere.* Bd.I und Bd.II (Heidelberg: Springer)
6.   Walker, A. and Teaford, M. (1989). Die Suche nach Proconsul. *Spektrum Wiss.*, 3, 102–113
7.   Wilhelm, F. (1987). *Der Gang der Evolution.* (München: Ch. Beck)
8.   Ziegelmayer, G. (1987). Phylogenetische Entwicklung des Menschen. In Wilhelm, F. (ed.) *Der Gang der Evolution*, pp. 193–213, Figure p. 197. (München: Ch. Beck)

21

Clinical aspects of sacroiliac function in walking

P.E. GREENMAN

Low back pain with or without leg pain continues to be a major social problem[18]. Sixty to eighty per cent of low back pain is identified as idiopathic and specific diagnosis eludes the most skilful practitioner. A common finding in these patients, in addition to their complaint of pain, is alteration of the functional mobility of the lumbar spine, pelvic girdle, and lower extremities. The role of sacroiliac joint function in both asymptomatic and symptomatic patients continues to be controversial[1,3,10,19,21]. Many authors have described methods of evaluating and treating the sacroiliac region for various pain syndromes[1,2,5,7,9,12,15,16,20,22,24-26,28,32]. In order to develop a rational diagnostic and therapeutic system of the sacroiliac syndrome, one needs comprehension of the anatomy and biomechanics of the joints of the pelvic girdle[7,17,31,33,36].

ANATOMY

The bony pelvis can be described as three bones and three joints. The three bones are the right and left innominate, consisting of the fused elements of the ilium, ischium and pubis; and the sacrum, consisting of the five or six fused sacral segments. The three articulations are the right and left sacroiliac joint and the symphysis pubis. Above and below the bony pelvis are three other articular structures, namely, the right and left hip joint, and the lumbosacral joint including its two facet joints and the lumbosacral intervertebral disc. The symphysis has a fibrocartilaginous disc and is stabilized by the superior pubic ligament and the arcuate pubic ligament found between the two inferior pubic rami. The sacroiliac joints have both a synovial component as well as extensive interosseus ligamentous structures. The synovial articular component is ventrally located and the opposing surfaces of the sacrum and ilium have extensive cartilaginous surfaces[4,38,41]. The cartilage on the sacral surface is considerably greater than that on the ilial side of the joint. The opposing surfaces vary widely and during the ageing process demonstrate progressive increase in grooving. The joint is described as being L-shaped with a short upper arm and a longer lower

186

arm joining at approximately S2. There is usually a change in bevel at the junction of the upper and lower arms with the ventral surface of the upper arm being narrower than the dorsal, and the lower arm being wider on the ventral surface than on the dorsal. There is also a convex–concave relationship of the opposing surfaces of the sacroiliac joint, with the sacral side having a concavity near the junction of the upper and lower arms and the ilial side having a convexity. The changes in bevelling and the convex–concave relationship provide much stability to the joint and its articular surface. The greatest stability to the sacroiliac joint results from its ligamentous structures. The ventral sacroiliac ligaments are quite thin and some anterior fibres of the iliolumbar ligament are continuous with the ventral sacroiliac ligament. The interosseous sacroiliac ligaments are very short and tight and prevent much of the movement between the sacrum and ilium. There are several layers of the dorsal sacroiliac ligaments. As they progress dorsally and become progressively longer, the fibres attach more medially on the sacral side and more dorsally on the ilial side. The long dorsal vertically oriented sacroiliac ligaments become continuous with the sacrotuberous and sacrospinous ligaments. The innervation of the sacroiliac joint is primarily from the S1 root.

The pelvic girdle responds to muscle action from above and below. The abdominal musculature attaches to the iliac crest and inguinal ligament, which is basically a reflection of the oblique musculature. The rectus abdominis muscle attaches directly to the pubis. Imbalance of right to left abdominal muscle groups can influence symphyseal function. Posteriorly there are two major muscles that influence pelvic girdle motion, the psoas major and minor and the quadratus lumborum. The psoas links the thoracolumbar junction with the hip joint and is a major long restrictor of lumbopelvic function. As the psoas traverses the pelvis, it joins with the iliacus, which takes its origin from the inner surface of the innominate. The psoas is one of the few muscles that cross the sacroiliac joint. Another highly significant muscle that crosses the sacroiliac joint on each side is the piriformis. Taking origin from the anterior surface of the sacrum via several digitations, it traverses the sciatic notch to insert on the greater trochanter of the femur. Another significant structure that passes through the sciatic notch with the piriformis is the sciatic nerve. Functional alteration of the piriformis can lead to sciatic-type pain and is called the piriformis syndrome[29,35]. The piriformis functions as an external rotator and abductor of the hip joint and also appears to be of significance in sacroiliac motion during the walking cycle.

The muscles of the pelvic and urogenital diaphragm are intimately related to the osseous pelvis. While these muscles appear to have little influence on pelvic girdle motion, alteration in pelvic girdle function does seem to affect the relative balance of the pelvic diaphragm. Frequently patients presenting with pelvic girdle dysfunction have symptoms involving the rectum, lower urinary tract, and pelvic genitalia. Urinary urgency, frequency, dysuria, dyspareunia, and rectal pruritis, for which no organic reason can be identified, are frequently seen.

The musculature of the lower extremities, particularly the muscles within the six compartments of the hip and thigh, strongly influence pelvic girdle motion. The action of these large and strong muscles during walking move the innominates through space. Alteration in function of the lower extremity muscles due to problems within the foot, ankle, knee, or hip joint can all influence mechanical behaviour of the pelvic girdle through each innominate bone.

BIOMECHANICS OF THE PELVIC GIRDLE

The pelvis responds to the load of the vertebral axis and trunk from above as it meets the upward force of the lower extremities through the hip joint. In the sitting position there is difference in the influence of the pelvis from below, since the weight is now supported by the ischial tuberosities. In both the standing and seated positions the pelvis may rotate forward or backward depending upon the relationship of the weight-bearing line from above meeting upward force from below.

Movement within the pelvic girdle is not great and depends upon integrated motion of the two sacroiliac joints and the symphysis pubis. Most of our knowledge about the movement within the pelvic girdle has been from radiographic methods in fresh and embalmed cadavers, and on humans. One study used the insertion of Steinman pins on the ilial and sacral side of the joint to measure movement[8]. Most studies have evaluated only one component of the motion within the pelvic girdle[6,11,13,14,23,27,30,34,37].

There are primarily two movements at the symphysis pubis. The first is a cephalad to caudal translatory movement occurring on prolonged one-legged standing[6,11]. When the movement at the symphysis pubis is physiological, one-legged standing on the opposite side, or prolonged two-legged standing, will return the relationship of the symphysis to symmetry. However, if something restricts the mobility at the symphysis pubis with either one side being more superior or the other more inferior, pubic dysfunction occurs. Associated with unlevelling at the symphysis pubis is altered muscle balance between the abdominals above, particularly the rectus abdominis, and the adductors from below. Imbalance of muscle length and strength from right to left at the rectus abdominis, or at the adductors of each thigh, also appears to be related to pubic symphysis dysfunction. The second movement at the symphysis is an alternating anterior and posterior rotation of each pubis during the walking cycle. This can be described as movement around a transverse axis, which biomechanically is actually an intersection of two axes of rotation for each innominate crossing at approximately the symphysis. When the symphysis pubis is found to be dysfunctional in its cephalad to caudal translatory motion, which unlevels the symphysis pubis, there appears to be altered mechanical behaviour of the rest of the pelvis during the walking cycle. During gait, the symphysis is basically the most stable point within the pelvic girdle. It oscillates up and down in a sinusoidal curve but translates little from side to side.

During gait, the two innominates alternately rotate forward and backward asynchronously with each other. The pelvis rotates left and right around a vertical axis and the rotation is opposite to the shoulder girdle, resulting in the normal cross pattern gait. This alternating anterior and posterior rotation of each innominate during walking is accompanied by anterior and posterior rotation of the pelvis and a changing of the centre of gravity of the trunk over the hip joints. This anterior–posterior rotation of each innominate involves a relationship at the symphysis pubis in front and at the sacroiliac joint behind. This motion can be described as iliosacral in that it is rotation of one innominate in relation to one side of the sacrum. There are other possible motions of one innominate on one side of the sacrum. These motions are dependent upon the shape of the sacroiliac joint. If the two joint surfaces are more parallel because of the lack of definitive bevel change, and from flattening of the convex–concave relationship, then the possibility of superior to inferior translatory movement is also possible. The basic stability of the iliosacral joint in this condition is less than average and occurs in approximately 15% of the population. Dysfunction of this translatory movement appears to be related to the superior and inferior innominate shear dysfunctions[15,25,32]. A third possible iliosacral movement appears to result in those iliosacral joints where the convex–concave relationship is reversed and the concavity occurs on the ilial side and the convexity on the sacral side. This provides for the possibility of rotation of an innominate medially or laterally around a vertical axis. Dysfunction within the medial or lateral rotation of an innominate can then occur and has been described as in-flare or out-flare dysfunction of an innominate.

Movement within the pelvic girdle can also be described as that which the sacrum does between the two innominates, the so-called sacroiliac movement. The sacral motion between the innominates about which we know the most is that described as nutation and counternutation[17,39]. Nutation is ventral nodding of the sacral base between the two innominates, and counternutation is posterior nodding. This motion can be described as occurring across a transverse axis. Biomechanical studies have defined a number of different transverse axes around which this motion appears to occur. The fact that several different transverse axes have been described should not be surprising, since the anatomy of each sacroiliac joint differs within each specimen study. This motion occurs primarily in two-legged standing with forward and backward trunk bending. While described as nutation–counternutation, there is a point near the middle of the range that can be described as neutral. Ventral nutation from neutral can be described as anterior nutation and dorsal nutation from neutral can be described as posterior nutation. During anterior nutation, the sacral base moves ventrally and the sacral apex dorsally. In posterior nutation, the sacral base moves dorsally and the apex ventrally. If both sacroiliac joints are symmetric, this anterior and posterior nutational movement remains symmetrical. However, in the presence of asymmetry of the right and left sacroiliac joint, a condition that is far more common than symmetry, asymmetrical anterior and posterior nutation can

189

occur. It is for this reason that occasionally one finds restriction of anterior or posterior nutational movement in one sacroiliac joint while not being present in the opposite. There is also a translatory component of sacral movement during the anterior nutation–posterior nutation movement[12,40]. During anterior nutation, there is some caudal translation of the sacral base and during posterior nutation a cephalad translation. Again depending upon the shape of the two sacroiliac joints, unilateral dysfunction of the sacrum when anteriorly nutated may also be described as an inferior sacral shear dysfunction.

A second movement of the sacrum between the innominates is that which accompanies the walking cycle[22,24]. This is the motion that has been researched less than nutation and counternutation of two-legged standing. However, if one clinically observes sacral movement during the walking cycle by placing the thumbs on each side of the sacral base and the long fingers on each side of the sacral apex and walking naturally, there appears to be a 'wobble' motion of the sacrum. This motion occurs alternately during left and right strides. Since the trunk is in the neutral position, and the lumbar spine is active while the lordosis is neutral, this sacral motion can be described as 'neutral' sacroiliac motion. This movement is obviously a polyaxial movement in three-dimensional space, but for descriptive purposes it has been identified as motion around an oblique axis. The left oblique axis has been described as being between the upper pole of the left and the lower pole of the right sacroiliac joint, and the right oblique axis as traversing from the right upper to the left lower pole. Motion around the oblique axis is described as rotation of the anterior surface to one side and side-bending of the superior sacral articular surface to the opposite side. The combined side-bending and rotational movements are described as torsional in nature. During walking the behaviour of the sacroiliac joints appears to be that of left torsional movement on the left oblique axis, returning to neutral, then switching to right torsional movement on the right oblique axis, returning to neutral, and then repeating the cycle with each stride. This left-on-left and right-on-right torsional movement can then be described as neutral sacroiliac mechanics. The sacrum can become restricted between the two innominates during either a left-on-left or right-on-right sacral torsional movement.

A third motion of the sacrum between the two innominates can be described as that which occurs with two-legged standing when the trunk is forward bent and then side-bent to one side. This is the position in which the lumbar spine has coupled motion of side-bending and rotation to the same side. Concurrently with this non-neutral lumbar position, there is movement of the sacrum in torsion around one of the oblique axes. In this example the rotation and side-bending are to opposite sides but now the sacral base moves posteriorly instead of anteriorly as it does during walking. If one forward bends and side-bends the trunk to the right, the sacrum rotates to the left, side-bends to the right, and posteriorly nutates the left sacral base. This motion is described as left-on-right backward torsional movement. Side-bending to the left while forward bent results in right-on-left posterior torsional movement of the sacrum with rotation occurring to the right, side-bending to the left, and posterior nutation of the right sacral base. Since these sacroiliac movements occur when non-neutral lumbar mechanics are operative, they can be described as non-neutral sacral mechanics.

Another significant motion in the lumbopelvic region is that which occurs at the lumbosacral junction. Motion of the inferior surface of L5 on the superior surface of the sacrum physiologically always appears to be in opposite directions. During trunk forward bending, L5 moves into forward bending and anterior translation while the sacral base moves into posterior nutation. During trunk backward bending, L5 rotates into backward bending and the sacral base moves into anterior nutation. When the sacrum rotates left during its torsional movement, it side-bends to the right and results in right rotation and left side-bending of L5. Therefore, as the sacrum rotates right, L5 rotates left; and when the sacrum side-bends right, L5 side-bends left, and vice versa. When L5 becomes dysfunctional in relation to the sacrum with rotation and side-bending to the same side, it is described as 'nonadaptive' lumbosacral dysfunction. The normal adaptive response of a functional lumbar spine is that of side-bending and rotating to opposite sides as a group in response to side-bending of the sacral base. As the sacrum rotates left and side-bends right, the lumbar spine side-bends left and rotates right. When the sacrum rotates right and side-bends left, the lumbar spine side-bends right and rotates left. The capacity of the lumbar spine to accomplish this alternating motion is an essential component of the normal walking cycle.

PELVIC GIRDLE DYSFUNCTIONS

Restriction of any of the motions described can occur owing to either chronic microtrauma or a single traumatic episode. In most instances there are restrictions of multiple movements within the pelvic girdle when it is dysfunctional. For descriptive as well as therapeutic purposes they can be described as dysfunctions at the symphysis pubis, iliosacral dysfunctions (one innominate in relation to one SI joint) and sacroiliac dysfunctions (the sacrum between two innominates)[22,24,25]. The diagnosis of these dysfunctions is made by a combination of asymmetry of anatomical landmarks; alteration in range of motion of one side of the pelvis to the other; and tissue texture abnormalities primarily at the inguinal ligament, overlying the sacroiliac joints, and related muscles and ligaments such as the gluteal muscles and the sacrotuberous ligaments.

The possible dysfunctions within the pelvic girdle are as follows:

– Pubic
  (1)   Superior
  (2)   Inferior

- Sacroiliac
  (1) Bilateral anterior nutation
  (2) Bilateral posterior nutation
  (3) Unilateral anterior nutation (flexion)
  (4) Unilateral posterior nutation (extension)
  (5) Anterior torsion (L-on-L or R-on-R)
  (6) Posterior torsion (R-on-L or L-on-R)

- Iliosacral
  (1) Anterior rotation
  (2) Posterior rotation
  (3) Superior (cephalic) shear
  (4) Inferior (caudal) shear
  (5) Medial rotation (in-flare)
  (6) Lateral rotation (out-flare)

Regardless of the system used to evaluate the pelvic girdle dysfunction, one or more of these motions will be found to be restricted. There are numerous manual-medical procedures that are used to address pelvic girdle dysfunction and, when successful, will be found to have restored one or more of the restricted motions found within the pelvis. It behoves the manual medicine practitioner to be aware of the multiple motion characteristics of the pelvic girdle to identify those that are lost and to restore them to physiological normality as much as possible. In addition to restoring pelvic girdle motion, one must also assure the capacity of the lumbar spine to function in synchronous neutral mechanics for walking, as well as assuring maximum function of the lower extremities including length and strength of the major muscles of the hip and thigh.

This discussion has been based upon our current knowledge of the anatomy and biomechanics of the pelvic girdle, coupled with the clinical observations of many authors. Several of the motions described are based upon a theoretical construct that attempts to explain the clinical observations. Because the amount of motion within the sacroiliac joints is quite small, they are difficult to measure *in vivo*. With expanding new technology for motion analysis, it is hoped that it will be possible to better describe the motions available and their axis systems, and better understand the motions available.

REFERENCES

1. Beal, M.C. (1982). The sacroiliac problem: review of anatomy mechanics and diagnosis. *J. Am. Osteopath. Assoc.*, **81**, 667–679
2. Beckwith, C.G. (1944). *J. Am. Osteopath. Assoc.*, **43**, 549
3. Bellamy, N., Park, W. and Rooney, P.J. (1983). What do we know about the sacroiliac joint? *Semin. Arthritis Rheum.*, **12**, 282–312

4. Bowen, V. and Cassidy, J.D. (1981). Macroscopic and microscopic anatomy of the sacroiliac joint from embryonic life until the eighth decade. *Spine*, **6**, 620–628
5. Bressler, H.B. and Deltoff, M.N. (1984). Sacroiliac syndrome associated with lumbosacral anomalies: a case report. *J. Manipulative Physiol. Ther.*, **7**, 171–173
6. Chamberlain, W.E. (1930). The symphysis pubis in the roentgen examination of the sacroiliac joint. *J. Am. Roentgen.*, **24**, 621
7. Clark, M.E. (1906). *Applied Anatomy*. (Kirksville, Mo: Journal Printing Co.)
8. Colochis, S.C., Worden, R.E., Bechtol, C.O. and Strohm, B.R. (1963). Movement of the sacroiliac joint in the adult male: a preliminary report. *Arch. Phys. Med. Rehabil.*, **44**, 490–498
9. Conti, J.J. (1980). An osteopathic approach to the treatment of low back pain caused by sacroiliac joint lesions, short leg problems, and lumbosacral angle increase. *Osteo. Med.*, **5**, 50–55
10. Cyriax, J. (1965). *Textbook of Orthopedic Medicine*, 7th edn. Vol.2. (New York: Harper and Row)
11. Dihlmann, Wolfgang (1980). *Diagnostic Radiology of the Sacroiliac Joint*. (Chicago: Year Book Medical Publishers)
12. DonTigny, R.L. (1985). Function and pathomechanics of the sacroiliac joint. *Phys. Ther.*, **65**, 35–44
13. Egund, N., Alsson, T.H., Schmid, H. and Selnik, G. (1978). Movements in the sacroiliac joints demonstrated with roentgen stereophotogrammetry. *Acta Radiol. Diagnosis*, **19**, 833–846
14. Frigerio, N.A., Stowe, R.R. and Howe, J.W. (1974). Movement of the sacroiliac joint. *Clin. Orthop. Related Res.*, **100**, 370–377
15. Greenman, P.E. (1986). Innominate shear dysfunction in the sacroiliac syndrome. *Manual Med.*, **2**, 114–121
16. Hoover, H.V. (1942). Dr Fryettes' spinal technic. *Yearbook Acad. Appl. Osteopath.*, **48**, 25–30
17. Kapandji, I.A. (1974). *The Physiology of the Joints, Vol.3, Trunk and Vertebral Column*, 2nd edn., pp. 53–67. (Edinburgh: Churchill Livingstone)
18. Kirkaldy-Willis, W.H. and Hill, R.J. (1979). A more precise diagnosis for low-back pain. *Spine*, **4**, 102–109
19. Maigne, R. (1972). *Orthopedic Medicine: A New Approach to Vertebral Manipulations*. (Springfield, IL: Charles C Thomas)
20. McGregor, M. and Cassidy, J.D. (1983). Post-surgical sacroiliac joint syndrome. *J. Manipulative Physiol. Ther.*, **6**, 1–11
21. Miltner, L.S. and Lowendorf, C.S. (1931). Low back pain: a study of 525 cases of sacroiliac and sacrolumbar sprain. *J. Bone Joint Surg.*, **13**, 16–28
22. Mitchell, F.L. (1948). The balanced pelvis and its relationship to reflexes. *Yearbook Acad. Appl. Osteopath.*, **48**, 146–151
23. Mitchell, F.L., Jr. and Pruzzo, N.A. (1971). Investigation of voluntary and primary respiratory mechanisms. *J. Am. Osteopath. Assoc.*, **70**, 149–153
24. Mitchell, F.L., Jr., Moran, P.S. and Pruzzo, N.A. (1979). *An Evaluation and Treatment Manual of Osteopathic Muscle Energy Procedures*, 1st edn. (Valley Park, Mo.: Mitchell, Moran and Pruzzo Associates)
25. Neumann, H.D. (1985). Manuelle Diagnostik and Therapie von Blockierungen dr Kreuzdarmbeingelenke nach F. Mitchell (Muskelenergietechnik). *Manuelle Med.*, **23**, 116–126
26. Nicholas, A.S. (1979). Dysfunction of the innominate complex. *Osteopath. Med.*, **4**, 65–77
27. Peckham, R.R. (1965). Associated bilateral sacroiliac movement. *Yearbook Acad. Appl. Osteopath.*, **65**, 117
28. Pitkin, H.C. and Pheasant, H.C. (1936). Sacroarthogenetic telegra. II. A study of sacral mobility. *J. Bone Joint Surg.*, **18**, 365–374
29. Retzlaff, E., *et al.* (1974). The piriformis muscle syndrome. *J. Am. Osteopath. Assoc.*, **73**, 799–807
30. Reynolds, H.M. (1980). Three-dimensional kinematics in the pelvic girdle. *J. Am. Osteopath. Assoc.*, **80**, 277–280
31. Sashin, D. (1930). A critical analysis of the anatomy and the pathologic changes of the sacroiliac joints. *J. Bone Joint Surg.*, **12**, 891–910
32. Schwab, W.A. (1933). Principles of manipulative treatment. The low back problem IX. *J. Am. Osteopath. Assoc.*, **10**, 216; **11**, 253; **12**, 292

193

33. Simkins, C.S. (1965). Anatomy and significance of the sacroiliac joint. *Yearbook Acad. Appl. Osteopath.*, **65**(2), 111–116
34. Solonen, K.A. (1957). The sacroiliac joint in the light of anatomical, roentgenological, and clinical studies. *Acta Orthop. Scand. Suppl.*, **27**, 1–115
35. Steiner, C., Staubs, C., Ganon, M. and Buhlinger, C. (1987). Piriformis syndrome: pathogenesis, diagnosis and treatment. *J. Am. Osteopath. Assoc.*, **87**, 318–323
36. Strachan, W.F. (1939). Applied anatomy of the pelvis and perineum. *J. Am. Osteopath. Assoc.*, **38**, 359
37. Strachan, W.F., Beckwith, C.G., Larson, N.J. and Grant, J.H. (1938). A study of the mechanics of the sacroiliac joint. *J. Am. Osteopath. Assoc.*, **37**, 576
38. Weisl, H. (1954). The articular surfaces of the sacroiliac joint and their relation to the movements of the sacrum. *Acta Anat.*, **22**, 1–14
39. Weisl, H. (1954). Ligaments of the sacroiliac joint examined with particular reference to their function. *Acta Anat.*, **20**, 201–213
40. Weisl, H. (1955). The movements of the sacroiliac joint. *Acta Anat.*, **23**, 80–91
41. Wilder, D.G., Pope, M.H. and Frymoyer, J.W. (1980). The functional topography of the sacroiliac joint. *Spine*, **5**, 575–579

22
The sacroiliac lesion – does it exist?

M.C.T MORRISON

We know the sacroiliac joint exists, but what is meant by the sacroiliac 'lesion' or sacroiliac 'strain'?

As a synovial joint it is subject to the same pathologies as any other synovial joint – which may affect the joint itself, its ligaments or the muscles involved. It has a nerve supply, the segmental innervation being shared with the lower lumbar spine and hip joints.

Is there a characteristic pain pattern for the sacroiliac joint? Can we differentiate by clinical examination between lower lumbar spine, sacroiliac and hip joints? If we manipulate, can be be sure we are moving the sacroiliac joint only?

A plea is made for a recognition of syndromes, without attaching a conjectural pathological label, in a language that can be understood and accepted by orthodox medicine and the manipulating fraternity.

The syndrome that I recognize – which is *reputed* to be a sacroiliac lesion is:

– History

Dull aching pain – usually definitely one side and lateral to sacroiliac joint
Radiates to groin and/or outer side of thigh
Worse standing, sitting and in bed; better 'on the move'

– Examination

Stands with iliac crests and spines on different levels, but leg lengths equal
Sits with crests and spines unequal
Pain on flexion and adduction of the thigh
Tender over, and lateral to, sacroiliac joint
Lumbar movements full and pain free
Normal SLR and no neurological signs

23

Differential diagnosis of muscle tone in respect of inhibitory techniques

V. JANDA

The understanding and concept of treatment of painful joints has been subjected to continuous change and development. Probably the most important is a holistic concept that regards a painful syndrome as an expression of dysfunction of the whole motor system and not as an affliction affecting one structure (= joint) only. From this point of view it is less important whether within the frame of the complex pathogenetical picture more stress is laid on muscles[1], soft tissue[2], chain reaction[3] or central nervous motor dysregulation[4], to mention only some important views. The important point is that each approach emphasizes the need to analyse and treat the whole body instead of limiting ourselves wrongly to one structure or segment.

However, in an attempt to describe or define new aspects, symptoms or relations, often an unprecise and vague terminology is used which makes understanding and communication very difficult. It is no exception for a too 'generous' terminology to lead to chaos and confusion that in turn slows down the acceptance of sound ideas and prevents the introduction of new rational and more effective therapeutic methods. The understanding of muscle dysfunction in pathogenesis of various pain syndromes may serve as a classic example.

Evidently the terminological chaos is due to the fact that our knowledge of function of many structures is very limited. There is a striking discrepancy between our clinical assessment ability and the possibility of measuring observations objectively and of course of finding an explanation based on sound physiological facts.

It is understood today that muscles in general play an extremely important if not a decisive role in the pathogenesis of various pain syndromes of the locomotor system. In view of their direct relation to joint dysfunction, there are a number of reasons to support the view that the muscles are most important in the initiation and maintenance of joint blocking[5]. One can share the view of Maigne[6] that 'the spasm of muscles undoubtedly constitutes a major factor in the genesis of the painful spine'. The main muscular factors accompanying joint dysfunction are:

(1)   There is always muscle spasm in the area of the painful lesion.
(2)   Pressure of the muscle in spasm increases the characteristic pain.
(3)   Muscles and fascia are the only tissues that are common to several segments and thus if strained may cause restriction of several contiguous segments.
(4)   Muscle fatigue is a predisposing factor that decreases the force available to meet demands.
(5)   Muscle tightness may influence joint position and thus lead to a strain of soft tissue and joints in positions and movements even within the normal range of movement.
(6)   Impaired central nervous motor programming due to stress, constrained movements and postures and/or chronic fatigue influences muscles, causing a consequent muscle imbalance and thus overstress in all structures of the musculoskeletal system. This situation can be considered one of the most important preconditions for the development of chronic pain syndromes.

Increased muscle tone can thus be considered as an important factor in the genesis of pain in the locomotor system. Despite this fact, not much attention has been paid to the differential diagnosis of this hypertonus, and 'spasm' without any further definition is almost the only term used. This gap necessarily causes a simplified approach to treatment followed by disappointing results.

Although the clinical differentiation of increased muscle tone due to impaired function is far from satisfactory, at present at least five types of increased muscle tone can and should be differentiated. With the exception of the last type, all of them are usually described just as 'spasm'. Increased muscle tone can occur owing to:

(1)   Dysfunction of the limbic system;
(2)   Impaired function at the segmental (interneuronal) level;
(3)   Impaired coordination of muscle contraction (trigger points?);
(4)   As a response to pain irritation;
(5)   Overuse (this is as a rule combined with changed elasticity of the muscle and usually described as muscle tightness).

MAIN CHARACTERISTICS

(1)   Muscles in spasm owing to dysfunction of the limbic system are usually not spontaneously painful. They are tender and sometimes even painful on palpation. Spasm can be found most frequently in the shoulder–neck area, then in the low back muscles and in muscles of the pelvic diaphragm. It is difficult to estimate by palpation the exact borderline between the hyper- and normotonic areas as the changes are gradual and the transitory area rather broad, about 5 cm. Examples of syndromes of this aetiology are some types of 'non-specific' low back pain, tension headache and many (pseudo)gynaecological disturbances.

(2)   Increased tone due to dysfunction on the segmental spinal level is not very common. It is characterized by an altered balance between physiological antagonistic muscles. One group of muscles develops spasm, whereas the antagonist shows inhibition, hypotonia and even weakness. Hypertonic muscles commonly ache spontaneously and are extremely tender or even painful on palpation. The symptomatology is similar to the 'muscles in spasm' in acute poliomyelitis and other neuroinfections. It is believed that it occurs owing to the impaired function of internuncial motoneurons[7]. Some cases of fibromyalgia are very probably of this origin.

(3)   Increased muscle tone due to incoordinated muscle contraction is characterized by increased muscle tone in part of a muscle while the rest remains normal. Even fibres in the vicinity of hypertonic fibres are inhibited, which can be recognized as a groove on deep-layer palpation. This type is very similar if not identical to trigger points as described for example by Travell and Simons[8]. Muscle fibres may ache spontaneously (active points) or may only be painful or tender on palpation (latent points). In this situation, synchronized activity of the motor unit can be expected. This phenomenon was first described by Clemmessen and Skinhøj[9] in poliomyelitis and probably is the expression of an attempt to meet overdue demands on muscle force. Guyton[10] reports this finding as common in workers carrying heavy loads.

(4)   Muscle spasm due to pain irritation is very common. It is evidently a defence reaction to immobilize the injured part of the body. The defence musculaire in appendicitis or paravertebral spasm in acute low back pain are the most frequent situations. This type of spasm is the only situation in which it is possible to register spontaneous EMG activity. This means that the whole reflex arch (the anterior horn cells included) is activated and that this spasm can to a certain extent be compared to sustained active muscle contraction. Discussion of clinical consequences that occur owing to exhaustion of the peripheral motoneuron and muscle fibres is beyond the scope of this chapter.

(5)   Muscle tightness should not be confused with muscle spasm, although both symptoms can appear simultaneously in the same muscle. In most cases, tight muscles perform a part of the general 'muscle imbalance' syndrome and are the result of chronic over-use. The tight muscle is as a rule not spontaneously painful but is tender on palpation. The irritability threshold of such a muscle is lowered and therefore the muscle is more readily activated. In early stages, the strength increases; in extreme and long-lasting tightness, however, the strength decreases as the active fibres are replaced by non-contractile tissue[11].

THERAPEUTIC METHODS

A detailed description of all possible treatment modalities would be beyond the scope of this paper. It should only be mentioned that in general the most effective methods that reduce either muscle spasm or muscle tightness are those based on the physiological principle of post-facilitation inhibition. We mention the 'hold relax' procedures of the PNF technique[12], muscle energy procedures[13], post-isometric relaxation[14] or even 'spray and stretch'[15,16]. The problem, however, is to estimate (a) the appropriate degree of muscle contraction and thus the number of motor units activated and inhibited consequently, and (b) the degree, quality and type of stretch. Here only basic recommendations can be given. In general it can be stated that (a) the more muscle fibres needing to be inhibited, the stronger is the resistance that should be applied to the voluntary contraction and (b) the more changes in elasticity and therefore the more degenerative changes in the muscle are expected, the stronger is the stretch that should be applied. Thus, in type 3 only a minimal stretch is needed, whereas in types 2 or 4 minimal or moderate stretch is needed. In type 5 the stretch must be strong, even vigorous, as not only the contractile fibres but the mechanical muscle properties have to be influenced[11]. The most effective methods for type 1 are general inhibitory techniques such as Schultz autogenic training, yoga and procedures based on similar ideas.

REFERENCES

1. Janda, V. (1969). Postural and phasic muscles in the pathogenesis of low back pain. *Proceedings of the XIth Congress of the ISRD, Dublin*, pp. 553–554
2. Ward, R.C. (1989). Myofascial release, Level I. Course handouts, Michigan State Univ., USA
3. Lewit, K. (1987). Muskelfazilitation und Inhibitions-techniken in Manuellen Medizine. *Manuelle Med.*, **18**, 19–22
4. Jull, G.A. and Janda, V. (1987). Muscles and motor control in low back pain. In Twomey, L.T. and Taylor, J.R. (eds.) *Assessment and Management, Physical Therapy of the Low Back*, pp. 253–278. (New York: Churchill Livingstone)
5. Good, A.B. (1985). Spinal joint blocking, *J. Manipul. Physiol. Ther.*, 8(1), 1–8
6. Maigne, R. (1979). *Orthopaedic Medicine*. (Springfield, Ill: C.C. Thomas)
7. Hník, P. and Skorpil, V. (1961). Pathophysiology of poliomyelitis. In Janda, V. (ed.) *Treatment of Poliomyelitis*. (Prague: Medical Publishing House)
8. Travell, I.G. and Rinzler, S. (1952). *Myofascial Pain and Dysfunction*. (Baltimore: Williams & Wilkins)
9. Clemmessen, S. and Skinhøj, E. (1947). *Acta Psychol. Neurol.*, Suppl. (Copenhagen)
10. Guyton, A.C. (1981). *Textbook of Medical Physiology*. (Philadelphia: Saunders)
11. Janda, V. (1984). *Pain in the Locomotor System. A Broad Approach to Aspects of Manipulative Therapy*, pp. 148–151. (Melbourne: Churchill Livingstone)
12. Kabat, H. (1952). The role of central facilitation in restoration of motor function in paralysis. *Arch. Phys. Med.*, **33**, 521–533
13. Mitchell, F.L., Moran, P.S. and Pruzzo, M.F. (1973). *An Evaluation and Treatment of Osteopathic Manipulative Procedures*. (Kansas City: Institute of Continuing Education)
14. Lewit, K. (1987). Chain reaction of the functional disturbances of the motor system. *Čas. Lék Čes.*, **26**, 1310–1312 (in Czech)
15. Travell, I.G. and Rinzler, S. (1952). The myofascial genesis of pain, *Postgrad. Med.*, **11**, 425–434
16. Mennell, M. (1975). The therapeutic use of cold. *J. Am. Osteopath. Assoc.*, **74**, 1146–1157

24
Practical approaches to the normalization of muscle tension

A.H. LAXTON

Abnormal muscle tension is associated both causally and consequentially with all disorders of the musculoskeletal system. Normal muscle tone consists both of 'passive elasticity or turgor of muscular (and fibrous) tissues and the active (though not continuous) contraction of muscle in response to the reaction of the nervous system to stimuli' (Basmajian). Abnormal muscle tension may, therefore, result from injury, disease or dysfunction of muscle, or from a multitude of factors impinging on the nervous system, or from both.

The motor system functions as an integrated whole. What is going on in one part can never be thought of as an isolated event. Any local lesion provokes more or less evident changes throughout the whole system and may, in its turn, have been secondary to remote causes.

The exponents of applied (and 'clinical') kinesiology have demonstrated that the body as a whole functions as a complex biocomputer the individual components of which exhibit a biphasic response, i.e. ON or OFF, that is outwardly demonstrable by changes in the strength or weakness of muscles tested. The motor system thus provides the display unit of this biocomputer and can be utilized in assessing the current state of the body. It can help in the localization of areas requiring therapy, and in assessing the effectiveness of therapeutic procedures. Its diagnostic and therapeutic consistency in skilled hands compels us to recognize how intricately interrelated are the chemical, structural and electromagnetic aspects of body function.

An understanding of normal physiology and of pathology, both functional and structural, enables us to select practical approaches to treatment from a variety of therapeutic modalities. Zohn[1] gives a balanced evaluation of the use of a wide range of physical treatments that deserves careful study. We cannot overemphasize *one basic principle in treatment – the need to ensure that injured tissues are given sufficient time and rest to heal, with nutritional needs being fully met and harmful substances avoided.* Whatever we may do therapeutically is but a helping hand along the pathway to healing and full recovery of function. This chapter will concentrate on just three pathological conditions which, however, are of major importance for our understanding of common musculoskeletal pain syndromes and for our choice of therapy.

PARTIAL DENERVATION OF MUSCLES

When peripheral nerves suffer minor trauma or deformation, e.g. in the intervertebral canal (narrowed perhaps by prolapse of an intervertebral disc or by swelling of a posterior vertebral joint), or where they penetrate tough fascial layers, there is liable to develop in the tissues supplied by those nerves a denervation hypersensitivity. Cannon's law states that 'when, in a series of efferent neurons, a unit is destroyed, an increased irritability to chemical agents develops in the isolated structure or structures, the effect being maximal in the part directly denervated'. This may happen even when efferent impulses are still able to pass along the nerve to the muscle being supplied. It has been shown that acetylcholine percolates throughout the muscle instead of being confined to the zone of innervation, leading to the development of 'hot spots' throughout the muscle. The result is that the muscle is liable to go into a state of 'contracture' (this is not a normal muscle contraction and is not associated with increased activity as shown by electromyography).

When the nerve damage is not severe, this is a reversible condition that merely requires time for recovery – in the case of a simple percussion injury it takes 2–4 weeks, and in the case of an indentation injury 4–8 weeks. In more severe injury there is disintegration of the myelin sheath and death of the nerve[2]. This pathology may account for some of those cases where there is pain and muscle contracture that clear spontaneously in 4–8 weeks whatever treatment (or none) is given. Lomo[3], a Norwegian physiologist, has shown that recovery from this denervation hypersensitivity may be hastened by electrical stimulation at 100 Hz via implanted electrodes. Gunn[4] has suggested that the 'current of injury' generated by simple needling acts in the same way. Here, then, is one practical approach to the normalization of muscle tension. It may be postulated that denervation hypersensitivity is also one of the initiating causes of 'reversible spinal dsyfunction' – to which we will return in due course.

MUSCLE SPINDLE HYPERACTIVITY

The muscle spindle is a complex structure functioning as a sensor that generates feedback to the associated muscle fibres around it. These control signals are simultaneously modulated by other influences such as signals from higher motor centres. The spindle is thus an integral part of the system that detects, evaluates and adjusts muscle length. Let us consider its nerve supply.

(a) At the centre of the spindle is the 'annulo-spiral receptor'. This has a large myelinated nerve giving rapid conduction to the spinal cord, passing without synapse to the anterior horn cells that serve the muscle in the vicinity of the spindle. It does not influence the higher cortical centres. This is very sensitive: very small changes in the length of the muscle affect its discharge pattern, and it tends to over-shoot – over-react – leading to a prompt emergency response.

(b)   On either side of the annulo-spiral receptor is the 'flower-spray receptor'. This has a smaller nerve. It maintains a gradual rate of discharge with no over-shoot. It is not monosynaptic. Its influence ascends to the cortex giving a steady report that is important so far as conscious activity is concerned.

        The spindle receptors discharge almost continuously with an impulse frequency proportional to the degree to which the spindle is being stretched. It may be mentioned in passing that the application to a muscle of a vibrator leads to an increase in afferent discharge from the spindle, producing an illusion that there has been joint movement leading to a stretching of the muscle that is being vibrated. This may lead to a reflex relaxation of that muscle.

(c)   Gamma efferent fibres. These very small fibres innervate small muscle components at the periphery of the spindle. Contraction of these muscle components stretches the main body of the spindle, with consequent stimulation of its sensory nerve endings. Thus, activation of the spindle sensory nerve endings may follow stretching of the spindle either (i) by stretching of the extrafusal fibres, i.e. the main muscle in which the spindle lies, or (ii) by contraction of its intrafusal fibres.

What, then is the function of the intrafusal muscle fibre? It adjusts the sensitivity of the spindle. It is possible for us to set a predetermined tension in the intrafusal fibres such that the discharge from the spindle receptors will reach a resting level only after there has been sufficient contraction of the surrounding (extrafusal) muscle to let the spindle off the stretch, with consequent slowing down of its afferent discharge (Figure 24.1).

How may this delicate function be disturbed? It is probable that a sequence of events occurs as follows:

(1)   The spindles in a muscle are silenced either:

        (a)   By prolonged relaxation of the muscle e.g. by maintaining a particular posture which keeps the muscle concerned in a shortened condition, or
        (b)   By the sudden stretch of its antagonist, e.g. in a fall, or as the result of a sudden impact.

(2)   There occurs a reflex 'turning up' of the 'volume control' by gamma efferent discharge to the intrafusal fibres of the spindle, making it more sensitive.

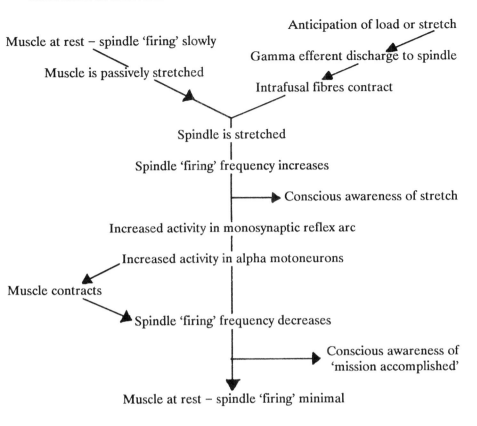

Figure 24.1 Function of the muscle spindle

(3)   At that point even a small stretch on the spindle (produced, for example, by initiating straightening-up of the back after a period in full flexion) leads to a hyperactive response from the spindle (comparable to the reverberating whine from an excessively turned-up volume control of a public address system).

(4)   Muscle shortening occurs associated with, and augmented by, weakness of the antagonist.

(5)   The result is a muscle, often 'marked' with a tender spot – probably associated with the hyperactive spindle. These are the tender spots noted by Jones[5] (the originator of 'counterstrain' therapy).

Table 24.1 Example of the pathogenesis of spindle hyperactivity

Contracting quadriceps	Relaxing hamstring
Muscles are subjected to a sudden passive stretch	Muscles are subjected to a sudden passive shortening
↓	↓
	Hamstring muscle spindles become 'silent'
	↓
Real strain of quadriceps	Reflex 'turning up of volume control' – hypersensitive spindles
↓	↓
Panic-type contraction of quadriceps to force leg forward to re-establish balance ⟶	Sudden stretch/lengthening of hamstrings triggering the hypersensitive spindles
↓	↓
End result	
Strained quadriceps – pain on active use *not* tenderness	Tender spot in hamstrings *Not* pain
Apparent weakness/disuse wasting	

Let us consider, with the help of Table 24.1, an example of what may happen to a person walking along a path when their foot suddenly hits an obstruction, e.g. an uneven paving stone. Once this acute muscle spindle hyperactivity syndrome has been triggered into action, it cannot easily be 'turned off' by the body. The only mechansim whereby the annulo-spiral efferent impulses can be shut off is by passive shortening of the muscle containing the malfunctioning spindle – in Table 24.1, the hamstrings.

We see that the mechanism for ongoing dysfunction is commonly not to be found in the muscle that has suffered real strain but in its opposing partner. Our treatment, therefore, needs to bear in mind the requirements of both muscle groups, and care must be taken to avoid further injury to the strained muscle that is in the process of healing. However, when that healing has been allowed to take place, persistent discomfort and weakness will suggest that there is still something wrong. Then is the time to palpate carefully the opposing muscle (although it is not painful or weak), seeking for a tender spot.

How can we respond therapeutically to this situation? We can 'shut off' the hyperactive spindle by markedly shortening the muscle containing it. This can be achieved by one of the following:

(i) *Spindle technique.* Put the muscle in a position of relaxation and then press together the body of the muscle on either side of the tender spindle.

(ii) *Jones' 'counterstrain' technique.* The adjacent joint is moved to the position that gives maximal shortening of the muscle containing the tender spot. This involves moving the joint in the direction that gives immediate ease and comfort until, usually at or close to a position of strain for the opposing muscle, the tender spot disappears. There has been 'release by positioning'. The joint is held in this position for 90 seconds and then very slowly returned to its neutral position. Jones claims that for each musculoskeletal dysfunction there is a tender point and, consistently, a position that relieves it.

REVERSIBLE SPINAL DYSFUNCTION

In health the spinal cord receives an afferent input from a multitude of sensory nerve endings both superficial and deep, some mechanoreceptors, some nociceptors. Under 'normal' conditions this input is processed through the neuronal circuits of our spinal 'computer', leading to an output via efferent nerves resulting in appropriate postural balance, desired activity and any reflex movement required for pain avoidance. Coordination of agonist and antagonist muscles is very finely synchronized.

If, however, the input is excessive or confused, then the output will be uncoordinated. Confusion may be caused in the first instance by a variety of somatic 'insults' that may be, for instance, postural or traumatic, and may not even be painful in themselves. These insults may indeed cause a mild strain of tendons, ligaments or joint capsules; but when these original noxious stimuli have ceased, and the mild strains have healed, it becomes evident that a self-perpetuating cycle of events has taken over that may continue indefinitely. There is disease though there is no structural pathology.

Physiologically there is established a state of 'chronic facilitation' (in a spinal segment or group of segments). Clinically this shows itself in the following ways:

(a)   Reduction in the threshold of pain and touch in the dermatome(s) involved;
(b)   Muscle hypertonicity;
(c)   Sympathetic hyperactivity – the segment behaves as if in a state of alarm.

This has repercussions on the functioning of the vascular system, viscera and endocrine glands[6].

This syndrome has, over the years, been given many different names, e.g. osteopathic lesion, chiropractic intervertebral subluxation, myofascial pain syndrome, secondary fibromyalgia, and reversible spinal dysfunction. Each 'name' is linked with an idiosyncratic approach to treatment. We need to evaluate carefully which approach has the maximum likelihood of benefit (with the minimum undesirable side-effects) in individual syndromes.

Travell and Simons[7] have described in detail the common occurrence of myofascial pain syndromes and trigger points. A trigger point (TP) is described by them as a focus of hyperirritability in a muscle or its fascia that causes the patient pain of a characteristic pattern (the 'target' area). An 'active' TP refers pain at rest, or with motion that stretches or loads a muscle. It is always tender and is located in a palpable band of muscle fibres. It prevents full lengthening of the muscle which is usually weakened. Local pressure produces referred pain that makes the patient jump (jump sign). Adequate stimulation of the TP also mediates a 'local twitch response' of the palpable band of muscle fibres. The TP can also initiate referred sympathetic phenomena that generally appear in the pain reference zone. The relationship between the site of a TP and its associated target area is constant, thus indicating fixed anatomical pathways.

The syndrome that Travell and Simons[7] so clearly describe and illustrate is none other than that described by osteopaths and chiropractors in time past, though they highlight the occurrence and significance of trigger points. Aetiological factors are the same – fatigue, stress and trauma. Are there any histological changes in the tissues in the region of TPs? Some workers have demonstrated a highly localized arterio-venous shunt, probably activated by sympathetic nerve stimulation and leading to ischaemic changes with release of algesic agents and an increase of interstitial (and, possibly, intracellular) fluid. The algesic agents initiate further stimuli that feed into a cycle of increasing motor and sympathetic activity, producing pain and muscle hypertonicity.

Travell advocates a particular treatment technique of 'stretch and spray' using chlorofluoromethane as a coolant spray (doubtless this will need to be replaced by an ozone-friendly alternative). She follows this with the use of hot packs. Her use of 'stretching' corresponds to the techniques developed by others and referred to as 'post-isometric relaxation' or indirect 'muscle energy' techniques.

As a second line of treatment, Travell advocates TP injection followed by ischaemic compression. This corresponds to the use of acupressure or *Shiatsu*. In a similar way, osteopaths noticed that pressure over a muscle in spasm, maintained for some 90 seconds, will often lead to relaxation of that muscle ('muscle inhibition').

Travell's third line of treatment is the identification and management of common perpetuating factors, e.g. structural adjustment, postural re-education, attention to nutrition, infection and infestation. Where there is underlying disorder, e.g. nerve compression, specific treatment needs to be directed at that.

There is clearly a striking similarity between trigger-point therapy and other therapeutic approaches. An injection of local anaesthetic, or of saline, or simply 'dry needling' (acupuncture) into the TP is often adequate to break the vicious circle of happenings that constitute the underlying 'reversible spinal dysfunction'.

Joint locking

Over the years there has been continuing disputation concerning the causation and consequences of joint 'locking'. Is it due to some innate problem in the joint itself? Or is it all due to abnormal muscle tension? In practice it is impossible to separate these two factors, though doubtless they vary in importance from case to case. We can, however, consider them separately.

Frictional factors at a joint interface

Cartilaginous surfaces are not perfectly smooth: there is dimpling or corrugation. During normal functioning, with lubrication by synovial fluid, this unevenness caues no obstruction to joint movement, although it may serve to limit side-slip of the opposing surfaces. However, when movement approaches the physiological maximum, the situation becomes unstable, corrective muscle pull becomes increasingly ineffective, and the articulating surfaces tend to side-slip in opposite directions: the eccentric positioning of the bones then leads to stretching of the capsule, with consequent compression and jamming of the dimpled/corrugated cartilaginous surfaces. These become rapidly deprived of the lubricating and nourishing synovial fluid that has been squeezed away (Figure 24.2).

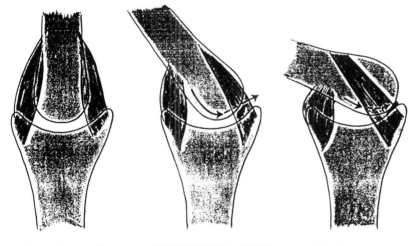

NORMAL JOINT	PHYSIOLOGICAL RANGE	PATHOLOGICAL POSITION
Muscles in balance	Some force tending to produce side–slip	Muscle balance lost
Capsule relaxed	Capsule relaxed	Evident side–slip producing eccentricity and joint locking
		Capsule stretched
		Loss of mobility

Figure 24.2 Suggested model of joint 'lock-sprain'

This hypothesis explains Lewit's finding of persistent mobility restriction in the cervical spine of patients even when the musculature had been relaxed with myorelaxant drugs under general anaesthesia[8].

It is clinical experience that effective relief is often obtained by manipulative treatment that appears to involve an initial increasing of deformity and distraction of opposing surfaces, thus allowing them to side-slip back into their normal apposition.

Some workers have postulated that the loss of mobility in joints is due to minute firm-edged particles of cartilage – called meniscoids – becoming jammed between the opposing joint surfaces. Whether or not such particles are generally present, it is difficult to see why they should float around freely yet block joints just at the moment when a patient has made the sort of awkward movement (e.g. of flexion and rotation of the trunk) that we know is often the movement that precipitates acute episodes of pain and muscle spasm.

Muscle hypertonicity and imbalance

It is often suggested in medical circles that tightening of muscles in the vicinity of joints is secondary to pathological changes in and around those joints, and that this tightening has a protective splinting action. This surely cannot be a true explanation in view of our observations that methods of treatment designed primarily to produce simple relaxation of such muscles often enables joints to regain freedom of movement with consequent relief of pain and the settling down of the whole painful episode – and all this without recourse to thrust techniques, injections, swallowing of tablets, etc.

Adhesions and pericapsular fibrosis

In a small proportion of cases it seems that chronic dysfunction and reduced mobility have been followed by the development of adhesions and pericapsular fibrosis. In such cases there is clear indication for sharp thrust techniques.

Effective manipulation may be administered by different operators, each with different concepts in their minds and each using different techniques, but all share a common objective – the re-establishment of normal mobility and function. The majority of manipulative and other non-manual approaches to treatment are directed at specific points of the reflex arc pathway that ultimately coordinates muscle contraction. Thus, the majority of effective treatments can be categorized as 'reflexotherapies'. Even 'thrust' techniques have a 'reflex' component.

Here, then, in summary, is a list of options from which each therapist can make a selection.

MANUAL TECHNIQUES FOR THE NORMALIZATION OF MUSCLE TENSION

1. *Pressure techniques*

    (a) Light pressure over the antagonist of a tight muscle maintained for seven seconds (Gaymans).
    (b) Firm pressure over a tight muscle for 30–60 seconds ('deep inhibition').
    (c) Pressure with a vibrator.

2. *Soft-tissue techniques*

    (a) Superficial and deep massage – including muscle-stretching by longitudinal or transverse massage.
    (b) Mobilization – passive joint movements ('articulation'). Rhythmic motion stimulates mechanoreceptors, producing a gate-closing effect on nociceptive impulses that would otherwise increase muscle tension.

3. *Thrust techniques*

    These may be effective both through
    (a) Reflex action on disturbed neuromuscular circuits, and
    (b) Release of mechanical 'joint-bind' ('fixation').

4. *Positioning techniques*

    (a) Functional technique. The affected joint is moved progressively to the position of overall maximal ease.
    (b) Spontaneous release by positioning ('strain and counterstrain'). This has already been discussed in detail.

5. *Muscle energy techniques*

    (a) Indirect. The subject attempts to make a movement away from the barrier, while the therapist resists. The subject then relaxes and the 'slack' is taken up. (This is the same as 'post-isometric relaxation'.)
    (b) Direct. The subject attempts to make a movement toward the barrier, while the therapist resists. Active contraction leads to reflex inhibition of the antagonist, thus allowing the therapist, during relaxation, to advance the part to the new, withdrawn barrier.

209

6. *Miscellaneous techniques*

    (a) Traction.
    (b) Impact therapy. The affected joint, suitably surrounded and supported by bags of sand or millet seed, is 'thumped' gently with another sand-bag[10].

NON-MANUAL TECHNIQUES FOR THE NORMALIZATION OF MUSCLE TENSION

1. *Dry needle techniques – acupuncture*

    (a) Musculotendinous portion of tight muscle (in region of Golgi tendon organ).
    (b) Motor point of antagonist.
    (c) Trigger points and other tender points.
    (d) Anywhere in muscles suffering from partial denervation
    (e) Master points and ear points.

2. *Magnet techniques*

    A similar effect to that obtained by the insertion of needles can be obtained by the application of small magnets to the skin. This can be useful when problems, temporarily alleviated by manipulation, keep recurring.

3. *Injection techniques*

    (a) Local anaesthetic, e.g. Huneke's 'neural therapy' (turns off excessive afferent stimuli).
    (b) Local steroid.

4. *Central reflex techniques*

    (a) Controlled respiration. In the cervical and lumbar regions expiration facilitates relaxation of the posterior spinal muscles.
    (b) Eye movements. Turning of the eyes to one side relaxes the spinal muscles that effect rotation of the spine to the opposite side.

5. *Postural re-programming techniques*

    e.g. 'Alexander technique'.

6. *General relaxation techniques*

(a) Conscious change from thoracic to diaphragmatic (abdominal) breathing.
(b) Conscious contraction of a group of muscles, followed by relaxation.
(c) Visual imagery.
(d) Counselling (e.g. Wilhelm Reich and Bioenergetic therapy)
(e) Meditation (e.g. yoga), prayer. These are particularly valuable when tension is arising from deep internal conflict – when the individual has difficulty in coming to terms with life itself.

It would clearly be impracticable and inappropriate to use regularly all of these approaches, but each option has its merits and can be useful. In general it can be assumed that each approach is most effective in the hands of the therapist who is using it regularly. Individual therapists seldom possess adequate knowledge and skills right across the therapeutic spectrum. There is, therefore, need for a multidisciplinary approach to back-pain research, to the evaluation of clinical therapies and to health care delivery if sufferers from musculoskeletal problems are to receive the treatment that, for them, will be most effective.

One organization committed to this sort of multi-disciplinary approach is The Physical Medicine Research Foundation[9].

REFERENCES

1. Zohn, D.A. (1988). *Musculoskeletal Pain*, 2nd edn. (Boston: Little, Brown)
2. Bradley, W.G. (1974). *Disorders of Peripheral Nerves*. (Oxford: Blackwell Scientific)
3. Lomo, T. (1976). The role of activity in the control of membrane and contractile properties of skeletal muscle. In Thesleff, S. (ed.) *Motor Innervation of Muscle*, Chap. 10. (London: Academic Press)
4. Gunn, C.C. (1978). Transcutaneous neural stimulation, acupuncture and the current of injury. *Am. J. Acupuncture*, 6(3), 191–196
5. Jones, L.H. (1981). *Strain and Counterstrain*. (American Academy of Osteopathy)
6. Korr, I.M. (1978). Sustained sympathicotonia as a factor in disease. In *The Neurobiologic Mechanisms in Manipulative Therapy*. (New York: Plenum)
7. Travell, J.G. and Simons, D.G. (1983). *Myofascial Pain and Dysfunction*. (Baltimore: Williams & Wilkins)
8. Lewit, K. (1978). The contribution of clinical observation. In *The Neurobiological Mechanisms in Manipulative Therapy*. (New York: Plenum)
9. Physical Medicine Research Foundation. (Odstock Hospital, Salisbury, UK)
10. Tracey, J.B. (1979). *Impact Therapy*. (Exeter, UK: John B. Tracey)

25
Metameric medicine and atlas therapy

A. ARLEN

METAMERIC DIVISION OF THE BODY; METAMERE FUNCTION AND DYSFUNCTION

The metameric organization of the embryo is maintained to a certain extent in the mature organism and is of basic significance in the development, recognition and treatment of a variety of pathological conditions (Figure 25.1)[18]. Metameric medicine converts this metameric organization into diagnostic and therapeutic practices, and also into new pathogenetic conceptual models.

A metamere is defined as the anatomical and functional regrouping of all components belonging to a myelotome and its associated spinal nerve pair: myotome, dermatome, sclerotome, viscerotome and angiotome. The myelotome forms the metamere neurotome together with the motor, sensory and vegetative component of its spinal nerve pair and the right and left sympathetic trunk ganglia[2,12] (Figure 25.2).

The individual metamere components are functionally interrelated, their autoregulation being controlled by the myelotome as site of metameric integration. Each metamere is also connected vertically, however, with all other metameres through intermetameric associative paths and the orthosympathetic nervous system.

As with all cybernetic regulatory systems, the neuroregulation of the metameric functional unit is susceptible to disturbance and can become impaired. Whereas the initial disturbance can originate in principle from any single metameric component, all other components are involved in the disturbance through metameric reflex activity, so that total metameric dysfunction develops, with increased motor and autonomic efferents and occurrence of muscular and sympathetic hypertonus[2,4].

The easily disrupted arthromuscular control loop appears frequently to provide the initial trigger for metameric dysfunction. As a result of an increase in tone in the myotome, the articular tension is also increased, the rate of afferent impulses from the joints becomes greater and, to complete the vicious circle, myotome activity is stimulated (Figure 25.3). This metameric dysfunction of the arthromuscular control loop, equivalent to the classic 'blockage', does not always involve complete immobilization of the joint but is rather a variable phenomenon embracing all degrees of impaired mobility up to and including immobility. This being the case, not only a complete 'block' but even a slight mobility impairment can cause nociceptive irritation leading to dysfunction of all metameric components. The way, if at all, that this metameric dysfunction is experienced subjectively will depend on the duration and intensity, age of the subject and other noxae.

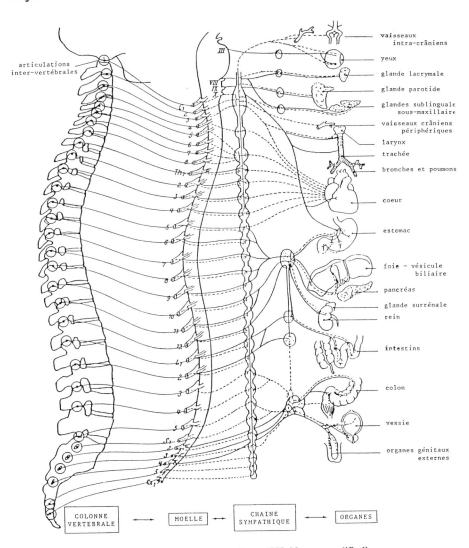

Figure 25.1 Metameric organization of the body (from F.H. Netter; modified)

213

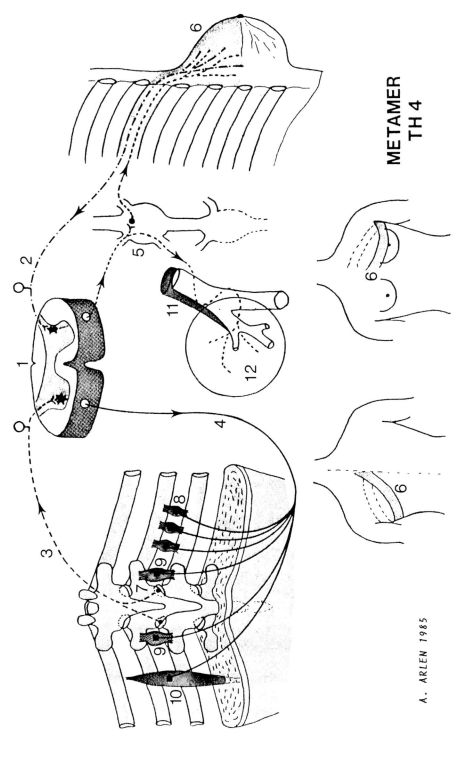

METAMER
TH 4

Figure 25.2 Simplified schematic representation of metamere Th4; 1. Myelotome, 2. Cutaneous afferent pathway. 3. Afferent pathway from intervertebral joints.

A. ARLEN 1985

214

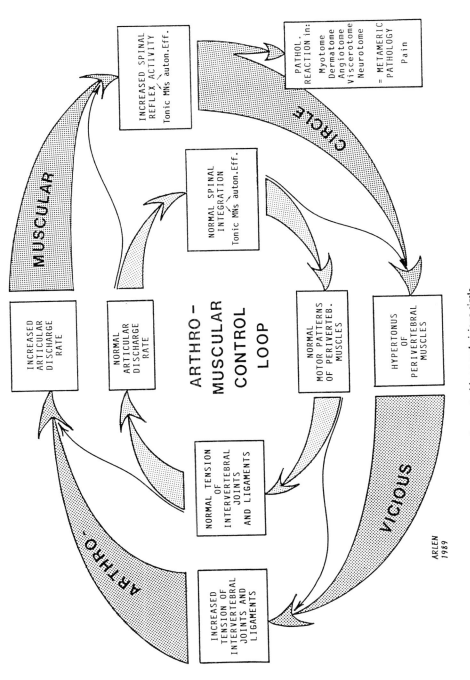

Figure 25.3 Diagram to illustrate the arthromuscular control loop and vicious circle

215

CLINICAL DEMONSTRATION OF METAMERIC DYSFUNCTION

Irrespective of its location, each metameric dysfunction is clinically recognizable and identifiable by characteristic palpable changes in the externally accessible metamere components, even when no subjective discomfort is felt:

1. Increased tone in the associated myotome;
2. Change in consistency and increased adherence in the dermatome, the distinction between a pathological and normal dermatome being readily identifiable (Figure 25.2);
3. Changed palpation resistance at the spinal process of the vertebra concerned, i.e. a certain elasticity, usually associated with tenderness on pressure.

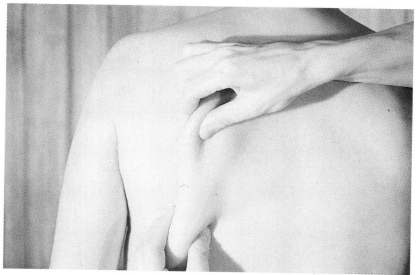

Figure 25.4 Palpatory metamere diagnosis of normal and pathological dermatomes

Palpatory metamere diagnosis is suitable particularly for the thoracolumbar region where the functional status of the individual metameres can be assessed within minutes and the vertebral level and intensity of the metameric dysfunction determined. The palpable signs of metameric dysfunction are identifiable as 'silent metameres' even at an early stage of development and often a long time before subjective symptoms occur[4]. The possibility of identifying dysfunction at a clinically latent stage through palpatory metamere diagnosis makes it extremely practical as a method of prophylactic early diagnosis.

RADIOLOGICAL METAMERE DIAGNOSIS IN THE CERVICAL REGION

Metameric dysfunctions of the type occurring in the thoracolumbar region can also be found in the cervical spine. In this instance, however, the topographic level and quantitative evaluation of the dysfunction are technically more difficult and less precise than in the thoracic region. For this reason, radiological function analysis of the cervical spine is an expedient method of differential metameric diagnosis[1,6]. It determines the intervertebral mobility, giving insight into the arthromuscular and hence metameric function. On the basis of the mobility impairment in the cervical spine, the level and severity of cervical metamere dysfunction can be determined with precision (Figure 25.5).

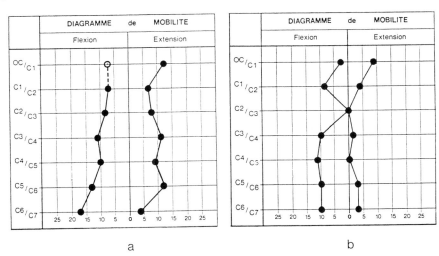

Figure 25.5 (a) Normal movement diagram (22-year-old male). (b) Movement diagram in a case of vertebro-basilar insufficiency (64-year-old female); severe multimetameric impairment of the extension movement of the cervical spine

METAMERE C1

Metamere C1 has a special significance for a number of reasons (Figure 25.6).

(1) As a result of the comparatively dense clustering, compared with the periphery, of receptors in the joints, muscles and ligaments of the craniocervical crossway[9,20,21], to which myelotome C1 corresponds as a projection and processing interface, this first metamere is of decisive importance as a coordinating and control organ. It modulates both the tonic control of the autochthonous muscles and the vegetative reflex activity of all peripheral metameres.

217

(2)   The superior cervical ganglion is anatomically and functionally dependent on metamere C1[16,17]. This ganglion is the source of a large number of adrenergic fibres that accompany the arterial trunks of the basilar and internal carotid systems as far as the arteriole and capillary region and the venous outflow[7,14,19]. Through the superior cervical ganglion, metamere C1 thus influences the entire cerebral vasomotor system.

(3)   Apart from the possibility of influence through the vasomotor control function of the superior cervical ganglion, there are also direct neural connections between the craniocervical receptor system and nuclear areas of the brain stem and reticular formation[11,13]. For their part, these structures are linked into a number of central nervous and peripheral function loops. In this way, metamere C1 becomes a higher-level key instance for the control of vital functions. Atlas therapy aims at intervening in this control. It is a form of metameric medicine that uses the atlas as the externally accessible point of attack, but has as its objective a 'remote-controlled' effect, through metamere C1, on both the peripheral metameres and the encephalic region.

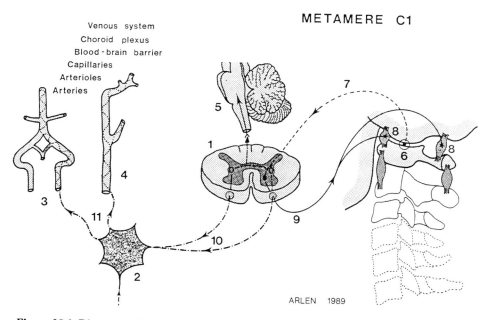

Figure 25.6 Diagrammatic representation of metamere C1. 1, myelotome C1; 2, superior cervical ganglion; 3, vertebro-basilar system; 4, carotid system; 5, brain-stem; 6, atlanto–occipital joint; 7, articular afferent pathway; 8, myotome C1; 9, motor efferents; 10, autonomic efferents; 11, postganglionic vasomotor fibres

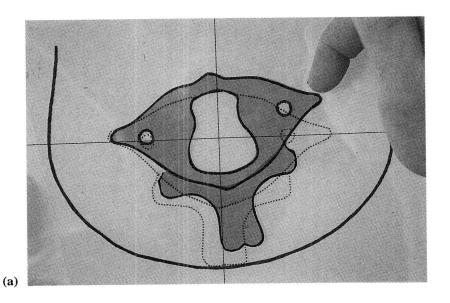

(a)

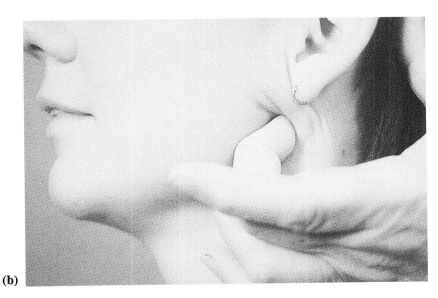

(b)

Figure 25.7 (a) Schematic representation of left anterior position of the atlas. (b) Thrust to the left transverse process of the atlas

ATLAS THERAPY

Atlas therapy consists of a sequence of thrusts applied with the middle finger to the transverse process of the atlas. The thrusts are directed and must come from the direction of the positional asymmetry of the atlas[5] (Figure 25.7).

Positional asymmetry or variance of the atlas is to be understood as the deviation from the symmetrical position of the atlas with respect to the occiput, without any rotation or lateralization. A 'normal' atlas position of this type is extremely rare, however, and asymmetry more or less the rule. It is highly likely that positional variance of the atlas is determined by genetically preformed motor patterns in the suboccipital muscles. It already exists in small children and remains throughout the subject's life. It is not to be confused with 'incorrect positioning' or a functional impairment of the atlanto-occipital joints. Impairments of these joints can occur simultaneously but without any relation to the positional variance.

An absolute prerequisite for atlas therapy is the determination of this asymmetry through precise palpatory and radiological diagnosis, as the direction of thrust depends on the position of the atlas. It should be pointed out, however, that the asymmetry serves merely as an indicator for the direction of the thrusts and is not in any way 'corrected' by atlas therapy. Nor is this therapy aimed primarily at correcting occipital joint disorders.

The position of the atlas is diagnosed by three-dimensional palpation to locate the site on both sides of the transverse processes within the triangle formed by the posterior edge of the ascending mandibular branch and the anterior edge of the mastoid process. The transverse processes can be palpated there as small, spherical structures. Their location within the triangle varies in accordance with the positional asymmetry of the atlas[5].

It is essential to combine palpatory and radiological localization to prevent deviations in the shape of the transverse processes from giving a false picture of the atlas position, which could have serious consequences in treatment.

Before the start of any atlas therapy, a pathological metamere is located through palpatory diagnosis in the thoracic region. Such metameres are identifiable through paravertebral hypertonus in the myotome and increased tension in the dermatome, together with 'spring-like' resistance and tenderness on palpation of the spinous process. This metamere is used as a reference and must be palpated again after each thrust, since a regression in the myotome and dermatome hypertonus should be palpable after every thrust of the correct dose and direction. This control of the peripheral metamere is mandatory. It confirms the correctness of the thrust direction and allows the intensity and number of thrusts per session to be adapted appropriately to each individual case. In the first atlas therapy session, a test thrust of low intensity is applied with subsequent peripheral metamere diagnosis to determine the tolerable thrust intensity for the patient in question.

Atlas therapy is administered with the patient seated and his/her head in a normal position at rest. Neither pretensioning nor immobilization are necessary. The therapy is not in the form of a single 'stroke' but rather a progressive series of thrusts with the peripheral metamere reaction being checked after each thrust.

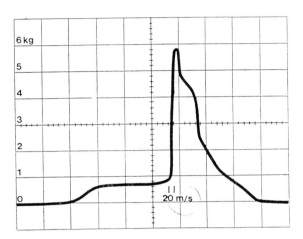

Figure 25.8 Graph of the thrust in atlas therapy

The success of atlas therapy depends on the thrust quality. It is essential that the thrusts are applied consistently from the direction of asymmetry of the atlas. They must be performed directly from the bony contact with the transverse process, without a 'run-up', and must be executed with an extremely rapid, dry and energetic but measured action (ca. 3–6 kg in 20 ms) (Figure 25.8).

A good deal of practice is generally required before the optimal thrust quality is achieved. The atlas therapist must develop and train his/her own motor processes to such an extent that he/she is in a position to administer each thrust precisely in the desired direction with extreme rapidity and in the required dosage without handedness-related weakness or habitual muscle patterns being noticeable. The atlas therapy technique is also relatively difficult to learn, and to facilitate the initial learning phase the Munster school of the SMIMM uses a simulator with visual control on a monitor, by which the speed and dosage of the thrust can be trained. Once a good thrust technique has been acquired, considerable experience is still required, however, to estimate correctly the thrust sequence and intensity and the treatment frequency.

The disadvantages of this difficult technique are far outweighed, however, by the advantages:

(1)   The indicated thrust intensity can be checked by means of a test thrust.

(2)   The effect of every thrust can be checked by means of peripheral metamere diagnosis.

(3)   Apart from structural changes or severe shape anomalies in the craniocervical transition, there are no contraindications, nor does hypermobility present any obstacle to atlas therapy.

(4)   In the case of an error in the positioning diagnosis, it is possible to attenuate the effect of a thrust from the wrong direction by providing a thrust from the opposite direction. (The error should not be played down, however, nor should the positioning diagnosis be made negligently or thrust technique deficiencies made light of as a result.)

(5)   Atlas therapy is an extremely low-risk form of treatment, if administered properly by a practitioner with sufficient experience.

POSSIBLE EFFECT MECHANISMS OF ATLAS THERAPY (Figure 25.9)

The way in which atlas therapy works involves a number of questions: What happens when the thrust is administered? Which paths convey the thrust effects centrally and into the peripheral metamere? Why is the optimal effect achieved when the thrust is applied from the direction of the positional asymmetry?

No satisfactory answer to these questions has been provided to date. It is not possible to determine with accuracy whether the thrust triggers stimuli, blocks afferent activity or both. One hypothesis is that the thrust interferes with the neuron switching programmes of the craniocervical receptor field.

The results of atlas therapy show at all events that it has an effect both peripherally on the reflex activity of all distal metameres and also centrally on the control processes in the encephalic region[3].

1. Peripheral, 'remote-controlled' action on cervical, thoracic and lumbosacral metameres

The most striking effect is to be noted in the autochthonous trunk muscles; during an atlas therapy session, hypertonus gradually regresses[4]. It might be supposed to be a result of this that the control of the tonic muscular system and arthromuscular function play a dominant role in the effect mechanisms in question. Atlas therapy appears to have a decisive influence on the spinal arthromuscular control loops and hence to affect both the metameric function units at all levels and the statics of the spinal column.

Not only can the reduction in tonus in the myotomes be palpated, it can also be measured objectively by electromyography[4] and, in an indirect way, by quantitative radiological investigation of cervical dynamics[1,6] (Figure 25.10).

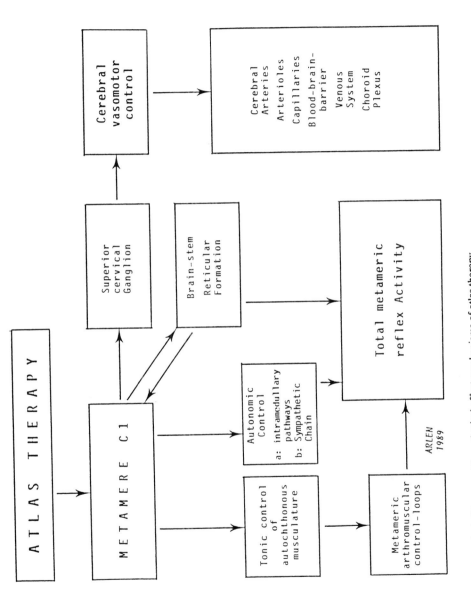

Figure 25.9 Diagram of hypothetical effect mechanisms of atlas therapy

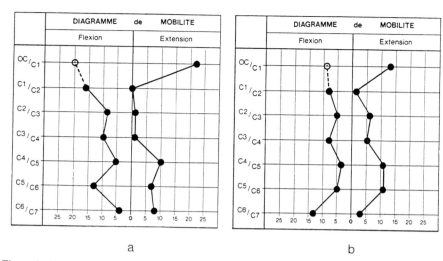

Figure 25.10 Movement diagrams in a case of post-traumatic Barré-Liéou syndrdome (31-year-old male): (a) before atlas therapy; (b) after atlas therapy

Atlas therapy impinges upon the dermatome with delayed effect, compared with the muscle reaction, and results in a reduction of the sympathetic tone. It shows that the thrust affects both motor and autonomic efferents and changes the function of the metamere as a whole. Dermatome changes following atlas therapy are palpable but can also be demonstrated sonographically in the form of a reduction of density[4].

The thrust effect could be transferred to the peripheral metameres via the associative intermetameric paths of the funiculus posterior system[8,10]. Other possible transmitters are the non-specific descending reticulospinal fibre system in the anterior funiculus lateralis, which connects with control loops at all metameric levels[15], or the periependymal system[8]. Some of the information might also be transferred by the sympathetic trunks.

2. Effect of atlas therapy on suprametameric centres

The special status of metamere C1 has already been discussed. The fact that the superior cervical ganglion is an integral component of the neurotome C1[16] gives good cause to suppose that the effect of atlas therapy on the CNS is transmitted as a result of the vasomotor control function of this ganglion. The extreme complexity of cerebrovascular control mechanisms and the fleeting nature of vasomotor phenomena have meant that indications of the efficiency of atlas therapy have been limited to the clinical observation that these thrusts can improve coordination and enhance vigilance[3]. Even these improvements could be conceivably interpreted as suggestive effects if it were not possible to demonstrate the parallel change in the peripheral metamere.

Recent animal experiments give support to the postulated effect of atlas therapy on the cerebral vasomotor system. Tests on the superior cervical ganglion in animals have shown that the adrenergic fibres coming from this ganglion interfere in the vasomotor modulation of the brain in the region of the major arterial trunks and the arteriolar and capillary system, choroid plexus and venous system. In this way the permeability of the blood–brain barrier is also affected by the superior cervical ganglion. Trigger and blocking tests showed that a complex interplay of vasoconstriction and vasodilatation occurs at all levels of the cerebrovascular system, designed to hold constant the flow volume and the intracranial pressure under changing conditions[7].

The influence of atlas therapy on this phenomenon has now been demonstrated with the aid of transcranial Doppler ultrasonography, which showed changes in the basilar and internal carotid flow. This study is not yet complete and initial results will be described in a forthcoming paper.

INDICATIONS FOR ATLAS THERAPY

In view of the global effect of metamere C1 on central and peripheral control functions, atlas therapy covers an extremely large indication spectrum. While the 'remote-control effect' enables it to be used for metameric dysfunction of the cervical, thoracic and lumbosacral regions, atlas therapy can also be applied to peripheral pain syndromes at all levels, multimetamere dysfunction syndromes and dystrophic conditions, as well as organic dysfunction at all metameric levels and peripheral circulation problems.

Atlas therapy also offers new possibilities for treatment of cerebrovascular syndromes and neurological systemic disease with vascular involvement. These contraindications to classical manual therapy are amongst its most gratifying and interesting areas of application and increase its significance in both geriatric care and paediatric development problems.

A more detailed discussion of the indications for atlas therapy will not be provided here since other contributions to this volume delivered by practitioners of the therapy will deal with indications and initial therapy results.

REFERENCES

1. Arlen, A. (1979). Biometrische Röntgen-Funktionsdiagnostik der Halswirbelsäule; ihr Aussagewert im zerviko-brachialen und zerviko-zephalen Syndrom. In *Schriftenreihe Manuelle Medizin*, Vol.5. (Heidelberg: Fischer-Verlag)
2. Arlen, A. (1980). Mastodynie, pathologie métamérique et statique rachidienne. *Sénologia*, 5(3), 230–236
3. Arlen, A. *et al.* (1985). Reversible Veränderungen der Hirnstamm-Potentiale nach manipulativer Atlastherapie bei zerviko-enzphalen Syndromen; erste Ergebnisse. In Hohmann,

D., Kügelgen, B. and Liebig, K. (eds.) *Neuroorthopädie 3, Brustwirbelsäulenerkrankungen, Engpass-syndrome, Chemonukleolyse, evozierte Potential.* (Berlin: Springer-Verlag)

4. Arlen, A. (1985). Zur Aetio-pathogenese der thorakalen Schmerzsyndrome. In Hohmann, D., Kügelgen, B. and Liebig, K. (eds.) *Neuroorthopädie 3, Brustwirbelsäulenerkrankungen, Engpass-syndrome, Chemonukleolyse, evozierte Potential.* (Berlin: Springer-Verlag)

5. Arlen, A. (1985). Leitfaden zur Atlastherapie. Ass. rech. méd. prév. santé, F-Munster

6. Arlen, A. (1988). Aussagen der Röntgenfunktionsanalyse zu posttraumatischen Funktions-störungen der oberen HWS. In Wolff, H.-D. (ed.) *Die Sonderstellung des Kopfgelenkbereichs. Grundlagen, Klinik, Begutachtung.* (Berlin: Springer-Verlag)

7. Baumbach, G., Busija, D., Werber, A. and Heistad, D. (1984). Role of autonomic innervation in modification of cerebral vascular responses. In MacKenzie, E.T., Seylaz, J. and Bes, A. (eds.) *Neurotransmitters and the Cerebral Circulation*, LERS Monograph Series Vol.2 (New York: Raven Press)

8. Clara, M. (1959). *Das Nervensystem des Menschen.* (Leipzig: Joh Amb Barth)

9. Cooper, S. (1966b). The small motor nerves to muscle spindles and to extrinsic eye muscles. *J. Physiol.*, **186**, 28–29

10. Delmas, J. and Delmas, A. (1962). *Voies et centres nerveux.* (Paris: Masson)

11. Fredrickson, J.M., Schwarz, D. and Kornhuber, H.H. (1966). Convergence and interaction of vestibular and deep somatic afferents upon neurons in the vestibular nuclei of the cat. *Acta Otolaryngol. Stockholm*, **61**, 168–188

12. Hansen, K. and Schliak, H. (1962). *Segmentale Innervation.* (Stuttgart: Thieme)

13. Hülse, M. (1983). Die zervikalen Gleichgewichtsstörungen. (Berlin: Springer-Verlag)

14. Kahrström, J., Hardebo, J.E., Nordborg, C. and Owman, C. (1986). Experiments on cerebro-vascular nerve plasticity and trophic vascular adaption in young and adult rats. In Owman, C. and Hardebo, C.E. (eds.) *Neural Regulation of Brain Circulation.* (Amsterdam: Elsevier)

15. Lang, J. (1985). Anatomie der BWS und des benachbarten Nervensystems. In Hohmann, D., Kügelgen, B. and Liebig, K. (eds.) *Neuroorthopädie 3, Brustwirbelsäulenerkrankungen, Engpass-syndrome, Chemonukleolyse, evozierte Potential.* (Berlin: Springer-Verlag)

16. Lazorthes, G. (1961). *Vascularisation et circulation cérébrales.* (Paris: Masson)

17. Lazorthes, G., Gouazé, A. and Salamon, G. (1976). *Vascularisation et circulation de l'encéphale*, Vol. 1. (Paris: Masson)

18. Netter, F.H. (1962). *Nervous System.* The CIBA Collection of Medical Illustrations, Vol. 1. (CIBA)

19. Owman, C., Andersson, J., Starko, J. and Hardebo, J.E. (1984). Neuro-transmitter amines and peptides in the cerebrovascular bed. In Mackenzie, E.T., Seylaz, J. and Bes, A. (eds.) *Neurotransmitters and the Cerebral Circulation.* LERS Monograph Series, Vol.2. (New York: Raven Press)

20. Voss, H. (1958). Zahl und Anordnung der Muskelspindeln in den unteren Zungenbeinmuskeln, dem M. sternocleidomastoideus und den Bauch- und tiefen Nackenmuskeln. *Anat. Anz*, **105**, 265–275

21. Voss, H. (1963). Untersuchungen über die absolute und relative Zahl der Muskelspindeln in weiteren Muskelgruppen (Mm. Scaleni und Rückenmuskeln) des Menschen. *Anat. Anz.*, **112**, 276–279

25

The method of autotraction in manual medicine

Guido BRUGNONI and Corrado LEUCI

The method of autotraction for the treatment of lumbago-sciatica has been elaborated at the Karolinska Hospital of Stockholm by Gertrud Lind. After her death, the method has been further improved and developed by Natchev from Stockholm, himself a pupil of Doctor Lind.

This method can be considered the perfecting and development of the realization that patients with back pain can be improved by suspension holding on to a bar. In our case this takes place on an appropriate table. There are three important elements:

(1)   The patient can lie on the bed, supine, supine with hip and knee at 90° of flexion, prone, or on the right or left side, depending upon which of these positions is least painful.

(2)   The traction is conducted in varying steps of inclination on a horizontal plane or even against gravity.

(3)   In particular, traction may be conducted while the patient pulls himself up; the moving parts of the bed allow specific movements modifying the vertebral posture.

PERFORMANCE OF THE TABLE

The bed has at its extremes two systems of bars on which the patient can pull with his arms and push with his feet. The patient is strapped by two belts, thoracic and lumbar, but there is no system of mechanical traction except for gravity.

The bed plane is divided into two parts that can move upwards and downwards. The cranial plane is able to rotate on its longitudinal axis. The entire plane of the bed can be tilted until it reaches a vertical position, this causing, if required, a gravity traction.

The purpose of these movements is to adapt the shape of the table to the pain-free position or, better, to the patient's back to attain a completely pain-free position on the bed, which is essential for starting the treatment. This position must be taken from one of the five possible positions, using varying degrees of inclination and plane rotation.

Treatment then begins, consisting of the movement of the two parts of the bed towards the apposite position, passing through the position 0° simultaneously with the patient's pulling with his arms and pushing with his legs on the bars against the resistance created by the abdominal belts. If after one of the bed movements the patient feels pain, it can be relieved by a contrary movement.

After the session, the bed is gradually tilted while the patient walks 'on the spot' on a platform, thus realizing a real 'gradual loading'.

Generally, after 4–6 sessions the patient shows an improvement resulting in the total absence of the original positions and feels no more pain.

A CASE REPORT

We have treated in the course of 1987, 68 cases of lumbar pain or pain of lumbar origin. Of these, 35 were men of average age 47 and 33 were women of average age 45.

Diagnosis

Sciatica by disc hernia ascertained by CT-scan	20
Pseudo-radicular sciatica with negative or without CT-scan	18
Acute lumbago	8
Chronic lumbago	10
Secondary spinal stenosis	5
Post-operative pain resulting from the operation for disc hernia	5
Double root	1
Posterior osteophytes pressing root 5L	1

We have classified the results as follows:

Good (recovery without further pain)	24 cases (35%)
Improved (net improvement with persistence of some symptoms)	23 cases (35%)
Unchanged (none or insignificant improvements)	11 cases (15%)
Non-treatable (forced to interrupt after 1–3 sessions)	10 cases (15%)

In no case did aggravation occur, and in only two cases was there re-occurrence of the pain lasting less than 20 days.

Follow up. After 4 months the results of the 58 patients treated proved stable; of the 23 cases belonging to the 'improved' classification, 7 continued to improve after a further treatment of vertebral manipulation and 3 showed spontaneous improvement; 2 patients had slightly worsened. Overall, therefore,

Good or improved 70%
Unchanged 30%

PRELIMINARY CONSIDERATIONS REGARDING THE METHOD

The method uses only painless positions and movements according to the 'no pain rule' of Maigne. If pain occurs during the course of a movement, it is possible to banish it by the reverse movement. The method is therefore especially suitable in acute forms, provided that the indications and contra-indications are respected as regards not only inflammatory and neoplastic illnesses but also pregnancy, some abdominal disturbances, heart disease, sequestrated disc hernia, syndrome of 'cauda equina' or bladder paresis, and bilateral sciatica due to serious neurological disturbances.

Main indications:
(a) Sciatica, acute, radicular or due to referred pain;
(b) Acute lumbago with or without postural scoliosis;
(c) Post-operative pain after an operation on discal lumbar hernia;
(d) Spinal stenosis, which, even if not a contra-indication, requires techniques with less effective results.

These are obviously cases in which the use of vertebral manipulation is more difficult and risky.

In chronic cases, especially those concerning lumbago alone, the method even if equally successful, requires numerous and long sessions. We believe that manipulation is by far more effective and rapid in these cases. It is therefore possible to use both methods; for example, in acute and subacute cases autotraction can be begun and, once an improvement has been achieved either in the pain or in the muscle spasm, it is advisable to proceed with manipulative treatment for better results.

Mechanism of action

As when considering vertebral manipulation, we are in the field of hypothesis, but we can consider various possible actions.

(a) Mechanical: modification of the behaviour between the disc and the posterior articulations and the root. Modification of the distribution of the loading inside the disc.

(b)   Reflex: on the muscle, relaxing, modification of the patterns and therefore of the balance of agonist and antagonist.

(c)   Circulatory: improvement of the inflammatory or congestive phenomena.

(d)   Action upon the 'gate control system'.

CONCLUSIONS

Autotraction often permits successful treatment, always without risk and in a short period of time, of the acute cases that are the most difficult to treat with manipulation.

By this method, prolonged bed-rest and the use of corsets and drugs are no longer necessary. It is very useful to use it in association with manipulative treatment, which often becomes possible after the first session of autotraction.

In our opinion, autotraction – which is still little studied and little known – may, if submitted to further experiment, produce even better results and integrate itself well in the therapeutic field of our specialization.

FURTHER READING

Maigne, R. (1974). *Douleurs d'Origine Vertebrale*. (Paris: L'Expansion)
Natchev, E. (1984). *A Manual on Auto-traction Treatment for Low Back Pain*. (Stockholm: Tryckeribolaget i Sundsvall)

27

The space truss as a model for cervical spine mechanics – a systems science concept

S.M. LEVIN

Modern-day bioengineers feel they know well how to deal with structures that are complex, like biological tissues. They break the complex structure down into simple elements, such as beams and columns. They analyse the behaviour of each element, and put all those behaviours together to see how the total structure will behave. Their present paradigm is that the musculoskeletal system is analogous to the framework of a modern high-rise building[12].

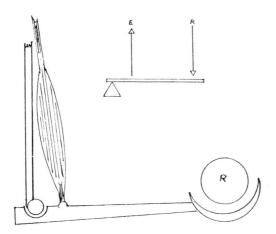

Figure 27.1 The arm as a lever

For a biological skeleton to be analogous to a skyscraper frame, the skeleton would have to be rigid-hinged, gravity-dependent, unidirectional, immobile, local loading and linear in its response to stresses. Biological structures are flexible-hinged, independent of gravity, omnidirectional, mobile, load-dispersing and non-linear in response to stress. Biological beams and columns are articulated, with essentially frictionless hinges. The stability of an articulated column is precarious at best and to be able to convert that column almost instantly to an articulated horizontal beam, as one would do to the spine in bending over, would be a nightmare of mechanical design.

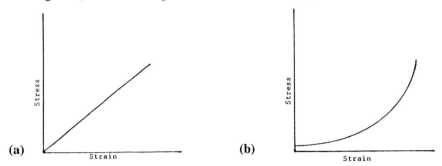

Figure 27.2 Linear (a) and non-linear (b) curves

Give a bioengineer the problem of calculating the force generated by the biceps muscle when loaded with a weight in the hand and he constructs a free-body diagram, with the forearm a simple lever and the elbow as a one-degree-of-freedom hinge (Figure 27.1). This is a standard reductionistic approach to biomechanics and completely ignores that fact that what happens at the elbow (or any other joint) has macro and micro consequences that affect the whole body which, in turn, affect the forces generated at the biceps muscle. Putting and keeping the elbow joint at a point in space is in itself an engineering feat that requires some stabilizing forces of several muscles to be active continuously in a feedback loop. The biceps is a two-joint muscle and as it contracts it creates a moment not only at the elbow but at the shoulder joint, which in order to be stabilized would need contraction of the triceps (amongst others), which would, in turn, create moments around the elbow which would require compensatory contractions of the biceps (amongst others), which would then feed back into the loop. Intertwining feedback loops with a complex interdependent system are readily apparent. Rather than a simple linear equation of static mechanics that can be expressed as a straight line on a graph, the equation of the forces at the elbow must be able to express a dynamic situation in a constant state of flux with nonlinear relationships that are not strictly proportional and cannot be graphically depicted as a straight line (Figure 27.2). The problems of three bodies acting on each other in space have not yet been solved with Newtonian mechanics and classical biomechanics has not been up to the task of simultaneously handling over two hundred bones and thousands of muscles. We have been presented with apparent solutions to local problems with little understanding of the underlying biomechanical design. Simple systems such as levers often result in complex behaviour. The forces needed to stabilize a multiple-hinged, rigid linked system, as the body would be in presently conceived linear, lever models, are bone breaking, muscle tearing, and energy exhausting.

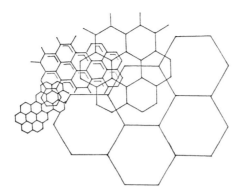

Figure 27.3 A hierarchy of hexagons

Systems science is a discipline that seeks solutions to problems in a more global, holistic, and deductive approach. All subsystems must be approached as part of a metasystem, a grand design. Like reflections in a room of mirrors, or hexagonal patterns on a tile floor (in which each tile is a hexagon unto itself, but at the same time is part and parcel of several other hexagonal patterns (Figure 27.3), natural systems are recursive and hierarchical, independent, and interdependent. Removing one mirror from the room or changing one tile on the floor changes everything and changes nothing. The new science of non-linear dynamic systems, 'chaos'[3,7], provides us with some mathematical tools in systems science and may provide further insights into the structure of biological systems. Dynamic non-linear systems are self-generating, with order arising spontaneously in those systems. There is self-similarity, or symmetry across scale, so that at any level of magnification or scale the structure is similar. As in the hexagonal tiled floor, there is recursion with pattern inside pattern. These complex systems may exhibit simple behaviour with rhythmic, self-regulating patterns. Systems science theory seems ideal for modelling complex biological structures that must be hierarchical in their complexity and consistent with evolutionary theories. After all, there must be some link in the mechanics of complex structures such as cervical spines of vertebrates, as well as form, if Darwinian theories are to be believed[11].

Present concepts of cervical spine mechanics of humans are based on a theory of a column or post supporting a load[9] (the post-and-lintel design of architecture) stablized by muscles and ligaments as 'guy wires'. Once the centre of gravity of the head falls outside the base of the post, the post becomes an articulated beam or complex cantilever, so that the simple act of head nodding or leaning over a desk significantly alters the mechanics. The proposed traditional mechanics of the cervical spine of cattle and other hoofed animals (ungulates) is based on a complex cantilever system, requiring a very tall spinous process of the first thoracic vertebra to act as a mast[1]. A unidirectional system like the mast must always be perpendicular to gravity forces. Since the T1 spine, as it exists in a giraffe, would be too short, the principle does not apply to all ungulates. Birds must have still another system that must allow for long, slender very flexible, articulated shafts, as many as twenty-six vertebrae long. These shafts would have to be rigid and strong at one moment in time, highly flexible the next, omnidirectional and supported by minimal muscle mass. Just about an impossible task in the lever system. The column–beam–lever system of classical Newtonian mechanics does not play well in the arena of flora, fauna and evolution.

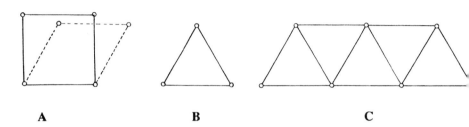

A   **B**   **C**

Figure 27.4 A – square frame; unstable with flexible hinges. B – simple truss; stable with flexible hinges. C – single plane truss system

D'Arcy Thompson, in his classic book, *On Growth and Form*[15], suggests that trusses (Figure 27.4) can be analogous models for structural support in vertebrates. Trusses have clear advantages over post-and-lintel construction as a structural support system for biological tissue. They have flexible, even frictionless hinges, with no coupled moments about the joint and the support elements are in tension and compression only with no bending moments. Loads applied at any point are distributed about the truss, as tension or compression rather than local loading as levers, as in column-and-beam construction. There are no levers in a truss. A truss, being fully triangulated, is inherently stable and cannot be deformed without producing large deformations of individual members. Since only trusses are inherently stable with freely moving hinges, it follows that any structure that has freely moving hinges and that is inherently structurally stable must be a truss. Vertebrates, meeting those criteria, must therefore be constructed as trusses. The tension elements of the body (the soft tissues – fascia, muscles, ligaments and connective tissue) have largely been ignored as constructional members of the body frame and have been viewed only as the motors. In loading a truss the elements that are in tension can be replaced by flexible materials, such as ropes, wires or in vertebrate systems, ligaments, muscles and fascia. The 'tone' alone of live muscle and fascia may be enough to sustain the low-energy triangle.

In developing a space truss metasystem model for the cervical spine we must conform to the natural laws of least energy, laws of mechanics and the peculiarities of biological tissue. Any non-conformity with any of these would make the model invalid. In the modular, hierarchical, finite-element analysis of a three-dimensional 'space' truss the finite element must be a three-dimensional 'space' truss and not a cube as it is in present lever models. The basic element of a single plane truss is a triangle. The basic element of a space truss must be a tetrahedron with four fully triangulated sides, an octahedron with eight fully triangulated sides, or an icosahedron with 20 fully triangulated sides. There are no other fully triangulated regular three-dimensional structures (polyhedra) (Figure 27.5). Buckminster Fuller[2] states that all naturally occurring structures must be composed of these polyhedra.

Because of its ability to fill space and form self-organizing systems with stable carbon molecules[5], the icosahedron seems to be the space truss most suitable for biological structures. Since, for biological structures, a truss must be omnidirectional, both in form and stress-resisting pattern, the tension icosahedron, first conceived by Kenneth Snelson[13,14], with the outer shell composed of tension elements separated by compression elements suspended within the tension network, appears to be the most suitable if not the only suitable structure (Figure 27.5d). As biological structures, icosahedron trusses are omnidirectional and once constructed, tension elements are always loaded in tension and compression elements are always loaded in compression, no matter what point of application or direction of load. As are biological structures, icosahedra are stable even with frictionless hinges and at the same time can easily be altered in shape or stiffness merely by shortening or lengthening one or several tension elements (in biological systems, the muscles). The icosahedron can be linked in an infinite variety of sizes or shapes in a modular or hierarchical pattern[13] with the tension elements, the muscles, ligaments, and fascia, forming a continuous interconnecting network and with the compression elements, the bones, suspended within the network. The structure will always maintain the characteristics of a single icosahedron so that a shaft, such as a cervical spine, may be built that is omnidirectional and can function equally well in tension or compression with the internal stresses always distributed in tension or compression with no bending moments and therefore, lowest energy costs.

A unique property of a tension icosahedron, as a structure, is that it has a 'J'-shaped, non-linear, stress–strain curve when loaded (Figure 27.2), so that as a structure the icosahedron seems to be a non-linear dynamic system unto itself. This property is not demonstrated in mechanical systems such as the column-and-beam construction or lever construction when using cubic or any other polyhedral shapes. J-shaped, non-linear, stress–strain curves seems to be the *sine qua non* of biological tissue[4,8]. This property has been demonstrated in bone, muscle, disc, fascia, nerve, composite biological structures, and just about any other biological tissue studied[8,16]. It seems sensible to use a structure that has analogous mechanical properties to biological tissue when one is doing biological modelling.

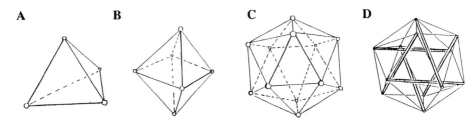

Figure 27.5 Three-dimensional trusses. A – Tetrahedron; 4 faces. B – Octahedron; 8 faces. C – Icosahedron; 20 faces. D – Tensioned icosahedron; compressive elements suspended in a tension network

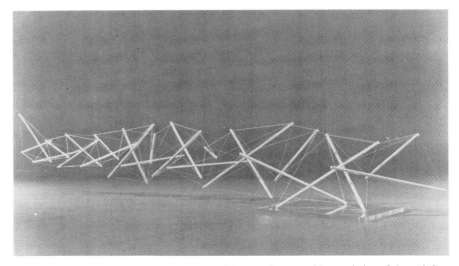

Figure 27.6 Model for Easy K 10" × 58" × 10" (Kenneth Snelson with permission of the artist)

Viewed as a model for the cervical spine of man or any invertebrate species, the tension icosahedron space truss (Figures 27.6 and 27.7), with the bones acting as the compressive elements and the soft tissues as the tension elements, even with multiple joints, will be stable in any position, vertical or horizontal, any configuration from ramrod straight to sigmoid curve, or any position or configuration in between. At the same time, it will be highly mobile, omni-directional, and low in energy consumption. It is a unique structure in that when used as a biological model the constructs would conform to the natural laws of least energy, laws of mechanics, and the peculiarities of biological tissues. The icosahedral space truss has been shown to be present in biological structures at the cellular, subcellular and multicellular levels[6]. In the cervical spine, each subsystem (the vertebra, the disc, the soft tissues), would be subsystems of the

236

cervical spine metasystem. Each would function as an icosahedron independently and as part of the larger system, as in the hexagonal tile analogy.

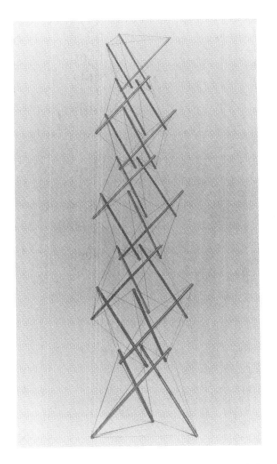

Figure 27.7 E – C Column 41' × 11' × 9'6" (Kenneth Snelson with permission of the artist)

The icosahedral space truss cervical spine model is a universal modular hierarchical system that has the widest application with the least energy cost. As the simplest and least energy-consuming system, it becomes the metasystem against which all other systems and subsystems must be judged and if they are not simpler, more adaptable, and less energy-consuming, rejected. Since this system always works with the least energy requirements, there would be no benefit to nature for cervical spines to function sometimes as a column, sometimes as a beam, sometimes as a truss, or to function differently for different species conforming to the minimal inventory–maximum diversity concept[10] and evolutionary theory[11].

The icosahedral space truss model could be extended to incorporate other anatomical and physiological systems. For example, as a 'pump' the icosahedron functions remarkably like cardiac and respiratory models, which themselves have been shown to be non-linear dynamic systems, and so may be an even more fundamental metasystem for biological modelling. As suggested by Kroto[5] the icosahedral template is 'mysterious, ubiquitous and all powerful'.

REFERENCES

1. Fielding, W.J., Burstein, A.H. and Frankel, V.H. (1976). The nuchal ligament. *Spine*, 1(1), 3–14
2. Fuller, R.B. (1975). *Synergetics*, pp. 314–431. (New York: McMillan Publishing Co.)
3. Gleick, J. (1988). *Chaos*. (New York: Penguin)
4. Gordon, J.E. (1988). *The Science of Structures and Materials*, pp. 137–157. (New York: W.H. Freeman)
5. Kroto, H. (1988). Space, stars, C and soot. *Science*, **242**, 1139–1145
6. Levin, S.H. (1986). The icosahedron as the three-dimensional finite element in biomechanical support. *Proceedings of the Society of General Systems Research Symposium on Mental Images, Values and Reality Philadelphia, PA, May 1986, St Louis*, Society of General Systems Research, 1986, pp. G14–G26
7. Mandelbrot, B. (1983). *The Fractal Geometry of Nature*. (San Francisco: Wm. Freeman)
8. McHelhaney, J.H. and Edward, B.F. (1965). Dynamic response of biologic materials. *Am. Soc. Mech. Engin.*, 65–WA–HUF-9
9. Nolan, J.P. and Sherk, H.H. (1988). Biomechanical evaluation of the extensor musculature of the cervical spine. *Spine*, 13(1), 9–11
10. Pearce, P. (1978). *Structure in Nature as a Strategy for Design.*, pp. xii–xvii. (Cambridge, Mass.: MIT Press)
11. Roth, J. and LeRoith, D. (1987). Chemical crosstalk. The Sciences. The New York Academy of Science, May/June 1987, pp. 51–54
12. Schultz, A.B. (1982). Biomechanics of the spine. *Proceedings of the Back Pain Association, London, October 1982*
13. Schultz, D.G. and Fox, H.N. (1981). *Kenneth Snelson*. (Buffalo: Albright-Knox Art Gallery)
14. Snelson, K. (1965). Discontinuous compression structures. US Patent #3169611, February 1965
15. Thompson, D. (1965). *On Growth and Form*. (London: Cambridge University Press)
16. White, A.A. and Panjabi, M.M. (1978). *Clinical Biomechanics of the Spine*, pp. 1–57. (Philadelphia, PA.: J.B. Lippincott)

28

Anamnesis as diagnostic tool in musculoskeletal medicine

Kaj REKOLA

The easiest way of all to reach a diagnosis is to ask the patient what is wrong with him and translate the answer into Latin. This gives us what we usually understand as a diagnosis, a symptomatic diagnosis such as lumbago or *syndroma cervicocranalis*. If we then ask him what he thinks has caused this complaint, the answer will lead us to an aetiological diagnosis. If no answer is forthcoming, we can add to the symptomatic diagnosis an epithet such as *cryptogenetica*, *idiopathica* or *essentialis*.

WHAT IS A DIAGNOSIS?

According to the *Oxford Advanced Learner's Dictionary*, diagnosis means determination of the nature of a disease by examining the symptoms[8]. One characteristic of musculoskeletal medicine is that symptoms can occur intermittently throughout the patient's life or in episodes of short or long duration, varying from a few days to a matter of years. In the case of back pains one might refer to the 'three-joint complex' model[16] proposed by Wedge (1983) to explain the natural course of degenerative back complaints. Acute musculoskeletal pain will usually originate from some acute damage or inflammation in the tissues, while chronic pain, frequently connected with straining, may be explained in terms of dysfunction, so that any change to acute symptoms may be attributed to inflammation or nerve structure compression.

The nature and pathophysiology of musculoskeletal pain and dysfunction is often highly complex. A functioning musculoskeletal apparatus needs an intact hierarchy of normal functions in the central nervous system, the peripheral nerves and the physiological joints, consisting of active and passive joint structures[5]. In addition, the physical and psychological environment in which the musculoskeletal apparatus is required to function inside the human being is of great importance. The external physical load on this musculoskeletal apparatus may be too great, or the patient's psychological or social circumstances may contribute to the common symptoms of pain and dysfunction. Research suggests

239

that the prognosis for most common musculoskeletal diseases is good, so that Andersson et al.[1], for instance, state that only 55% of patients with acute back conditions are on sick leave for longer than 10 days, and no more than 20% for longer than a month.

PAIN MECHANISMS

At the acute stage the nociceptors are activated and give rise to the clinical nociceptive reflex findings easily recognizable in clinical examinations – local tenderness, pain and restrictions on movement, muscle spasms – and general and segmental findings arising from activation of the autonomic nervous system. In the case of subacute or chronic pain the acute nociceptive reflex undergoes adaptation, and there are few clinical findings, at least in conventional orthopaedic examinations. As Vällfors notes in her thesis, conventional clinical findings are absent in as many as 70% of patients with chronic back pain[16].

DIAGNOSTIC TECHNIQUES

What techniques are available, then, for reaching a musculoskeletal diagnosis? How reliable and reproducible are they? And how cost-effective as far as the patient is concerned? In other words, what is their predictive value with regard to the correct diagnosis and the prognosis for the patient, and are the resources devoted to them and the possible risks involved, e.g. the radiation risk, justified in terms of the fundamental purpose of the diagnosis, which is to help the patient to regain a healthy state?

The traditional methods employed for obtaining a musculoskeletal diagnosis involve a clinical interview and physical examination, together with radiological examinations to the extent that failure to use these could be regarded as an error of judgement. But what scientific proof exists of the appropriateness of such diagnostic practices?

Many research reports and reviews in the medical literature have shown that little proof exists, and indeed doubts have been cast on the whole validity of routine, non-specific radiological examinations, the results of which have been shown to correlate chiefly with the age of the patient. Radiological examinations could evidently be reduced to a mere fraction of their present number by employing them only for the verification or exclusion of working hypotheses based on clinical tests[4].

According to the Quebec Task Force report, only anamnesis, i.e. a clinical/medical history, and physical examination could be shown to be of use in cases of acute or chronic back pain (admittedly in non-randomized, controlled experiments[6]). It may be mentioned for comparison purposes that the same report claims that computed tomography could be shown to provide additional prognostic information (in a randomized clinical experimental framework) only for the diagnosis of spinal stenosis.

There are also some reports that cast doubts on the reliability and reproducibility of findings made in physical examinations[17].

WHAT DO WE NEED A DIAGNOSIS FOR?

In the words of Sackett, 'the act of clinical diagnosis is an effort to recognize the class or group to which a patient's illness belongs, so that, based on our prior experience with that class, the subsequent clinical act we can afford to carry out and the patient is willing to follow, will maximise that patient's health'[14]. It is not always possible to state an exact diagnosis in musculoskeletal medicine, nor is such a statement necessarily needed. In acute situations, a *prognosis* is sufficient rather than the traditional diagnosis, i.e. an opinion on whether the state of the patient calls for immediate intervention (e.g. the *cauda equina* syndrome) or whether one can afford merely to keep an eye on the situation and wait for the condition to cure itself spontaneously. In the latter case it is possible to continue diagnostic procedures later or initiate treatment on an experimental basis.

DIAGNOSTIC STRATEGIES IN MUSCULOSKELETAL MEDICINE

Sackett, in his book *Clinical Epidemiology*[14], distinguishes the following diagnostic strategies:

(1)   *Pattern recognition* in which instantaneous identification of a previously learned picture or pattern of a disease gives the clue to the diagnosis. This strategy may be applicable to acute lumbago or scoliosis attributable to disc prolapse, but because of the complexity of the musculoskeletal system and the relative scarcity of typical clinical pictures, it can be utterly misleading. It may also result in bias in the subsequent diagnostic process. One only has to think of all the possible aetiologies for pain in the upper extremities, for instance, of which Mumenthaler's textbook[12] mentions about 100!

(2)   *Multiple branching, or arborization strategy* in which algorithms are employed. This is often quite useful for going through the hierarchy of the musculoskeletal apparatus in order to identify the lesion responsible for the symptoms and rule out other pathologies.

(3)   *The strategy of exhaustion* involves a painstaking search for all medical facts about the patient, followed by sifting through the data for a

diagnosis. This is typically used by novices, but as the pain may be generated in many tissues and organs, it can be used in a systematic manner even by the experienced specialists in manual medicine, especially when a differential diagnosis is needed.

(4) *Hypothetico-deductive strategy* sets out from the earlier clues regarding the patient, formulates a shortlist of potential diagnoses or actions, and then performs those clinical and paraclinical manoeuvres that will serve best to reduce this list. This is the most time-effective strategy when used by experts.

HISTORY-TAKING (CLINICAL INTERVIEW)

The purposes of a clinical interview are:

– To gather information on the patient and his disease;
– To create a therapeutic relationship;
– To try to comprehend the contributory factors in the patient's environment;
– To construct a list of the patient's problems;
– To develop a diagnostic and therapeutic strategy for solving these problems[7].

In this problem-centred approach the pain itself, or the dysfunction caused by pain or a functional disturbance, should be analysed separately in order to create a balanced overall view of the patient's problems.

AIDS TO ANAMNESIS

The information obtained from the interview should be exact and reproducible, and the descriptions of symptoms both qualitative and quantitative. Aids available for this include questionnaire forms, diagrams to assist in locating the site of pain, word lists for identifying the nature of the pain and visual analogue scales (VAS) for depicting its intensity[9,11,13].

The interview naturally begins with certain open questions, allowing the patient to speak freely of his problems. How far one can proceed by this means depends on the nature of the problem or disease, how acute it is and how verbally gifted the patient is. Sooner or later, however, attention must be turned to more specifically directed questions that follow in principle the normal anamnesis technique employed in medicine[2,3].

TRENDS IN SYMPTOMS

Evaluation of the temporal trend in the pain and/or functional disability experienced is a matter of considerable importance. If the situation seems to be improving, it may be advisable to adopt a 'wait and see' strategy, whereas a problem that is constantly becoming worse, and all the more so where the patient is able to express this both qualitatively and quantitatively, can justify more thorough-going diagnostic tests, especially if there are few actual clinical findings. Where a symptom has remained essentially unchanged for some time, the primary cause is unlikely to be any very serious disease such as a malignant tumour, for instance.

Resting pain

Pain that is felt when resting, and especially at night, waking the patient in the middle of the night or preventing him from sleeping, can give important clues. A milder pain may emerge in a resting state, in the quietness of the night, when the proprioceptive and psychic stimuli that affect the modulation of pain decrease. If the pain is associated with a certain posture it may originate from the mobile structures in the back, whereas if it is not governed by posture at all one might suspect an inflammatory process, systemic disease or malignity. Being woken by back pain in the early hours of the morning, for instance, is regarded as typical of spondylitis, although it should be remembered that endogenous depression, which in itself is known to simulate various somatic symptoms or at least exacerbate subjective suffering due to pain, can also wake the patient at similar times.

Early morning symptoms

After the stress of the previous day, the back is usually in its best condition following a night's rest. Getting out of bed nevertheless usually requires twisting and bending of the lower back, which may provoke pains and force the patient to develop special manoeuvres to enable him to get up in a painless manner. The nerve compression symptoms present in cases of disc protrusion are frequently at their worst in the morning, when the disc has increased in volume following the night's rest. The back may feel stiff when washing in the morning if there is inflammation in the articular facets of the spine, e.g. in osteoarthritis or arthrosis. This stiffness often goes quickly after one or two loosening-up exercises, but morning stiffness caused by rheumatic inflammations can typically last for several hours.

Increased pain caused by stress

The spine is subjected to stress of different kinds in a variety of situations in the course of the day. In conditions involving instability, the static stress brought about by standing or sitting can provoke pain. If the pain is local, the reason may be irritation of the nociceptors in the capsules of ligament structures or articular facets; if it is a radial pain with numbness and 'pins and needles', this may be evidence of structural or dynamic spinal stenosis. Local pains of the instability type can usually be relieved by gentle movements and changes of position, but spinal stenosis can provoke claudication symtoms. The symptoms mentioned above can be quantified in terms of the time taken to provoke them in each type of stress situation.

Symptoms caused by bending forward are common, and the manoeuvre may be totally impossible under conditions of radicular compression. In other cases, straightening of the back may be painful, and the patient may need a helping hand when instability of the lower back is present.

The stress generated in coughing or defecation, for instance, increases intrathecal pressure, upon which a prolapse or tumour pressing on the nerve tissue can cause radiating pain in the region of the affected nerve root.

In addition to factors provoking pain, it is important to enquire about factors and postures that relieve the pain. Where the patient is suffering from a mechanical skeletal disturbance, it is natural that he will be able to find certain positions in which the pain is reduced or the symptoms disappear entirely. This is typical of cases of a slipped disc. If this antalgic position is biomechanically logical, it can increase the probability of the diagnosis.

Traumas

Acute musculoskeletal pains are often a consequence of minor traumas sustained during everyday activities, frequently sufficiently minor that the patient will not spontaneously even mention them. Also, the symptom may only make itself felt some hours later, so that the patient may not perceive any connection between the two. For this reason it is important to ask the patient to recall even quite small potentially traumatic events.

Other conditions

From the point of view of differential diagnosis, it is always necessary to bear in mind the possibility of referred pain from some internal organ, since these are known to simulate skeletal pains, and vice versa, and it should be remembered that a symptom may be derived from both an internal and a skeletal cause simultaneously. Also, anticoagulant therapy can cause haemorrhages in the joints

244

of the spine or around the nerves and thereby give rise to pains and neurological deficiency symptoms.

Age over 50 years, trauma, loss of weight, cortisone therapy, heavy consumption of alcohol (involving a risk of osteoporosis or inebriation trauma) and previous malignant disease are all warning signs that require more careful clinical examination and a more liberal use of diagnostic laboratory and visualization techniques[4].

Correspondingly, where children are concerned, it should be remembered that musculoskeletal pain in childhood can often be associated with some more serious disease, an infection, tumour or inflammatory disease such as rheumatoid arthritis.

The obtaining of a full anamnesis is the most critical and most demanding part of the clinical diagnostic routine.

SUMMARY

The problems reported by patients seeking medical advice for musculoskeletal diseases involve questions of pain and dysfunction, which may be intermittent in character and can vary greatly from day to day and at different times of the day in response to external stress factors. Especially in the case of chronic pains, the objective findings gained from a physical examination, laboratory tests and radiological investigations are frequently minimal and show a poor correlation with the patient's symptoms. Thus, the clinical interview becomes the most important, and often the only, diagnostic method available. If carried out properly, however, it can be regarded as highly objective and reliable, and can provide information relevant to the prognosis and treatment that could not be obtained by any laboratory test or imagery technique, namely, a portrait of the patient as a person. As we are all well aware, it is often more important to know what kind of person has a disease than to know what disease that person has.

In order to be successful, the gathering of an anamnesis requires a great deal of the physician: intellectual alertness, interest in the problems of even the most difficult of patients, clinical experience and interpersonal communication skills. The mostly somatic symptoms of pain reported by patients to their doctors frequently have hiding behind them extremely complex sets of problems of which the patients themselves may not be aware. It is from these complexes of problems that one has to try to identify the crucial factors detracting from the patient's health and that can be influenced by some kind of therapy. The notion of '*Aktualitätsdiagnose*' put forward by Guttman fits this situation very well[11]. If enough attention were paid to these factors it could have a profound effect on the worsening health-care costs crisis observable almost everywhere, part of which is attributable to the ever more expensive biomedical technology being made available. A greater volume of critical evaluative research is needed to indicate the relative significance of different imagery techniques, for example, beside the oldest of all diagnostic and therapeutic methods, the performing of an anamnesis and clinical examination by a physician. Current scientific research would seem to demonstrate increasingly clearly that these latter have been able to hold their own at the forefront of medical technology.

REFERENCES

1. Andersson, G.B.J., Svensson, H.O. and Oden, A. (1983). The intensity of work recovery in low back pain. *Spine*, **8**, 880–884
2. Bouchier, I.A.D. (1982). The medical interview. In Bouchier, I.A.D. and Morris, J.S. (eds.) *Clinical Skills*, 2nd edn., pp. 1–10. (London: W.B. Saunders)
3. Cyriax, J. (1975). The diagnosis of soft tissue lesions. In Cyriax, J. (ed.) *Textbook of Orthopedic Medicine*, Vol.1, pp. 64–68. (London: Baillière Tindall)
4. Deyo, R.A. (1987). Reducing work absenteeism and diagnostic costs for backache. In Hadler, N.M. (ed.) *Clinical Concepts in Regional Musculoskeletal Illness*, pp. 25–37. (Orlando: Grune & Stratton)
5. Frisch, H. (1987). *Programmierte Untersuchung des Bewegungsapparates*, 2nd edn., pp. 20–25. (Berlin: Springer-Verlag)
6. Goresky, C.A. (ed.) (1987). Approche scientifique de l'evaluation et du traitement des affections vertebrales chez les travailleurs. *Med. Clin. Exper.*, **10**, 15
7. Guckian, J.C. (1987). Establishing an effective patient – physician relationship. In Guckian, J.C. (ed.) *The Clinical Interview and Physical Examination*, pp. 4–24. (London: J.B. Lippincott)
8. Hornby, A.S. (1974). *Oxford Advanced Learner's Dictionary of Current English.* (London: Oxford University Press)
9. Huskisson, E.C. (1974). Measurement of pain. *Lancet* (Nov. 9) 1127–1130
10. Lewit, J. (1987). *Untersuchung und Diagnose Funktionsstörungen des Bewegungssystems* (vertebrage Störungen). In Lewit, J (ed.) *Manuelle Medizin im Rahmen medizinischen Rehabilitation*, 5th edn., pp. 129–132. (Munchen: Urban Schwarzenberg)
11. Ljunggren, A.E., Jacobsen, T. and Osvik, A. (1988). Pain description in patients with herniated lumbar intervertebral discs. *Pain*, **35**, 39–46.
12. Mumenthaler, M. (1980). *Der Schulter-Arm-Schmerz*, pp. 1–12. (Bern: Verlag Hans Huber)
13. Reading, A.E. (1989). Testing pain mechanisms in persons in pain. In Wall, P.D. and Melzack, R. (eds.) *Textbook of Pain*, pp. 260–280. (Edinburgh: Churchill Livingstone)
14. Sackett, D.L., Haynes, R.B. and Tugwell, P. (1985). *Clinical Epidemiology: A Basic Science for Clinical Medicine*, pp. 3–15. (Boston: Little Brown)
15. Vällfors, B. (1985). Acute, subacute and chronic low back pain. *Scand. J. Rehab. Med. Suppl.*, **11**, 50
16. Wedge, J.H. (1983). The natural history of spine degeneration. In Kirkaldy Willis, W.H. (ed.) *Managing Low Back Pain*, pp. 3–8. (New York: Churchill Livingstone)
17. Viikari-Juntura, E. (1987). Interexaminer reliability observations in physical examinations of the neck. *Phys. Ther.*, **67**, 1526–32.

29
A new technique of proprioceptive re-education in manual medicine

Ivano COLOMBO and Corrado LEUCI

Many hypotheses have been proposed on the mechanics of vertebral manipulations. In recent years, several European authors[1-6] have emphasized the hypothesis that the manipulative act causes a reflex proprioceptive stimulation, acting through and on the articular proprioceptors in which the intervertebral articulations are very rich.

We refer to the precise and thorough article by Gatto[6], in which the functional anatomy of the articular structures of the spine are clearly explained and an outline of the mechanics of spinal manipulation is given. The article underlines in particular the importance of manipulation; stimulation of the mechanoreceptors of the capsule and articular structures can reduce the pain owing to a reflex response ('gate theory').

Accepting these hypotheses, and with many years of practical knowledge and experience in the field of manual medicine, we felt that manipulative treatment could be followed and completed by a proprioceptive re-education, and that emphasizing and stimulating adequately the neurological circuits of proprioceptive activity could activate a better rehabilitation of the vertebral dysfunction that always follows a painful syndrome, especially when it lasts for a long time.

In addition some years ago (1976) we achieved satisfactory results from electrically stimulating the extensor muscles of the cervical spine, thus activating the proprioceptive afferents, in hemiplegic patients with serious trunk control disturbances. In fact, the static functions and the upright position are principally based on functional systems that are prevailingly reflexes, starting with the labyrinth, the muscular and articular proprioceptors and also esteroceptive excitations. The complex of these reactions produced by the afferential proprio-esteroceptive and labyrinthic pool activates static–dynamic muscular reactions that permit the upright position and walking. These reactions can be classified into three groups:

(1)   static reactions;
(2)   righting reactions;
(3)   balance reactions.

They are obviously linked and their separation is purely didactic.

We should not forget that the spine is the most important element of the body. In phylogenic and ontogenic evolution, the morphological and functional modifications of the spine (orientation of vertebral bodies, appearance of different curves, etc.) work equally with the institution of the erect position. In the erect position the most important physical element is represented by the force of gravity: which is opposed by muscular activity providing equilibrium that, in man, being a biped animal with a small base of support, is particularly unstable. The precise muscular play for the control of the erect position of walking is controlled by the sensory system, in which the proprioceptive system has a very important role.

The spine should be considered not only as an organ that supports but also as a functional complex generating an afferenting pool of primary importance in everyday life.

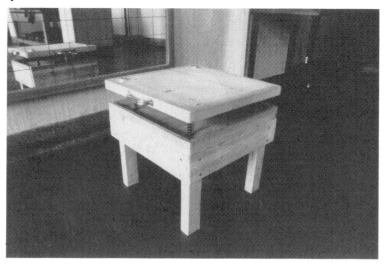

Figure 29.1

The traditional re-education for all painful pathology of the spine (techniques by Charriére, postural re-education, stretching, techniques by Mezière, etc.) are certainly useful and universally used, but need a long period of training to which the patient very often does not adjust, because of scarce sensitivity, lack of time or simple laziness. Therefore, we thought of using a 'floating' chair that permits us to obtain results and in a very short period of time (Figures 29.1,29.2,29.3). In 1984 Gatto and Bargero[8] published an interesting article on the proprioceptive re-education of the patient with spinal problems at the cervical and lumbar level. We agree with them on the usefulness of these methods, which represent a remarkable progress in technical re-education compared with the traditional methods. The 'floating' chair also seems useful in that it is a technique of mass re-education involving the entire trunk and the labyrinthine righting reflex.

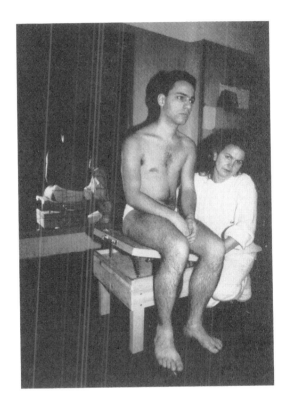

Figure 29.2

Electromyographic studies show a symmetrical and rhythmic activity of the paravertebral muscles and a global and synergic muscle activity of the whole trunk. The rhythmic and alternating action of the trunk muscles, which is principally static and of postural control, repetitive and rhythmic, does not arouse pain in the patient, facilitates the resolution of the painful stiffness and, by feigning the rhythmic muscular movement that is characteristic of walking, accustoms the patient to a return to everyday activity. In particular, the floating on the frontal surface is more useful for the recruitment of muscular activity.

TECHNIQUE

The patient is seated on the floating chair, placing his feet flat on a stool. The patient is asked to hold on to handles on both sides of the chair and to begin a floating movement, first on orthogonal planes then also a rotating movement, changing the direction of the rotation.

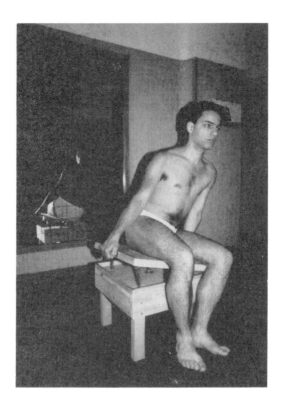

Figure 29.3

The sitting position is well accepted by the patient even if he is still frightened of using the muscles of the trunk. Each training session lasts 20 minutes, daily for 10 days.

RESULTS

We have treated 50 patients recovering from surgical treatment of lumbar disc hernias (20 days post-operative). We also have treated 20 patients with severe lumbar pain. The results are shown in Table 29.1.

All the patients showed very good tolerance during the treatment and did not feel vertebral pain or an increase in symptoms. The improvement of the spinal function has been more than satisfactory both subjectively and objectively.

Table 29.1

		Pathology		
	Number of patients	Good	Fairly good	Bad
Post-operative	50	48	1	1
Chronic lumbago	20	15	4	1

CONCLUSIONS

We believe this floating chair can be valid in aiding proprioceptive re-education for patients with spinal pain in their functional re-education, both because it is cheap and easy to use and also because the patient feels he is an active agent in his rehabilitation training.

REFERENCES

1. Fiandesio, D. (1975). Medicina manuale in reumatologia. *Conferenza al Convegno Incontro di Reumatologia*, Ospedale Civile, Alessandria
2. Wyke, B. (1976). Neurology of the cervical spine joints. *Physiotherapy*, **65**, 72
3. Wyke, B. (1979). Neurological mechanisms in the experience of pain. *Acupuncture Electrother. Res.*, **4**, 27
4. Wyke, B. (1980). Neurological aspects of low back pain. In Jayson, M. (ed.) *The Lumbar Spine and Back Pain*, 2nd edn. (Tunbridge Wells, Pitman Medical)
5. Astegiano, P.A. (1981). Le manipolazioni vertebrali. Meccanismo di azione di un esercizio passive e segmentario con risultati di ordine meccanico e reflesso. *Atti del 12° Congresso della SIMFER. Il Ciocco*, Vol. II, p. 79
6. Gatto, R. (1983). Modello d'azione della tecnica manipolativa sui recettori articolari. *Eur. Medicophysica*, **19**(4), 223
7. Colombo, I. and Cossu, M. (1976). L'elettrostimolazione dei muscoli estensori del capo: tecnica di facilitazione neuromuscolare per il controllo della stazione eretta nel grave neuroleso contrale. *La Riabilitazione*, **9**(1), 3
8. Gatto, R. and Bargero, V. (1984). La rieducazione propriocettiva della colonna vertebrale. *Eur. Medicophysica*, **18**(4), 191

Section III
FREE PAPERS

30
Cranial and visceral symptoms in mechanical pelvic dysfunction

Lennart SILVERSTOLPE and Gustaf HELLSING

During 1988, 373 cases of mechanical pelvic dysfunction were investigated and cranial nerve and/or visceral disorders and symptoms were found in 89 of them (23.9%, mean age 43.4 years). Sixty-one were female and 28 male. The age range was 18 to 68 years and 26 to 81 years, respectively. Table 30.1 shows distribution of cranial nerve and visceral disorders and symptoms in this group. Table 30.2 gives more detailed information about symptoms of cranial, visceral and spinal disorders. A great variety of symptoms at different levels of the CNS may thus be caused by mechanical pelvic dysfunction.

Table 30.1 Distribution of cranial nerve and visceral disorders and symptoms found in 89 out of 373 patients with mechanical pelvic dysfunction syndrome

Signs and symptoms	n	%
Visceral	2	2
Cranial	72	81
Visceral and cranial	15	17

The applied treatment[1] – massage and stretch with the forefinger of the sacrotuberous ligament at its upper part (coccyx level) – is performed until S-reflex and tender point have disappeared[2]. Repositioning of the compensatory scoliosis and mobilization of locked vertebrae is then performed all the way up to C1 according to Gaymans and Lewit[3,4]. Apparently complete recovery was achieved in 74 (83.2%), improvement in 13 (14.6%) and no improvement in 2 cases (2.2%). Mean observation time was 11.6 months and mean number of visits 2.7.

Sixteen professional singers, referred because of vocal disturbances, were included in the material (mean age 31.2 years, 3 male 24–57 years, 13 female 20–57 years). All of them were unable to reach their earlier pitch. The voice was hoarse and rough and the support from the abdominal musculature was reduced. Table 30.3 shows symptom distribution in this material. It is noteworthy that deviation of the tongue at thrusting was occurring in all patients despite their efforts to thrust straight out.

Table 30.2 Cranial, visceral and spinal symptom distribution in the patient group of Table 30.1

Symptoms	Male	Female	Total
Cranial			
Nausea	13	18	31
Vertigo	18	28	46
Headache	19	28	47
Swallow breathing	11	16	27
Craniomandibular disorders	14	33	47
Deviation of tongue	10	37	47
Blurred vision	16	24	40
Loss of hearing	11	17	28
Phonasthenia	12	36	48
Visceral			
Dysphagia	8	17	25
Globus sensation	17	28	45
Abdominal tenesmus	2	15	17
Sensation of perineal prolapse	0	6	6
Dysuria	2	12	14
Spinal			
Cervical			
Neck	21	35	56
Shoulder	20	32	52
Arm	14	29	43
Thoracic symptoms	11	12	23
Lumbar symptoms	4	12	16
Sacral symptoms	10	19	29
Leg	8	27	35

All patients of Table 30.3 were improved and normal pitch was achieved after treatment of the sacrotuberous ligament. During the treatment the patients experienced a sudden movement in the larynx. The unsymmetrical vocal cord vibration and its normalisation was verified by external palpation. Mean observation time was 11.8 months.

Another study of 17 cases with mechanical pelvic dysfunction and additional signs and symptoms of craniomandibular disorder is in the process of being published. These patients were consulting for lower back pain as the main complaint but also had symptoms of craniomandibular disorders. Mean age was 40 years (range 27–64), 12 were female and 5 male. Symptom duration had been more than 5 years for 11 patients, 1–5 years for 4 patients and less than 1 year for two patients.

Table 30.3 Symptom distribution among 16 professional singers, which belong to the patient group of Table 30.1. They were referred because of vocal disturbances

Clinical symptoms	n	Left	Right
Neck pain	8		
Chest pain	3		
Low back pain	8		
Vibration differences	Reduced at	left side	right side
between vocal cords	16	7	9
Deviation in jaw opening	16	7 to the left	9 to the right
Deviation of tongue	16	7 to the left	9 to the right

Table 30.4 Influence of pelvic treatment upon deviation of jaw at opening, tongue at thrusting, and upon clicking and crepitation of the temporomandibular joint in 17 patients with symptoms of craniomandibular disorders

	Before	After
Deviation of jaw	14	1
Deviation of tongue	9	0
Clicking	5	2
Crepitation	6	3

The lower back pain of all 17 patients was relieved. Moreover, 16 of them, including 6 patients who had been resistant to earlier local therapy by dentists, were improved regarding their mandibular pain/dysfunction by manual treatment of the sacrotuberous ligament. Enhancement of jaw opening ability after therapy was noted for all but three patients and amounted to a mean of 9.5 mm. Range of increase was 2–25 mm with small increments mainly in four patients who already opened more than 50 mm before treatment.

Table 30.4 demonstrates that marked mandibular deviation at jaw opening occurred in 14 patients before treatment but after in only one of them. Deviation of the tongue at thrusting disappeared in all 9 cases as it did in the 16 singers of the previously described study. It may thus be a sign of significant clinical interest. To our knowledge, observation of tongue thrusting has not been recommended in earlier literature of clinical examination of cases with craniomandibular disorders. During treatment clicking disappeared completely in three joints (Table 30.4). In four joints (3 patients) crepitation clearly decreased and disappeared completely within a few weeks. Reciprocal clicking of the temporomandibular joint is considered a significant sign of condylar slipping behind the disc at closure and reduction under the disc at opening[5]. Crepitation has been demonstrated, in radiographic and arthroscopic studies, to be a significant sign of temporomandibular joint osteoarthrosis[6,7]. It is considered to be a friction phenomenon caused by destructive changes on the articulating surfaces. Disappearance of unilateral clicking and crepitation in the two described cases, and of bilateral clicking and crepitation in one case, is therefore remarkable. Decreased muscular tension leading to reduction of loading forces in the joint and smoother movements is a hypothetical explanation.

The predominant subjective reaction of the 16 successfully treated patients was one of great relief of tension and pain in the orofacial area. All reported facilitation of mandibular movements; also two of the patients whose maximum opening did not increase.

The study showed that certain symptoms of craniomandibular dysfunction may disappear practically immediately during local treatment of mechanical pelvic dysfunction. This indicates that mechanical pelvic dysfunction may change the inflow from structures in the pelvic region and cause chronic disturbance also at brainstem level. Experimental data supporting this theory are scarce in the literature. It has, however, been demonstrated that electrical stimulation of spinal nerves from widespread areas of the body can evoke reflex responses in the masseter muscle[8].

The compensatory scoliosis of patients with mechanical pelvic dysfunction involved the cervical area in all cases studied. Neck pain, tender cervical vertebrae and reduced cervical mobility were noted. The close proximity of the cervical level to the temporomandibular joint and mandibular structures is of particular interest regarding development of craniomandibular disorders.

To summarize, mechanical pelvic dysfunction seems to be a possible background to development of pain and dysfunction of different structures not only at spinal but also at cranial and visceral levels.

REFERENCES

1. Midttun, A. and Bojsen-Möller, F. (1986). The sacrotuberous ligament pain syndrome. In Grieve, G.P. (ed.) *Modern Manual Therapy of the Vertebral Column*, pp. 815–818. (Edinburgh: Churchill Livingstone)
2. Silverstolpe, L. (1989). A pathological erector spinae reflex – a new sign of mechanical pelvic dysfunction. A proposal of treatment. *Manual Med.*, **4**, 28
3. Gaymans, F. and Lewit, K. (1975). Mobilisation techniques using pressure (pull) and muscular facilitation and inhibition. In Lewit, K. and Gutman, G. (eds.) *Functional Pathology of the Motor System.* (*Rehabilitàcia Supplementum*, **10–11**, 47) (Bratislava: Obzor)
4. Lewit, K. (1985). *Manipulative Therapy in Rehabilitation of the Motor System.* (London: Butterworths)
5. Farrar, W. (1978). Characteristics of condylar path in internal derangements of the temporomandibular joint. *J. Prosth. Dent.*, **39**, 319
6. Kopp, S. (1977). Clinical findings in temporomandibular joint osteoarthrosis. *Scand. J. Dent. Res.*, **85**, 434
7. Holmlund, A. and Hellsing, G. (1989). Arthroscopy of the temporomandibular joint. A comparative study of clinical and arthroscopic findings. *J. Prosth. Dent.*, **62**, 61
8. Cadden, S.W. and Maillou, P. (1987). The extent of the spinal reflex control of jaw-closing muscles in man. *J. Physiol.*, **390**, 259P

31
A study of the contribution of pain to rotation of vertebrae in the aetiology and pathogenesis of lateral spinal curvature

M. WISŁOWSKA

Idiopathic spinal curvature found in children and adults is characterized by side-curving in the frontal plane, changes in configuration and dimensions of normal curvatures of spine, and the appearance of rotation of the vertebra around the vertical axis of the spine[1,4]. Rotation is the most difficult deformation to eliminate both by conservative and surgical treatment[2,5-8]. In order to study the mechanism of this rotation in the lumbar spine, observations of lumbar spinal mechanics were made in other diseases. The rotation of vertebra in the lumbar section of the vertebral column in acute pain within the abdominal cavity has been researched.

Medical examinations were carried out on 45 patients aged 20–60 years in The Institute of Clinical Medicine in the Urological Division. Thirty patients with radiographically confirmed nephrolithiasis were examined. Fifteen of them had right-sided nephrolithiasis and 15 left-sided; radiographs were made during acute paroxysm of nephrolithiasis. No rotational or side-bending deviations of the lumbar spine were noted. Radiographic examinations of the lumbar spine did not reveal any degenerative or congenital defects; radiographs of hip ilia were at the same height in the frontal plane; heights of the ilia were determined by measuring the distance from the base of the fifth lumbar vertebra to the upper edge of the sacroiliac joints. The distance was the same on both sides. In most cases with nephrolithiasis, rotation of lumbar vertebrae was observed. For comparison, 15 patients were examined with other diseases of the kidney, 15 with acute cholelithiasis, and 15 with acute radicular syndrome. In order to compare lumbar rotation in these disease states with that in idiopathic scoliosis, 10 children with scoliosis of unknown origin were examined by similar methods.

Rotation of vertebrae becomes visible in radiographs of A–P lumbar spine as follows: the shadow of the bottom of the pedicle of the curved vertebra (from the side to which the turn has occurred) widens and moves away from the lateral edge of the vertebra, while the shadow of the bottom of the pedicle of the curved vertebra from the opposite side to the direction of the turn narrows and moves

259

nearer the lateral edge of the vertebra[2,3]. Simultaneously there is a shift of the bottom of the acantha from the axis of symmetry of the vertebra in the opposite direction to the turn of the vertebra. The right direction is indicated as negative, the left as positive.

(a)

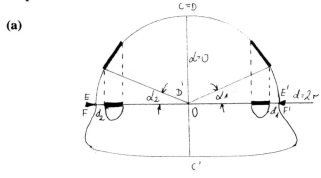

(b)

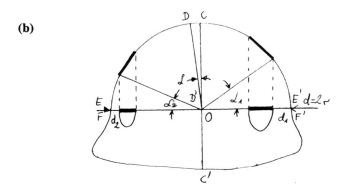

(c)

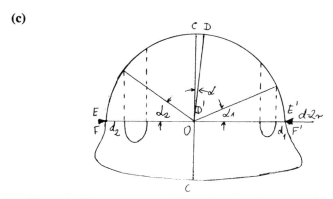

Figure 31.1 The method for measurement of the angles of rotation concerning vertebrae

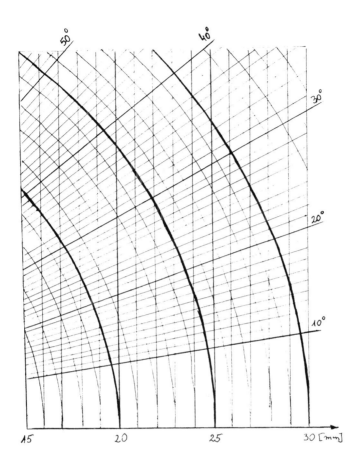

Figure 31.2 Nomograph

A method for accurate measurement of the relatively wide angles of rotation has been worked out (Figure 31.1). The principle of the method is the measurement of the distance between the border of the vertebra and a proximal edge of the bottom of the pedicle of the curve of the vertebra from the side to which the turn has occurred as well as from the opposite side, taking into account the width of the vertebra. In order to take the reading of the magnitude of the rotation angle, we used a nomograph, i.e. the alignment chart (Figure 31.2). The nomograph presented was made on a scale of 10:1; this enlargement made it possible to determine the rotation angle. In order to determine the angle of rotation from the nomograph, one lays out the radius of a circle in millimetres. On the nomograph, the given magnitude of the radius corresponds with the sector of the circle. From the magnitude of the radius on the horizontal

261

axis, one subtracts the distance (in millimetres) between the border of the vertabra and the proximal edge of the bottom of the pedicle from the side to which the turn has occurred. From the a/m magnitude on the horizontal axis one draws up the normal and at the point of its intersection with the sector of the circle for the given radius of circle to obtain the α_1 angle, which can be read on the vertical axis.

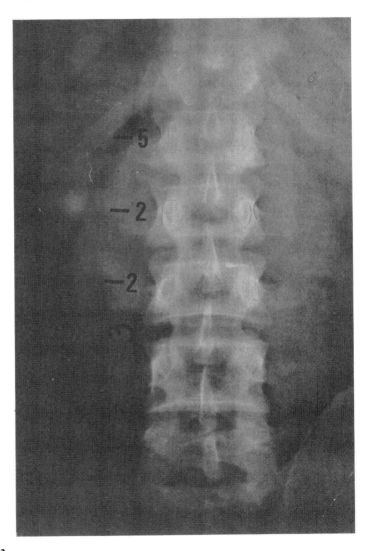

Figure 31.3

One similarly determines the α_2 angle: from the magnitude of the radius, one subtracts the distance between the border of vertebra and a proximal edge of the bottom of the pedicle of the vertabral curve from the side opposite to the turn of vertebra. The result of a subtraction between α_1 and α_2 angles divided by 2 gives the α angle of rotation.

If rotation is in the left direction the angle is greater than zero (positive) and if the rotation is in the right direction the angle is less than zero (negative). If there is no rotation, the angle is zero.

For example, consider the A–P picture of the lumbar spine of a 26-year-old patient, who had right-side nephrolithiasis. The rotation angle of the first lumbar vertebra was −5°, of the second −2° and the third −2° (Figure 31.3).

The magnitude of the rotation angles for individual groups of patients are presented in Tables 31.1 to 31.6.

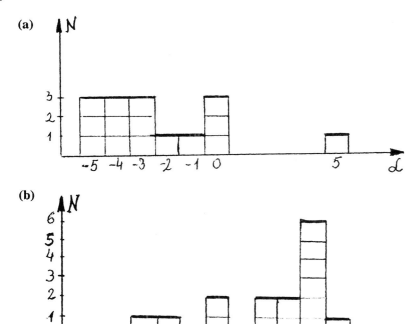

Figure 31.4

Table 31.1 Magnitudes of rotation angles (in degrees) of lumbar vertebrae of patients with right-si nephrolithiasis

No.	Age	Sex	Diagnosis	Vertebra	d	d_2	d_1	α_2	α_1	α	Direction
1	51	f	Neph. dex.	I	51	2.5	1	26	16	−5	R
				II	53	2	1	22	16	−3	R
				III	53	1.5	1	19	16	−1	R
2	55	m	Neph. dex.	I	45	1	0.5	17	12	−2	R
				II	47	1	0.5	17	12	−2	R
3	40	m	Neph. dex.	I	54	3.5	1.5	29	19	−5	R
				II	55	2	1	22	16	−3	R
				III	59	1.5	1	18	15	−1	R
4	28	f	Neph. dex.	I	38	2	1.5	26	24	−1	R
				II	40	2	1.5	26	24	−4	R
				III	44	1	0.5	17	12	−2	R
5	32	m	Neph. dex.				without rotation				
6	26	m	Neph. dex.	I	46	2	1	24	17	−3	R
				II	48	3	1	28	17	−5	R
				III	50	2	1	23	16	−5	R
7	24	f	Neph. dex.	I	42	2	1	25	18	−3	R
				II	43	1.5	1	22	18	−2	R
				III	44	1	0.5	18	12	−3	R
8	45	f	Neph. dex.	I	51	0	0.5	0	11	5	L
				II	51	0	0.5	0	11	5	L
9	45	f	Neph. dex.	I	41	1.5	0.5	22	13	−4	R
				II	46	2	1.5	24	21	−1	R
				III	48	1.5	1	21	17	−2	R
10	47	f	Neph. dex.	I	44	3	1.5	30	27	−4	R
				II	47	4	2.5	34	27	−3	R
				III	49	2	1.5	23	20	−1	R
11	31	f	Neph. dex.	I	48	2.5	1	27	17	−5	R
				II	49	1	0.5	17	12	−2	R
				III	52	1	0.5	16	11	−2	R
12	34	m	Neph. dex.	I	45	2	1	24	17	−3	R
				II	50	2	1.5	23	20	−1	R
				III	52	2.5	2	25	23	−1	R
13	31	f	Neph. dex.				without rotation				
14	28	f	Neph. dex.	I	40	1.5	0.5	22	13	−4	R
				II	44	1	0.5	17	12	−2	R
				III	46	1	0.5	17	12	−2	R
15	33	f	Neph. dex.				without rotation				

[a]L = left-sided rotation; R = right-sided rotation

Table 31.2 Magnitudes of rotation angles (in degrees) of lumbar vertebrae of patients with left-sided nephrolithiasis

No.	Age	Sex	Diagnosis	Vertebra	d	d_1	d_2	α_1	α_2	α	Direction[a]
1	51	f	Neph. sin.	I	39	1	1.5	18	23	−2	R
				II	43	1	2.5	18	28	−5	R
				III	51	0.5	1.5	11	20	−4	R
2	32	m	Neph. sin.				without rotation				
3	36	m	Neph. sin.	I	48	1.5	0.5	20	12	4	L
				II	52	1.5	0.5	19	11	4	L
				III	56	2	0.5	22	11	5	L
4	42	f	Neph. sin.	I	45	1	2	17	24	−3	R
				II	47	1	2	17	24	−3	R
				III	51	1	2	16	23	−3	R
5	47	m	Neph. sin.	I	48	1	0.5	17	12	3	L
				II	52	1	0.5	16	11	3	L
6	29	m	Neph. sin.				without rotation				
7	52	m	Neph. sin.	I	48	3	1.5	29	20	4	L
				II	49	1.5	1	20	16	2	L
8	33	f	Neph. sin.	I	41	1.5	1	22	18	2	L
				II	54	2.5	1	25	16	4	L
9	30	f	Neph. sin.	I	41	2.5	1	28	18	5	L
				II	42	2	1	25	18	3	L
				III	44	1.5	1	22	18	2	L
10	36	m	Neph. sin.	I	50	1.5	1	20	12	2	L
				II	52	15	1	20	16	2	L
				III	53	1	0.5	16	11	3	L
11	30	f	Neph. sin.	I	40	3.5	2	34	26	4	L
				II	45	5	3	39	30	5	L
				III	46	3	2	30	24	3	L
12	35	m	Neph. sin.	I	52	3	2	28	23	2	L
				II	52	3.5	1.5	30	20	10	L
				III	57	3	1	26	15	5	L
13	53	f	Neph. sin.	I	46	2	1	24	17	3	L
				II	47	3	1.5	30	21	4	L
				III	50	1	1.5	16	11	2	L
14	23	m	Neph. sin.	I	44	1.5	0.5	21	12	4	L
				II	48	2	0.5	24	12	6	L
				III	48	2	0.5	24	12	6	L
15	54	m	Neph. sin.	I	50	2	1	23	16	4	L
				II	53	2	0.5	22	12	5	L

[a]L = left-sided rotation; R = right-sided rotation

Table 31.3 Magnitudes of rotation angles (in degrees) of lumbar vertebrae of patients with neopla (tumour) and other kidney diseases

No.	Age	Sex	Diagnosis	Vertebra	d	d_1	d_2	α_1	α_2
Right-sided rotation									
1	33	f	Post. oper. ren.	I	45	1	2	17	24
			dex. propter Ca.	II	45	0.5	1	12	17
2	44	f	Pyelonephritis	I	43	1.5	2	22	26
			chr. ext.	II	44	1.5	3	22	30
3	51	m	Hydroneph. ren. sin.	I	55	0.5	2	11	22
				II	59	0.5	2	11	21
4	54	m	Ca. ren. sin.	I	46	1	2	17	24
				II	48	1	2	17	24
5	37	m	Ca. ren. sin.	I	46	1.5	3.5	21	32
				II	46	1	2.5	17	26
				III	50	1	2.5	17	27
6	52	m	Pyeloneph. acuta	II	48	2.5	3	26	29
				III	50	2	3	24	28
7	29	f	Ca. ren. dex.	I	47	0	0.5	0	10
				II	49	0.5	1	11	17
Without rotation									
8	36	f	Ca. ren. dex.						
9	22	m	Pyeloneph. chr. exc.						
Left-sided rotation									
10	58	f	Ca. ren. sin.	I	41	1	0.5	18	12
				II	45	1.5	0.5	21	12
				III	47	2	0.5	26	12
11	54	m	Ca. ren. dex.	I	46	2	1	24	17
				II	49	2	0.5	24	12
12	20	f	Syndroma Orlandi	I	43	2	1	26	17
				II	45	2	1	26	17
				III	46	2	0.5	24	13
13	22	m	Pyeloneph. chr.	I	49	2	0.5	24	12
			exc.	II	51	2	0.5	23	12
14	57	f	Ca. ren. dex.	I	41	1	0.5	18	13
				II	44	1	0.5	17	12
15	55	m	Pyeloneph. chr. exc.	I	51	4	2	32	23
				II	52	3	1	27	16

e 31.4 Magnitudes of rotation angles (in degrees) of lumbar vertebrae of patients with cholelithiasis

Age	Sex	Diagnosis	Vertebra	d	d_1	d_2	α_1	α_2	α	Direction[a]
4	m	cholecystitis	II	54	2.5	1.5	25	19	3	L
		calculosa	III	56	2.5	1	25	16	4	L
5	f	cholecystitis	I	48	3	5	29	38	-4	R
		calculosa	II	49	2	2.5	23	26	-1	R
3	f	cholecystitis	I	43	1	3	18	31	-6	R
		calculosa	II	44	1	2	18	25	-3	R
			III	50	0.5	1	12	17	-3	R
4	f	cholecystitis calculosa			without	rotation				
3	f	cholecystitis	I	44	0.5	1	12	18	-3	R
		calculosa	II	46	0.5	2	12	24	-6	R
			III	48	0.5	2	12	23	-5	R
4	f	cholecystitis	I	49	3	1.5	29	20	4	L
		calculosa	II	50	3	1.5	29	20	4	L
			III	52	2	1	23	16	3	L
2	m	cholecystitis	I	48	1.5	3	21	29	-4	R
		calculosa	II	50	1.5	3	21	29	-4	R
			III	54	1	2	16	22	-3	R
2	f	cholecystitis	I	42	2	3	25	31	-3	R
		calculosa	II	45	2	3	24	30	-3	R
			III	48	2	3	23	29	-3	R
7	f	cholecystitis	I	48	0.5	2	12	23	-5	R
		calculosa	II	53	0.5	2	11	22	-5	R
			III	56	1	2	16	22	-3	R
8	f	cholecystitis	I	42	1	2	18	25	-3	R
		calculosa	II	45	1	2	17	24	-3	R
			III	49	0.5	2	12	23	-5	R
7	f	cholecystitis	I	48	1	2	17	23	-3	R
		calculosa	II	48	2	3	23	29	-3	R
			III	54	1	2	17	22	-2	R
6	f	cholecystitis calculosa			without	rotation				
0	f	cholecystitis	I	42	1	2.5	18	28	-5	R
		calculosa	II	42	1.5	3	22	31	-4	R
			III	44	0.5	1	12	18	-3	R
0	f	cholecystitis	I	40	0.5	0	12	0	6	L
		calculosa	II	45	2	1	24	17	3	L
1	f	cholecystitis	I	44	5	2.5	39	28	5	L
		calculosa	II	44	2.5	1	28	17	5	L
			III	48	2.5	1	28	17	5	L

eft-sided rotation; R = right-sided rotation

Table 31.5 Magnitudes of rotation angles (in degrees) of lumbar vertebrae of patients with sharp spinal radix p

No.	Age	Sex	Diagnosis	Vertebra	d	d_1	d_2	α_1	α_2	α	Directi
1	50	f	Isch. rad. LV/SIsin	I	39	1.5	2.5	23	29	−3	R
				II	43	1.5	2.5	22	28	−3	R
2	57	m	Isch. dex. rad. LV	I	47	3	2.5	29	26	1	L
			discopathia LIV/LV	II	51	4	2.5	32	24	4	L
				III	54	3	2	28	22	3	L
3	37	m	Isch. dex. rad. LV discopathia LIV/LV				without rotation				
4	57	m	Isch. dex.				without rotation				
5	23	m	Isch. sin. discopathia LV/S1	III	48	1.5	1	21	17	2	L
6	31	f	Isch. sin.	I	39	1	0.5	18	13	2	L
			discopathia LIV/LV	II	42	1	0.5	16	12	2	L
				III	43	1	0.5	16	12	2	L
7	31	m	Isch. dex.	I	57	4	5	31	35	−2	R
				II	57	2.5	4	25	31	−3	R
				III	60	0.5	1	11	15	−2	R
8	50	f	Isch. dex.				without rotation				
9	39	f	Isch. sin.	I	38	1	2.5	18	29	−5	R
				II	42	1.5	3	21	31	−5	R
10	47	m	Isch. dex. rad. SI	I	51	1	2.5	17	28	−5	R
			discopathia LV/SI	II	51	0.5	1	12	17	−2	R
11	51	f	Isch. dex.	I	41	2.5	1.5	28	21	3	L
			discopathia LV/SI	II	42	2	1.5	25	21	2	L
12	53	f	Isch. sin. rad. SI	I	46	0	0.5	0	12	−6	R
			discopathia LV/SI	II	50	1	2	17	23	−3	R
13	39	m	Isch. sin.	I	46	0.5	1	12	17	−2	R
			discopathia LIV/LV	II	47	1	0.5	17	12	2	L
				III	51	1	0.5	16	11	2	L
14	30	f	Isch. sin.				without rotation				
15	47	f	Isch. dex.	II	47	2	1	24	17	3	L
			discopathia LV/SI	III	49	1.5	0.5	21	12	4	L

[a]L = left-sided rotation; R = right-sided rotation

Table 31.6 Magnitudes of rotation angles (in degrees) of lumbar vertebrae of patients with idiopathic scoliosis

No.	Age	Sex	Cobba angle at lumbar segment	Direction of bend of lumbar spine	Vertebra	Angle of rotation	Direction[a]
1	11	f	24	L	I	20	L
					II	20	L
					III	20	L
2	12	m	12	R	I	−11	R
					II	−9	R
					III	−9	R
3	13	f	13	R	I	−20	R
					II	−10	R
					III	−3	R
4	14	m	17	R	I	−14	R
					II	−15	R
					III	−20	R
5	14	f	11	L	I	7	L
					II	18	L
					III	8	L
6	11	f	8	L	I	14	L
					II	13	L
					III	8	L
7	12	f	8	L	I	7	L
					II	7	L
					III	9	L
8	13	f	8	L	II	9	L
					III	10	L
9	13	f	18	L	I	7	L
					II	12	L
					III	9	L
10	14	f	9	L	I	12	L
					II	17	L
					III	13	L

[a]L = left-sided rotation; R = right-sided rotation

Rotation angles for nephrolithiasis, cholelithiasis and radicular syndrome range from 0° to 6°. The rotation in disease other than radicular syndromes demonstrated no lateral spinal curvature. The rotation angles in the case of idiopathic scoliosis are from 7° to 20°. In 15 cases of right-sided nephrolithiasis there were 11 cases of right-sided spinal rotation, 1 case of left-sided rotation and in 3 cases no rotation was noted. In 15 cases of left-sided nephrolithiasis, there were 11 cases of left-sided spinal rotation, 2 cases of right-sided rotation and in 2 cases no rotation was noted.

We have observed that in 70% of the patients studied with nephrolithiasis there is rotation of vertebrae towards the involved kidney. In the comparative population it has also been found that other kidney diseases, acute cholelithiasis and acute radicular syndrom cause rotation, but correlation is much weaker.

Angles of rotation in left and right nephrolithiasis were statistically analysed. Data presented in histograms (Figure 31.4) show that the magnitudes of rotation angles in the case of left and right nephrolithiasis are similar, but of opposite directions.

In conclusion we propose that:

(1)   Irritation of the nervous system resulting from abdominal cavity pain may cause the appearance of symptomatic rotation of lumbar vertebrae.

(2)   In cases of acute nephrolithiasis there exists a correlation of the direction of rotation of vertebrae with involved kidney.

REFERENCES

1. Bizjak, F. and Gracanin, F. (1980). Mehanizmi nastajanja idiopatske skolioze. Report to Research Community of Slovenia. Grant N0-M-30/8759.
2. Gregersen, G.G. and Lukas, D.B. (1967). An in vivo study of the axial rotation of the human thoracolumbar spine. *J. Bone Joint Surg.*, **49**-A, 247
3. Lukas, R. (1952). Beitrag zur Bestimmung von Rotationgraden an Wirbelkorpen mittels Winkelmesser. *Z. Ortopedie*, **2**, 286
4. Maurcy, J., Guingland, M. and Dimnet, J. (1983). Representation tridimensionelle des scolioses, interet en reeducation. *IVe Congress National de la Soc. Fran. de reeducation fonctionnelle de readaptation et de medicine physique, Dijon.*
5. Ober, J.K. and Przedpelska-Ober, E. (1983). *Analiza czynników biomechanicznych w etiopatogenezie skoliozy idiopatycznej. Wczesne wykrywanie i zapobieganie progresji bocznych skrzywien kregoslupa.* (Warsaw: PAN, PZWL)
6. Schulze, K.J. (1983). Die Wirbelrotation bei der Scoliose – eine pathologisch-anatomische Studie. *Beitr. Orthop. Traumatol.*, **30**, 1
7. Tanaka, H. *et al.* (1982). The experimental study of scoliosis in bipedal rat in lathyrism. *Arch. Orthop. Trauma. Surg.*, **101**, 1
8. Troup, J.D.G. (1977). *Biomechanika ledzwiowego odcinka kregoslupa. Biomechanika w patogenezie zespolu bólów w dolnym odcinku kregoslupa u ludzi pracy.* (Warsaw: PZWL)

32
Pelvic dysfunction

K. LEWIT

There is hardly any problem in manual medicine that causes so much confusion and controversy as the pelvis with the sacroiliac joints. Not only do our views differ from those of the medical profession who do not practise manipulation, but the pelvis and the sacroiliac joints remain controversial among specialists in manipulation, even within the osteopathic profession, as can be seen from Beal's[1] excellent review paper. Opinion varies, from those who consider the sacroiliac joint to be the key to spinal problems, to those who almost disregard it[1-6].

The reason apparently lies in the fact that, unlike the rest of the spinal column and the extremity joints, where the concept of 'subluxation' or 'malalignment' has been abandoned in favour of movement restriction (i.e. disturbed function), 'dislocations', 'upslips' and 'downslips'[5,6,8] and other malpositions of the pelvis *and* the sacroiliac joints are still diagnosed and treated.

This is not by chance: the pelvis being a much larger structure than individual vertebrae, minute shifts between the ilia and the sacrum occur, and can be palpated by well-trained hands. They can also be corrected by appropriate techniques. As there are many landmarks on the ilia and the sacrum, the sophisticated examiner can find very numerous possible 'lesions', each with its specific adjustment, and can obtain excellent results. The snag is that slight asymmetry is in no way easy to palpate, and can be irrelevant; inter-examiner evaluation then becomes very problematic.

The basic problem is one of interpretation. Correct understanding of clinical findings should offer us a clearer approach to both diagnosis and therapy that is also more in keeping with the theory of manual medicine. The principle cause of confusion appears to be the fact that all disturbances of pelvic function are attributed to lesions of the sacroiliac joints.

Bearing this in mind, it is possible to distinguish three distinct conditions:

(1) Pelvic distortion;
(2) Sacroiliac dysfunction or blockage;
(3) Symphyseal shift.

PELVIC DISTORSION[8,9]

This lesion is particularly frequent in children and adolescents, and need not cause any symptoms. It can be detected by experienced examiners by mere inspection. The most pertinent findings are palpatory: on one side, usually the left, the spina iliaca posterior superior (SIPS) is lower and on the same side the spina iliaca anterior superior (SIAS) is higher. On the other side the situation is reversed; the iliac crest may be level, but need not be. If there is a difference it may be difficult to decide whether there is also pelvic obliquity. On inspection there is pelvic shift towards the side of the higher SIPS (usually the right); the buttock appears flatter, being more prominent on the other side. This is also borne out by asymmetry of the waist (Figure 32.1).

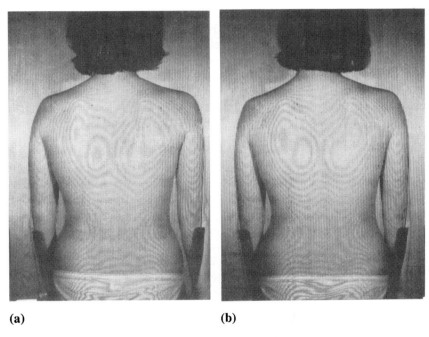

(a)   **(b)**

Figure 32.1 Moiré picture of patient D.V., pelvic distortion (a) before and (b) after mobilization of occiput/atlas: before treatment the lines in the lumbosacral region are oblique and after treatment horizontal; the waist is asymmetrical before and symmetrical after treatment; the lines on the shoulder blades differ slightly and the right shoulder is relatively less raised than before treatment

The underlying mechanism cannot be relative rotation of the ilia round a horizontal axis through both sacroiliac joints, as the palpatory findings would suggest, because this would cause rupture of the symphysis. The most plausible mechanism is that described by Cramer[10]: the primary lesion consists of a torsion of the sacrum caused by asymmetrical nutation, producing rotation of one innominate round a frontal axis through the acetabulum and of the other innominate round a sagittal axis through the acetabulum (Figure 32.2).

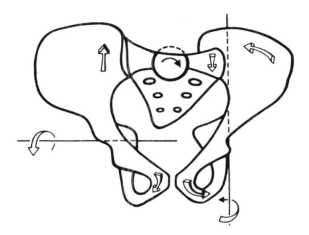

Figure 32.2 Cramer's diagram of pelvic distortion: there is primary torsion of the sacrum owing to asymmetrical nutation; as a consequence, one innominate rotates round a frontal and the other round a vertical axis

Whatever the mechanism, palpatory asymmetry may be considerable, suggesting 'subluxation'. Manipulation aiming at reposition was therefore carried out[11] with good results in apparent agreement with the subluxation concept. It sometimes happened, however, that mistakenly 'adjustment' in the opposite direction was carried out – with the same result! If manipulation took place because of some other clinically relevant lesion in any part of the spinal column, in particular at the craniocervical junction[12], adjustment of the pelvis was also observed (Figure 32.3). The same results were obtained by local anesthesia or dry needling of the sacroiliac ligaments and by local anesthesia in root syndromes. It became obvious that pelvic distortion (typically 'to the left') was a non-specific response of the pelvis to various changes in the motor system. Understandably, no specific symptoms exist – they depend on the underlying cause that determines the clinical manifestations.

There are, however, clinical signs that require further elucidation: these are the 'overtake phenomenon' and the 'spine sign'[13]. Characteristically we find in pelvic distortion that on forward bending (standing or sitting) the lower overtakes the higher SIPS. If the patient lifts his knee on one side or bends it, the distance between the SIPS and the spinous process of S_1 or L_5 changes under normal conditions. There will be no or little change at the lower SIPS in pelvic distortion. Both these phenomena are usually interpreted as signs of sacroiliac dysfunction. Downing[14], however, noted that the overtake phenomenon may be only temporary and may disappear after about 20 seconds. The same is true of the spine sign in pelvic distortion[8]. We may therefore speak of a 'false' overtake phenomenon and spine sign due to increased tension on the side of the lower SIPS.

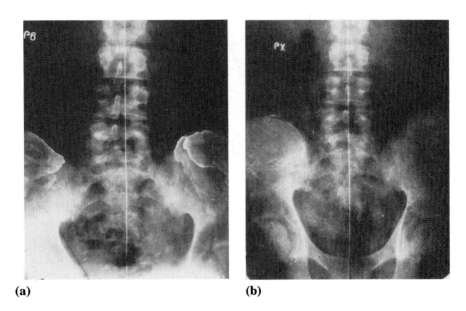

(a)   **(b)**

Figure 32.3 A–P radiographs of a patient with pelvic distortions. (a) Before treatment of occiput/atlas: the lumbar spine deviates to the left. (b) After treatment the sacrum and the lumbar spine are straight

SACROILIAC MOVEMENT RESTRICTION (BLOCKAGE)

The clinical picture is fairly characteristic: low back pain, mainly one-sided, with radiation in the S_1 segment. Both stooping and retroflexion may be restricted, and so is pelvic rotation on side-bending. The most typical pain points are on the sacrum laterally above and below the SIPS and at the symphysis. The pelvis is *level* as a rule, unless there is pelvic obliquity due to another cause. The overtake phenomenon and the spine sign are positive and permanent, the former being positive only in one-sided blockage. Both should be considered screening tests, as is passive adduction of the knee with the leg bent at the hip and the pelvis fixed from above, showing restriction on the blocked side.

The most specific signs, however, are direct springing (movement palpation) of the joint: (1) by producing nutation movement of the sacrum against the ilium with the patient prone, by springing the SIPS in a ventrocranial and the tip of the sacrum in a ventrocaudal direction (Figure 32.4)[6]; (2) by producing a wing-like movement of the ilium with the patient lying on his side, gapping the sacroiliac joint (Figure 32.5). Even these tests may be inconclusive, because the joint may be restricted only in its upper or lower half. In such cases there is restriction combined with tenderness only of the upper or lower part, which are examined and treated by springing pressure above or below the SIPS with the patient lying on his side (Figures 32.6 and 32.7).

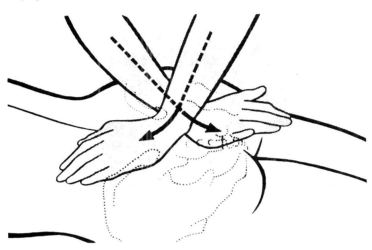

Figure 32.4 Mobilization of sacrum against ilium, the patient prone, the operator's hands crossed

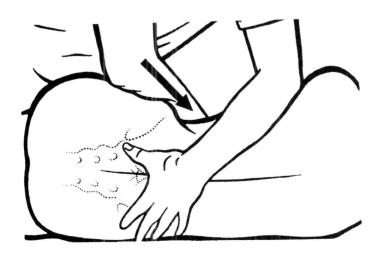

Figure 32.5 Gapping the sacroiliac joint

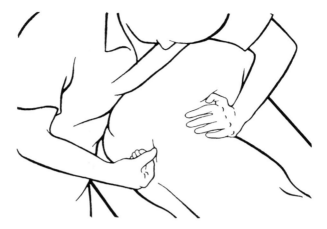

Figure 32.6 Mobilization of the upper part of the sacroiliac joint

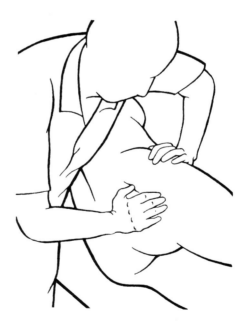

Figure 32.7 Mobilization of the lower part of the sacroiliac joint

At this point it is important to warn against the danger of failing to distinguish between lumbosacral and sacroiliac lesions, which both radiate in the S_1 segment. If there is spasm of the iliac muscle, lumbosacral involvement is more likely[15]; specific examination of the lumbosacral joint should then be carried out.

SYMPHYSEAL SHIFT[4,16,17]

As in pelvic distortion we find 'malalignment', but whereas the latter is examined mainly standing or sitting, this condition has to be looked for in the recumbent position; with the patient supine we have to palpate the symphysis from above, i.e. from the abdomen, and then we note that it is lower on one side (usually on the right) and that it is tender on one or even both sides. If this is the case, we find a corresponding trigger point in the straight abdominal muscle. As a rule this is linked to a relative shift of the ischial tuberosities occurring almost with the same frequency: (a) the ischial tuberosity on the same side is higher (lower) than the symphysis; or (b) on the side on which the symphysis is lower, the tuberosity is higher.

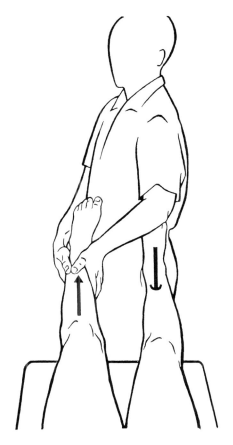

Figure 32.8 Correction of shift of both the symphysis and ischial tuberosity in the same direction by pulling one leg down and pushing the other up

Curiously this shift is only rarely found when the patient is examined standing. Again this lesion seems not to be correlated with sacroiliac dysfunction. In about two thirds of our cases with symphyseal shift there was no sacroiliac movement restriction, nor had specific mobilization of the sacroiliac joint any influence on the position of the symphysis and the ischial tuberosity, nor had adjustment of the symphysis any effect on a restricted sacroiliac joint.

In order to find out more about this type of lesion, 92 consecutive cases were examined in 1988 and 1989, 62 female, 30 male, the average age being 43 years (from 6 to 72 years). In 39 cases the symphysis and the ischial tuberosity were lower (higher) on the same side: in 32 cases lower on the right and 7 times lower on the left. They were shifted in an opposite direction in 53 patients and in this group the symphysis was lower on the left (the tuberosity higher on the left) only twice.

The symphysis was tender on palpation in 52 cases. Sacroiliac movement restriction was found (on one or both sides) only in 31 patients while there was normal mobility in 61. From the course of the disease it was possible to infer that the symphyseal (and tuberal) shift was clinically relevant in 42 cases, the relevance was doubtful in 27, while the condition was quite irrelevant in 21 cases.

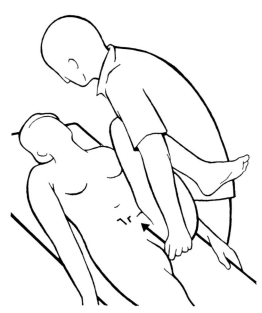

Figure 32.9 Correction of the syphysis that is lower and of the ischial tuberosity that is higher using a rotational manoeuvre

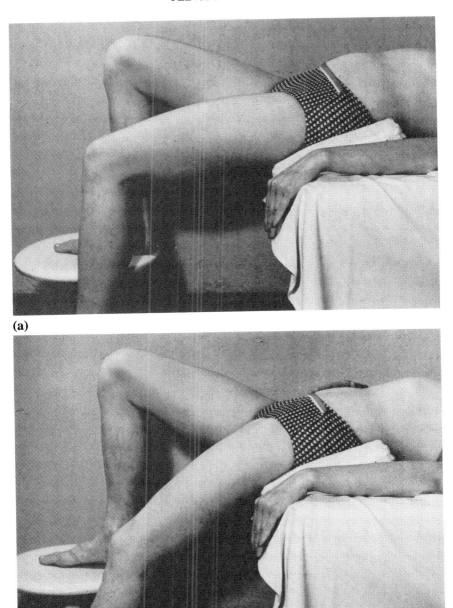

(a)

(b)

Figure 32.10 The symphysis is higher and the ischial tuberosity lower on the same side; correction by gravity-induced PIR of the abdominal muscles producing forward rotation of the innominate

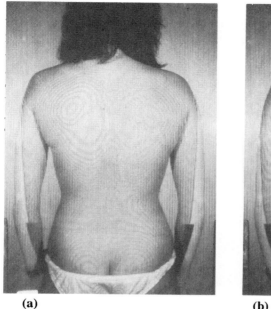
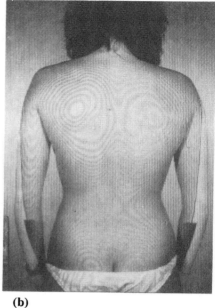

(a)   (b)

Figure 32.11 Moiré pictures of patient B.B. before (a) and after (b) correction of symphyseal shift by torsion manoeuvre: only slight changes at the buttocks, slight improvement in symmetry of the waist line; the greatest change is at the level of the shoulder blades

The main symptoms were low back pain in 43, pain in the lower extremities in 13, diffuse back pain in 5, headache in 7, vertigo in 5, pain in the groin (pelvis) in 4, pain in the hip joint in 3, abdominal pain in 2, neck pain in 2, pain in the upper extremity in 2, a painful calcaneal spur in 2, coccygeal pain in 1, carpal tunnel syndrome in 1 and a painful styloid process at the wrist in 1 patient; 1 was without symptoms.

Treatment of symphyseal shift is technically simple: if the symphysis *and* the ischial tuberosity are higher (lower) on the same side a simple traction movement is applied by which the operator pulls one leg, with his hands round the ankle, and pushes against the other outstretched leg with his thigh, by twisting his pelvis (Figure 32.8). If the symphysis is lower and the tuberosity higher on the same side, the patient lies supine and bends his leg and thigh on that side, so as to bring his knee to his chest. The operator pushes the patient's knee still further towards the patient's chest with his shoulder, while pulling the ischial tuberosity in a ventrocranial direction with his other hand, i.e. rotating the innominate backward (Figure 32.9). If the symphysis is higher and the tuberosity lower on the same side, we want to rotate the innominate forward. This is achieved with the patient supine, his buttocks on the edge of the plinth, the buttock of the treated side supported by a cushion. The leg of the treated side hangs over the edge of the table while the other leg is supported. The patient is told to lift the knee of the free-hanging leg slightly above the horizontal and to breath in slowly, then to hold his breath, let the leg drop, and to breath out. This is repeated 2–3 times. The operator may exert slight pressure from above while the patient lets his knee drop (Figure 32.10).

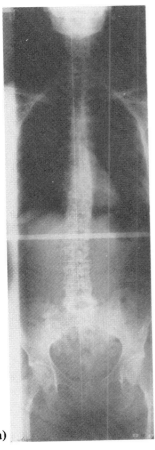 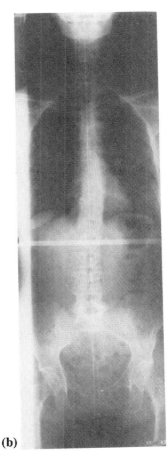

(a)   (b)

Figure 32.12 X-ray of the entire spine (a) before and (b) after correction of the symphysis: improvement of scoliotic curvature and no side-deviation of the head from the plumb-line after treatment

The most striking effect is that both tenderness at the symphysis and trigger points in the m. rectus abdominis clear up at once.

To get a better understanding of what is happening, 12 patients were examined by X-ray using also fluoroscopy. The patients were examined supine, standing and putting their weight on both legs, on the right and then the left leg.

Pictures of the entire spinal column were made before and after manipulation. The most striking effect was on body statics (Figure 32.12) which as a rule, markedly improved; this can be seen even clinically (Figure 32.11). The findings on the pelvis, however, were inconclusive: palpatory findings did not correlate with the X-ray (Figure 32.13) either at the symphysis or at the ischial tuberosity, although, at the latter, differences of about 1 inch could be palpated. This applied both to the apparent changes before and after manipulation and to the differences palpated recumbent or standing (Figure 32.14).

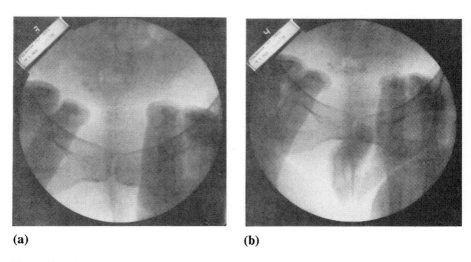

(a)   (b)

Figure 32.13 X-ray of the symphysis and the palpating fingers before (a) and after (b) 'correction': although the position of the bones has not changed, there is less difference in the position of the fingers after treatment

The only reasonable explanation is that mainly soft tissue changes are palpated and modified by our therapy. This has been borne out by recent experience, when mere soft tissue techniques (e.g. pressure on the sacrotuberous ligament) produced the same 'adjustment' on palpation.

The effect on body statics can best be explained by relieving spasm of the abdominal muscle causing a forward drawn position if on both sides and lateral shift if one-sided.

Interestingly, trunk rotation was at times improved after treatment of symphyseal shift, in particular if there was no thoracolumbar movement restriction.

Thus, by distinguishing three different lesions of the pelvis each with its specific therapeutic approach, it is possible to deal with each in a relatively simple way and avoid the confusion of mixing up movement restriction of the sacroiliac joints with certain changes of position in the pelvic girdle that are clinically relevant. This should not exclude some less common modifications and combinations that may occur, in particular after traumatism[16].

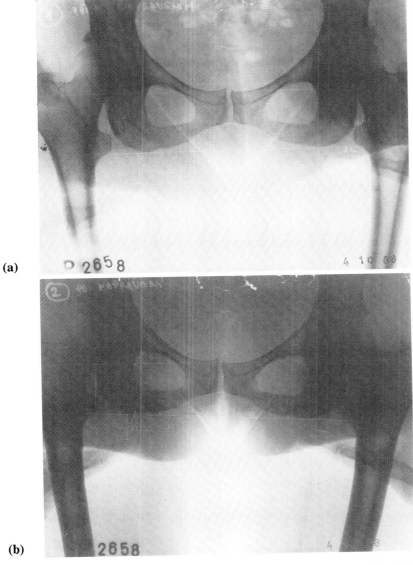

(a)

(b)

Figure 32.14 X-ray of the pelvis with the thumbs palpating the ischial tuberosities, (a) before and (b) after treatment: although the position of the bones has not changed, the position of the thumbs has markedly changed

ACKNOWLEDGEMENTS

Recent progress in the subject of this paper was made possible only by the constant support of the Central Railway Health Institute and its director, Dr V. Okres, and in particular by the X-ray department of the Institute headed by Dr L. Stejskal.

REFERENCES

1. Beal, M.C. (1982). The sacroiliac problem: Review of anatomy, mechanics and diagnosis. *J. Am. Osteopath. Assoc.*, **81**, 667–679
2. Bourdillon, J.F. and Day, E.A. (1987). *Spinal Manipulation*, pp. 58–72. (London: Heinemann)
3. Maigne, R. (1968). *Douleurs d'origine vertébrale et traitments par manipulations*. (Paris: Expansion Scientific Francaise)
4. Mitchell, F.L. Jr., Moran, P.S. and Pruzzo, N.A. (1979). *An Evaluation and Treatment Manual of Osteopathic Muscle Energy Procedures*. (Valley Park, Mo.: Mitchell Moran and Pruzzo Assoc.)
5. Neumann, H.D. (1985). Manuelle Diagnostik und Therapie von Blockierungen der Kreuzdarmbeingelenke nach Mitchell F. *Manuelle Med.*, **23**, 116–126
6. Stoddard, A. (1961). *Manual of Osteopathic Technique*. (London: Hutchinson)
7. Ankermann, K.J. (1982). Die iliosacrale Diskordanz (CISD) eine funktionelle reversible Fehlstellung des Iliosakralgelenks. *Z. Physiother.*, **34**, 377–381
8. Lewit, K. (1987). Beckenverwringung und Iliosakralblockierung. *Manuelle Med.*, **25**, 64–70
9. Kubis, E. (1970). Manualtherapeutische Erfahrungen am Becken. *Manuelle Med.*, **8**, 63–64
10. Cramer, A. (1965). Iliosakralmechanik. *Asklepios*, **6**, 261–262
11. Peper, W. (1953). *Technik der Chiropraktik*. (Heidelberg: Haug)
12. Gutmann, G. (1967). Halwirbelsäule und Manuelle Therapie. In Geiger, Th., Gross, D. (eds.) *Therapie über das Nervensystem, Vol. 7 Manuelle Therapie-Chirotherapie*, pp. 310–343. (Stuttgart: Hippokrates)
13. Dejung, B. (1985). Iliosakralgelenksblockierungen – eine Verlauf studie. *Manuelle Med.*, **23**, 109–115
14. Downing, C.H. (1935). *Osteopathic Principles in Disease*. (San Francisco: Orosco)
15. Schmid, H.J.A. (1985). Iliosacral Diagnose und Behandlung 1978–1982. *Manuelle Med.*, **23**, 101–108
16. Greenman, P.E. (1986). Innominate shear dysfunction in the sacroiliac syndrome. *Manual Med.*, **2**, 114–121
17. Greenman, P.E. and Tait, B. (1988). Structural diagnosis in chronic low back pain. *Manual Med.*, **3**, 114–117

33
Pyriformis muscle syndrome

Franco COMBI, Ivano COLOMBO and Corrado LEUCI

Lumbar pain, with referred symptoms in the gluteal region and legs, is one of the most common presenting complaints in physical medicine. These symptoms are also frequently found without positive results in the usual tests for nerve root involvement (Lasegue, Wassermann, Valleix) or instrumental diagnostic tests (computerized axial tomography, computerized axial tonography with contrast liquid, nuclear magnetic resonance) showing disc pathology.

If one excludes these pathogeneses one must consider that other pathologies exist that present local and referred symptoms similar to nerve root irritation of vertebral origin. One should keep in mind a particular case with painful symptoms in the gluteal region and posterior part of the legs, which has not been written about in great detail – the pyriformis muscle syndrome.

ANATOMY

The pyriformis muscle is a pelvitrochanterian muscle that has 3 bands originating from the edge of the second and third sacral foramina and the grooves near the foramina. It emerges from the pelvis through the greater sciatic notch, splitting it into an inferior and superior section (infrapyriformis and suprapyriformis canals). The tendon of insertion is attached to the superior margin of the intertrochanteric crest, just below the apex of the greater trochanter.

The blood vessels and nerves that emerge from the pelvis cross the suprapyriformis and infrapyriformis canals. The superficial and deep branches of the gluteal artery and the superior gluteal nerve cross over the suprapyriformis canal. The inferior gluteal artery, pudendal nerve, small ischial nerve – which divides into the inferior gluteal nerve (supplying gluteus maximus) and the cutaneous nerve of the leg (sensory nerve) – and the great ischial nerve (mixed nerve) cross over the infrapyriformis canal.

The course of the sciatic nerve, when it emerges from the pelvis, can vary anatomically:

(a)   In approximately 10% of cases the peroneal part penetrates the pyriformis muscle, while the tibial branch passes below it;

(b)   In 2–3% of cases the peroneal branch passes above the superior border and the tibial branch goes below the inferior margin;

(c)   In rare cases (0.8%) the whole sciatic nerve crosses over the pyriformis muscle, which is an external rotator and abductor of the hip with slight extension.

AETIOLOGY

The main cause of this syndrome is the contracture of the muscle and pinching of the vascular–nervous vessels owing to the applied anatomy described above.

It can occur in two cases:

(1)   Within the endopelvis on the anterior surface of the sacrum, causing sacral plexus compression (irritation can be due to an over stretched ampulla recti, a heteroplastic process of an ovarian cyst, or an extrauterine pregnancy), in which case the medial part of the contracted pyriformis muscle can be palpated via the rectum;

(2)   Owing to contracture and peduncle compression at the exit of the pelvis in the infrapyriformis canal (owing to prolonged trunk flexion, which increases muscle tone, or external compression of the buttock, for example by a wallet in a back pocket).

Another pathogenic cause of this syndrome could be contracture of the muscle itself with an unbalanced pelvis.

In his definition of sciatic nerve root irritation, R. Maigne mentions the pyriformis muscle as being one of the muscles 'that can be palpated like a large rope, hard and taut, across the buttock'.

The anatomico-physiological points described justify the assumption that a contracted pyriformis muscle can cause referred pain in the sacroiliac region, buttock, hip, posterior surface of the thigh as far down as the popliteal fossa and the upper part of the posterior surface of the leg, and in rare cases, all of the posterior surface as far as the sole of the foot. The longitudinal referred pain down the back of the leg is similar to that of disc involvement at the S1 level and a differential diagnosis is often very difficult.

The following points are signs of a pyriformis muscle syndrome:

– They are usually peripheral sensations, which vary from day to day or with changes in posture, rather than true painful symptoms;

– They never entirely cover the S1 area and rarely go beyond the popliteal fossa;

- The Lasegue test is not painful; if it is positive the pain disappears with passive external rotation of the hip (which fixes the muscle so that the peduncle ceases to be taut and trapped);
- The Lasegue test gives a different pain response, varying from day to day, unlike sciatic pain with disc involvement;
- The tendon reflexes are normal;
- The computerized axial tomograph, radiculograph, and nuclear magnetic resonance tests of the spine are all normal;
- Pain increases with prolonged sitting.

On objective examination one finds:

- A contracted pyriformis muscle, palpable as a hard and sensitive fusiform structure, situated transversely in the middle of the buttock. A second painful point is less frequently revealed on digital pressure of the lateral part of the buttock and in the supra- and retrotrochanteric regions.
- Painful and limited internal rotation of the hip (normal X-rays) that can be isolated or associated with limited abducton.
- Lombalgia is rare, and when present is of secondary importance.

DIFFERENTIAL DIAGNOSIS

Excluding, for practicality, syndromes due to disc–nerve root conflict, lombalgia due to posterior joint pain, and referred pain from visceral pathology, the most common syndromes to distinguish are as follows:

- *Quadratus lumborum muscle syndrome.* When the contracture involves the lateral, superficial fibres, the pain spreads downwards to the iliac crest and greater trochanter, sometimes to the lower abdomen and groin. When the contracture involves the medial, deep, fibres the pain spreads further back, towards the sacroiliac joint and the medial part of the buttock. Contracture of both the quadrati lumbori gives pain in the dorsal region and all of the buttock.

- *Myofascial gluteus muscle syndrome.* Contracture of all of the gluteal muscles gives rise to pain in the ischial region.

- *Fibrocystic gluteus muscle syndrome.* The referred pain is felt in the same region as the last syndrome.

- *Lumbar ligament syndrome.* Pain at the lumbosacral angle with possible irradiation to the ala of the ilium and inguinal region.

287

- *Sacroiliac ligament syndrome.* Pain in the sacral region with referred pain in the posterior part of the thigh.

- *Peripheral pain syndrome due to painful hip joints.* The pain can radiate to various parts:
  - inguinal region, anterior part of the thigh, knee or upper third of the tibia;
  - greater trochanter and anterior part of the thigh;
  - lower part of the buttock, posterior part of the thigh as far as the popliteal fossa.

THERAPY

Firstly the mechanical factors causing the contracture of the pyriformis muscle must be corrected (unbalanced pelvis due to one leg shortening, small half pelvis, external factors such as wallet compression). Decreased pain and the return to normal function all depend on the resolution of the contracted pyriformis muscle.

The most effective direct treatments, according to use, are fundamentally three:

(1) Injection of 2 ml procaine at 1% plus 3 ml of normal saline into the focal point;
(2) Stretch and spray;
(3) Ischaemic compression.

Injection. This injection with anaesthetic is the elective treatment because it is effective and practical. Resolution is almost immediate. One must repeat Lesser's manoeuvre each time to avoid leaking into the obturator artery.

Stretch and spray. The technique is based on the analgesic effect and inhibition of reflex responses caused by the cold and consequent relaxing of the passive distension of the contracted muscle.

Ischaemic compression. Good results on its own or combined with the stretch and spray technique. It is a simple technique and consists of digital compression on the most painful point of the muscle.

CONCLUSION

Cases of pain in the gluteal region and posterior part of the thigh, when there is no nerve root involvement, can be incorrectly treated by vertebral manipulation, spinal injections and physiotherapy, if diagnosed incorrectly. For this reason we felt it was important to bring attention to the pyriformis muscle syndrome, so that it has its rightful place in the differential diagnosis of low back pain.

34
Iliosacral lesion and the quadratus lumborum syndrome

J.P. RANDERIA

In this short contribution I wish to discuss the importance of the pelvic girdle and its relationship to the spine and the lower extremity. "The pelvic girdle is the cross-roads of the body, the architectural centre of the body, the meeting place of the locomotive apparatus, the resting place of the torso, the temple of the reproductive organs, the abode of the new life's development, the site of the two principal departments of elimination, and, last but not least, a place upon which to sit"[2].

The iliosacral lesion is quite separate from the sacroiliac lesion. In the iliosacral lesion it is the ilium, or rather the innominate bone which includes the ilium, ischium and pubis, that moves. These lesions are usually bilateral. If one ilium moves posterior in its relationship to the sacrum, the opposite ilium, to compensate for this, usually moves anteriorly. Thus, we get what looks like a pelvis twist with the corresponding lesion at the symphysis pubis. The muscles, ligaments and fasciae of the spine are responsible for the sacral movements, while the prime movers of the ilium are the muscles, ligaments of the lower extremity. The pelvis is thus the crossroads between the spine and the lower extremity. The amount of subluxation of the sacroiliac joints is very small. They are reinforced by the powerful ligaments: the sacroiliac, lumbosacral, iliolumbar, sacrotuberous and the sacrospinalis.

INVOLVEMENT OF THE QUADRATUS LUMBORUM MUSCLE

Origin: The quadratus lumborum muscle arises by the aponeurotic fibres from the iliolumbar ligament and the adjacent portion of the iliac crest for about 5 cm.

Insertion: It is inserted into the medial half of the lower border of the last rib and by four small tendons into the apices of the transverse processes of the upper four lumbar vertebrae and at times the fifth lumbar vertebra.

Nerve supply:D12, L1, 2,3 lumbar nerves.

Action: It helps to steady the twelfth rib from the pull of the diaphragm during inspiration.

The iliosacral lesions cause tension in the quadratus lumborum muscle resulting in lesion of the twelfth rib. The involvement of the thoracolumbar region, and the lumbar vertebrae through the quadratus lumborum muscle in time causes irritation of the psoas muscle, resulting in psoas pathology. The transverse processes of the lumbar vertebrae on the side of the lesion are pulled forwards and downwards, thus locking the spine and putting severe strain on the sacroiliac joint. The ilium is rotated posteriorly.

DIAGNOSIS

Loss of motion is the criterion in diagnosis of the osteopathic lesion and not the pain. A painful sacroiliac joint is often caused by a fifth lumbar lesion. Detection of mobility by palpating directly over the sacroiliac joint is impossible.

With the posterior ilium the crest is high, the anterior–superior iliac spine is high, the posterior–superior iliac spine is low, and if not complicated by a lumbar lesion on that side the leg will be shorter. With the anterior ilium, the iliac crest is low, the anterior superior iliac spine is low, the posterior superior iliac spine is high, with a long leg on that side.

LOCAL AND DISTAL SYMPTOMATOLOGY

It is possible to have sacroiliac lesion associated with iliosacral lesion. Any lesion of the ilium would affect the fourth and fifth lumbar vertebrae through the iliolumbar ligament, as well as put severe strain on the hamstring muscles resulting in pain about the knee. Tension in the iliotibial tract and the tensor fascia lata produces tenderness and pain on the lateral aspect of the thigh and at its insertion into the lateral tibial condyle. Tension in the quadratus lumborum D12, L1, 2,3 with the twelfth rib lesion may cause referred pain to the groin and inguinal region.

The pathology in the lumbar spine affects the sacroiliac joints. Thus, in dealing with a pelvic lesion we may have to look to the lumbar area for the primary condition, or the pelvic lesion may be a primary lesion, as from trauma or in women after delivery, etc., or it may be caused by conditions in the lower extremity, e.g. primary short leg, fallen arches, anatomical malformations, dropped cuboid, etc.

Lesions of the ilium cause lesion at the pubic symphysis. In the posterior ilium there is riding up of the crest of pubis on that side with pain and local

290

tenderness. There may be radiation of the pain in the groin, perinium and down the medial side of the thigh. Where there is sacrococcygeal strain either by trauma or by sacroiliac lesion due to sacrotuberous and sacrospinalis ligaments, the correction of the sacroiliac lesions helps a great deal in easing the tension of the coccyx. Iliac lesion could affect the hip joint mechanism resulting in time in its degeneration. The involvement of the gluteal muscles especially the pyriformis may affect the sciatic nerve, causing sciatica. Specific osteopathic manipulation of the sacroiliac joints has helped in relieving such pain.

TREATMENT

Before attempting correction of the pelvic lesions one has to ascertain the primary and secondary lesions. Treating the secondary lesions by soft-tissue articulation and correction to restore the free movement would help to reduce the strain on the primary lesion. Exercises to correct the postural deformities as well as occupational deformities should be given. After mobilizing all compensation, attempt to correct the primary lesion. Homoeopathic medicines – colocynth, nux vomica, rhus-tox, bryonia, etc. – in high potencies have been of great help.

SUMMARY

An attempt has been made to show the importance of the sacroiliac joint in the production of low back pathology. The pelvis is the cross-roads between the spine and the lower extremities. The pelvic lesion involves the thoracopelvic group of muscles (i.e. the quadratus lumborum), the lumbofemoral group (i.e. the iliopsoas) and the pelvic–femoral group (i.e. the gluteal and hamstring muscles). The latissimus dorsi muscle may also be mentioned.

Because of extensive nerve supply, the pain may be referred to a wide area.

Local and remote symptomatology is discussed and diagnosis outlined. General methods of treatment are discussed.

REFERENCES AND FURTHER READING

1. Gray, H. (1958). *Human Anatomy*
2. Mitchell, F.L. (1965). *Structural Pelvic Function*. (Carmel, CA: Academy of Applied Osteopathy)
3. Randeria, J.P. (1974). The role of the psoas muscle in low back pathology. *J. Man. Med.*, **4**

35
The cervico-lumbar syndrome

H. BIEDERMANN

Low back pain literature fills entire walls – an indication of the clinical importance of the problem. Two thirds of the cases commonly considered as 'vertebrogenic' are localized in the lumbar region[3], and almost everybody will undergo a attack of low back pain some time[15].

Being of considerable interest to all of us, many diagnostic and therapeutic approaches have been made to this problem. Alas, it has proved to be quite elusive. The intervertebral disc played its role as a main villain for some decades, and since the 1950s we have known about the importance of ligamental overstrain[10,13]. To remind readers of the importance of lumbar blockages or malfunctions of the sacroiliac joints seems a little superfluous. But still there are problem cases that this pathogenic framework does not seem to cover, especially as the enthusiasm for operations faded with every long-term study published.

DEFINITION

We define the cervico-lumbar syndrome as a clinical entity in which lumbar symptoms are mainly triggered and maintained by functional disorders of the occipito-cervical joints. Best proof is *ex juvantibus* the subsiding of the patient's complaints, but some anamnestic and clinical signs attract our attention to this cause.

In the 1930s DeKleijn and Nieuwenhuyse published on the influence of the neck afferents on vertigo[4]. Gutmann documented the importance of this region in dorso-lumbar ailments in 1957[6]; the underlying neurophysiological mechanisms are much better understood today, as anatomical[2], biomechanical[17] and neurophysiological research[5,14,18] help us to replace educated guesses by logical reasoning. Short pathways to the formatio reticularis, and close connections with the centres responsible for the programming of the postural muscles[8] explain the immediate effect of blockages between C0 and C3 on postural stability[1].

The significance of functional disorders of the cervico-occipital joints for headaches, brachialgia or pain in the neck and upper thorax is accepted and documented; their influence on lumbar syndrome is less well known.

The problem in the differential diagnosis stems from the 'monolayer' approach: we are used to ask for one principal reason, and, being visual animals, we look for a visible proof. Furthermore, we prefer a local reason to something farther away, especially when mechanical factors are involved.

Very often, the upper cervical spine is the leading factor in the generation of lumbar pain but acts through a local 'relay station'. This role can be taken over by all the classical reasons for sciatic pain, e.g. lumbar osteochondrosis, ligamentous insufficiency, morphological asymmetry or even the degenerated disc. Treating these local co-factors can also be successful, but it takes time. We do not wish to discourage this local therapy but to complement it with the treatment of the upper cervical spine to maximize efficiency and minimize morbidity.

A QUANTITATIVE TEST

Having known for some time that lumbar syndromes respond favourably to the manipulation of the occipito-cervical joints, we decided to check the effect by examining the patients of the 'spinal column consultation' of our out-patient clinic. We asked the patients to compare their situation before and 3–4 weeks after the treatment (when they came back for the follow-up examination). After that, additional therapies were applied, for example physiotherapy, local injections, electrotherapy, re-education of motor patterns, etc. We decided to form groups based on the first interview and to define the patients suffering from a cervico-lumbalgia by several parameters (Table 35.1).

Table 35.1 Criteria for the selection of patients with 'cervico-lumbar syndrome'

- Age between 15 and 45 years (mean, 26 years)
- Purely 'lumbar' symptoms
- No signs of radicular irritation
- No accompanying diseases
- No morphological findings on radiographies
- Manipulation of upper cervical spine the only treatment

The patients were sent by local practitioners (73%) or came themselves on the advice of friends or relatives (27%). Taking into account that the allotment was somewhat arbitrary, as there are no sharp distinctions between the groups, the overall distribution was as follows. Children below the age of 15 were excluded because their complaints are in almost every case not confined to the low back (including them would have made our success rate much higher[7]); patients over 45 years of age were excluded because morphological changes are

293

almost certain beyond that age and tend to dominate the clinical picture.

As it is almost impossible to devise a strict methodology with a double-blind approach we decided to compare the isolated effect of manual therapy of the upper cervical spine on the subjective wellbeing of the patients.

The main mechanism through which the occipito-cervical joints exert a pathological influence along the entire length of the spine and beyond* is the alteration of postural coordination by wrong input. The asymmetrical tonic neck reflexes, normally subsiding in the first year[5], can be documented in some of these patients[11]. The younger the patient, the more malleable are his/her motor patterns, and the farther the effects of disturbances in the upper cervical spine.

Table 35.2 Patients of the 'spinal column consultation' between 1/86 and 12/88

Main diagnosis	n	%
Cervico-lumbar syndrome	81	12.0
Low back pain of ligamentous or statical origin	168	24.9
Root syndromes (cervical or lumbar)	32	4.7
Dorsalgia	35	5.2
Cervico-cephalgia	183	27.1
Cervico-brachialgia	127	18.8
None of the above	49	7.3
Total	675	100.0

Table 35.3 Age distribution of patients with 'cervico-lumbar syndrome'

Age group (y)	n	%
15–20	21	25.9
21–25	17	21.0
26–30	13	16.0
31–35	8	9.9
36–40	8	9.9
41–45	14	17.3

Mean = 26

The examination of the radiographs often reveals signs of old traumata, and quite regularly the patients will not remember this incident, even after intense questioning. Typical signs for old traumata are:

*Diffuse knee-pains in adolescents are typically caused by functional disorders of the upper cervical spine unless there is trauma or tumour.

294

- Distinct dislocation of atlas and/or axis in the frontal plane;
- Signs of segmentally isolated rotation between occiput and atlas and/or between atlas and axis;
- Interruption of the harmony of the orientation of the vertebrae, i.e. sudden bends or marked steps, sometimes accompanied by discrete signs of soft-tissue lesions;
- Pseudo-physiological posture of the head, i.e. head tilted to one side with or without rotation, when asked to look straight.

Trauma plays an important role in the genesis of a typical cervico-lumbar syndrome. The causal connection is not always easy to trace, as long intervals without any symptoms are quite common. What for many patients does not count as a 'real' trauma is quite enough to stigmatize the cervical spine. The stress and mutilation the cervical spine undergoes during labour adds to that[12], and of the 81 patients in our group 31 remembered a complicated birth.

The vertebral column is *not* a string of vertebrae, with – at best – the occipito-cervical joint as *primus inter pares* but a hierarchically structured organ. Its performance is determined by the integrity and stability of the static base at L5/S1 *and* the optimal function of the sensomotor centre at C0/C1. The intricate interaction between these two poles determines the performance of the vertebral spine and thus the central component of man's musculoskeletal system. These ideas are nothing new, and are well accepted in these general terms.

As soon as these general truths are used in a concrete clinical concept, the disagreement starts: one group tends to treat all painful and/or mechanically restricted segments, whereas others try to find the main culprit, starting the therapy there. Adhering to the latter concept, I try to start with the pivotal regions of the vertebral spine before looking more closely at the segments in between. Lewit repeatedly stressed the importance of establishing a priority list of segments of the vertebral spine: most important is the craniocervical junction, followed by the lumbosacroiliac junction, and the other levels of the spinal column following behind . . . *"Therefore such a disturbance should never be overlooked even if the symptoms are manifest at the other end of the spinal column, or even in the extremities"*[13] – easier said than done.

TREATMENT

We used impulse (thrust) manipulation based on the functional analysis of radiographs of the cervical spine as the only treatment. In our group of 81 patients all further therapy was discouraged between the first examination and the follow-up. Thereafter we made concessions to patient's preferences, prescribing electrotherapy, fango, physiotherapy, etc. Our analysis is therefore based on the patients' response to our questions 3 weeks after therapy. This excludes all cases where additional therapy was inevitable, thereby distorting the picture. Our main comparison is with the (unsuccessful) therapy the patient underwent before they were admitted.

CLINICAL PICTURE

The 'typical' patient with a cervico-lumbar syndrome is in good physical shape continues his professional and private activities and has already consulted various generalists and specialists (mostly orthopaedics, neurologists, specialist in sports medicine (Ø 3.5)). In roughly half of the cases a significant trauma can be established in the case history, but only very few (under 15%) mention this trauma spontaneously.

Symptoms are centred around the low back. The younger patients also mention pain in the knees, and dorsal pain. When asked if anteflexion and/or rotation of the head influenced the symptoms, 38% answer positively. Some patients remember periods of back pain during childhood that subsided spontaneously or after physiotherapy. In these cases a trigger-event can often be found, be it a new trauma, occupational changes like new jobs, or exceptionally demanding work (renovation of a house or sports events). These event preceded the symptoms by days or weeks.

Table 35.4 Therapies applied prior to admittance to our consultation. Mean duration of previous therapy: 20 months

Local heat (e.g. fango, IR)	83%
Electrotherapy, microwave, etc.	65%
Lumbar manipulation	42%
Kinesitherapy (active)	36%
Kinesitherapy (passive)	78%
Medicaments	
Oral (mostly antiphlogistica)	76%
Injections (local and i.m.)	41%

Many show signs of impaired function of the cervical spine, like restricted range of movement, and painful trigger points at the processus transversi of the upper cervical vertebrae. Often the deep palpation of the m. psoas is painful uni or bilaterally (Kubis' test), and the lateral abduction of the hip is restricted (Patrick test). Restricted mobility of the lumbar spine (Schober's sign) or a *pseudo*-Lasegue is noted.

PRACTICAL CONSEQUENCES

We examine and treat the cervical spine of *all* younger patients, regardless of the character of their complaints. The same is true for the lumbo-sacral region, which is always examined and treated, even if the symptoms are purely 'cervical'.

We begin with the occipito–cervical joint, and – if not forced by circumstances – prefer to delay the evaluation of postural imbalances for the lumbo-sacral area till the effect of the cervical manipulation is clear, normally after 3 weeks. Very often, clinically diagnosed leg-length differences, blockages of the lumbo-sacral joints, or gait anomalies disappear after the treatment of the occipito-cervical joints.

This therapeutic approach saves a lot of expense, and saves the patients quite some time. Since the public is more aware of the side-effects of drugs, patients are especially grateful to no longer depend on them. But it is *not* a universal cure for all forms of low back pain; it does not replace the well-known and effective therapies. The optimization of the biomechanics of the upper cervical spine clears the ground, and removes obstacles to help other methods to reach their goal. Prevention of unfavourable posture during work and leisure supplements any successful therapy of the low back pain.

Table 35.5 Effect of one manipulation of the upper cervical spine; patient's reply at control 20–30 days after treatment

	n	Percentage
Without problems and 'a lot better'	52	64
Improvement	15	19
The same	14	17
Total	81	100

Table 35.6 Clinical findings before and immediately after manipulation of the cervico-occipital joints

Symptoms	Before		After	
	n	%	n	%
'Cervical' symptoms (asked for)	55	68	–	–
Traumata of cervical spine	43	54	–	–
Functional disability of the cervical spine	67	85	23	29
Lumbar imbalance	28	35	18	22
Blockage of lumbar sacroiliac joints	55	68	34	42
Patrick test ≥ 1/3 reduced	47	58	18	22
Rubis' test positive	60	75	40	50
Pseudo-Lasegue (> 40°)	42	54	21	26

THE FUTURE

Having pointed out the methodological pitfalls of our study, we are about to objectify the measurements by using a dynamic 4-quadrant-weight scale connected to a computer[16]. Given sufficient funding (applications are under way) we hope to repeat this series in the next 2 years.

SUMMARY

Case histories and statistical material are presented to emphasize the pathogenic potential of the upper cervical spine on 'common' low back pain and radicular symptoms of the lumbar spine. Acting mostly as an amplifier of a local disorder it proves in many cases that this pathogenic factor is most easily treatable especially in younger patients, even without complaints of cervical symptoms. Neurophysiological and anatomical information supporting this is reviewed. The importance of a correct radiological and postural analysis of the individual case is stressed.

Examination and manipulation of the upper cervical spine can have a decisive or supporting role in the successful treatment and should be routinely considered, at least with patients aged under 40 and/or with cervical trauma in the anamnesis.

REFERENCES

1. Brügger, A. (1977). *Die Erkrankungen des Bewegungsapparats und seines Nervensystem* (Stuttgart: Fischer)
2. Christ, B., Jacob, H.J. and Seifert, R. (1988). Über die Entwicklung der zervikookzipitale Übergangsregion. In Hohmann, D. *et al.* (eds) *Neuro-Orthopädie*, Vol.4. (Berlin: Springer Verlag)
3. Junghanns, H. (1986). *Die Wirbelsäule unter den Einflüsssen des täglichen Lebens, der Freizeit des Sports,*, Wirbelsäule in Forschung und Praxis Vol, 100. (Stuttgart: Hippokrates)
4. DeKleijn, A. and Nieuwenhuyse, A.C. (1927). Schwindelanfälle und Nystagmus bei einer bestimmten Stellung des Kopfes. *Acta OtoLaryng.*, **11**, 155–164
5. Flehming, I. (1979). *Normale Entwicklung des Säuglings und ihre Abweichungen.* (Stuttgart Thieme)
6. Gutmann, G. (1972). Kasuistik zum Problem der muskelreflektorischen Steuerung m Fernwirkung. *Man. Med.*, **10**, 121–124
7. Gutmann, G. (1987). Das Atlas- Blockierungs-Syndrom des Säuglings und des Kleinkinde *Man. Med.*, **25**, 5–10
8. Gutmann, G. and Véle, F. (1969) Die Gelenke der oberen HWS und ihre Einwirkung au motorische Stereotypen. In Wolff, H.D. (ed) *Wiss Grundlagen der Manuellen Medizin* (Heidelberg: Fischer-Verlag)
9. Gutmann, G. and Biedermann, H. (1984). *Die Halswirbelsäule: Allgemeine funktionell. Pathologie und klinische Syndrome.* (Stuttgart: Fischer)
10. Hackett, G.S. (1957). Referred pain and sciatica in diagnosis of low back pain disability. *J. An Med. Assoc.*, **163**, 183–189
11. Hülse, M. (1983). *Die zervikalen Gleichgewichtsstörungen.* (Berlin: Springer-Verlag)
12. Kurrek, H. (1982). Die mikrozirkulatorische Belastung des menschlichen Gehirns bei de Geburt. Speech at Münster University, Physiological Institute

13. Lewit, K. (1985). *Manipulative Therapy in Rehabilitation of the Motor System*. (London: Butterworths)
14. Norré, M.E. (1976). Der Zervikalnystagmus und die Gelenkblockierungen. *Man. Med.*, **14**, 45–51
15. Rothman, R.H., Simeone, F.A. and Bernini, P.M. (1982). *Lumbar Disc Disease – The Spine*. (Philadelphia: W.B. Saunders)
16. Stevens, A., Roselle, N. and Jacobs, C. (1982). A test bench for the spine. *Osteo. Ann.*, **10**, 572–578
17. Suh, C.H. (1981). Computer-aided spinal biomechanics. In Haldeman, S. (ed.) *Modern Developments in the Principles and Practice of Chiropractic*. (New York: Appleton-Century-Crofts)
18. Thoden, U. and Mergner, T. (1988). Propriozeptoren der oberen Kopfgelenke: Bedeutung für Augenbewegungen und Schwindel. In Hohmann, D. *et al.* (eds.) *Neuro-Orthopädie 4*. (Berlin: Springer-Verlag)

36

Clinical application of the basic physical principles for the use of mobilization and manipulation

E. RYCHLÍKOVÁ

It is not possible merely to demonstrate mechanically the basic therapeutic procedures of mobilization and manipulation, and simply to correct the actions of colleagues who are learning these procedures. Without understanding, and especially without the use of basic physical principles in mastering these procedures, it is very difficult to achieve their maximum effect and therapeutic value.

Just as it is difficult to find two absolutely identical individuals, it is equally difficult to find two individuals who have absolutely the same size fingers, feet, muscles and other bodily proportions. For this reason, the overall effect of manipulative procedures can be realized on two individuals only roughly to the same degree. Besides this, there is a biological difference between manipulation carried out by a woman or a man.

We must therefore seek generally valid principles that characterize the process and permit us to comprehend it.

If we are to carry out the mutual shift movement of two opposing joint facets, the following prerequisites must exist from a physical point of view:

(1)   The object we are concerned with must be correctly stabilized.
(2)   The correct conditions must be established for the effect of the force; these are generally characterized as force acting as a vector.
(3)   Since we are dealing with a procedure lasting for a specific period of time, it is necessary for its successful realization to establish a time characteristic or a time limit for the effect of the force or its change in time (brief pressure, gradually increasing pressure, suddenly acting, decline, etc).

STABILIZATION OF THE OBJECT

In carrying out the mobilization and manipulation of the joint, the aim of the external force is to bring about such a movement in the joint as will result in the mutual movement of the bones making up the joint. This mutual movement is very small. A condition for achieving movement in the joint is that one bone forming part of the joint must be fixed in an optimal position to act on the other bone. Fixation in an optimal position is referred to as *mechanical stabilization*. In short, the mechanical stabilization of the object is an absolute condition for carrying out the manipulation. Stabilization is shown schematically in Figure 36.1.

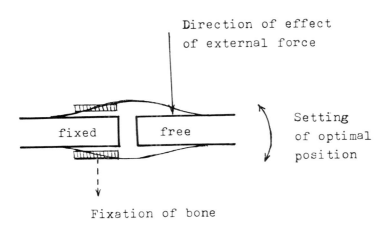

Figure 36.1 Schematic representation of the stabilization and effect of force

As well as mechanical stabilization, it is absolutely necessary to ensure *psychological stabilization*. This means achieving maximal relaxation of the patient.

WHAT IS UNDERSTOOD AS THE CORRECT CONDITIONS FOR THE EFFECT OF FORCE

The process of manipulation or mobilization *per se* is, from a general point of view, the effect of force on a particular area. As is generally known, force is a vector and for it to have effect it is necessary to know the location, direction and magnitude of that effect. These three parameters are important for the success of the action.

LOCATION OF THE FORCE EFFECT

The location is very important in the success of mobilization and manipulation. In manipulation, even a very small shift from the optimal point of effect considerably increases the need to use greater force for a given manipulation. In manipulation, the use of great force leads to the transfer of the effect to a broader area than is necessary, and thus to losing the effect of the directed manipulation.

Figure 36.2 presents a schematic view of a joint. The force is to be aimed at the free part of the joint. In our case, if we put pressure on point A, we basically affect the mutual movement of the joints areas, with a minimal rotation effect because the length of the arm is close to zero.

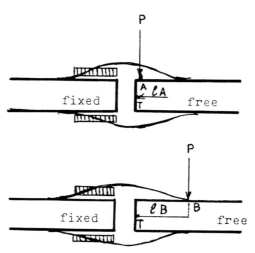

Figure 36.2 Location of the effect of the force

If the force is put on point B, the rotation component is considerably greater in the proportion of the ratio $l_A{:}l_B$. For example, if l_A is 2 mm and l_B is 12 mm, we see that the rotation component is increased six times at point B, with the use of the same force, as at point A.

This general discussion shows how moving the point of force by a few millimetres can considerably change the effect on the joint and thus also influence the success of the manipulation. In reality, the phenomenon is far more complicated, since it involves a space phenomenon (three-dimensional) and not, as our schematic diagram shows, only a flat, two-dimensional one. To this we must add the anatomical arrangement and peculiarities of the joint.

DIRECTION OF THE FORCE EFFECT

Beginners in our field have considerable difficulty in selecting the right direction of the force and pressure. It is interesting that bad habits acquired during the learning of manipulation have their roots in the wrong direction of the effect of the force. It is difficult to rid oneself of these habits; what is more, such people act very rigidly when carrying out the manipulation because they do it very painstakingly and thus with considerable effort.

If we again use for our illustration a simplified two-dimensional diagram (Figure 36.3), then force P, if it acts upon point C in the direction of the arrow, diffuses its effect into the axis of the bone, that is, in the X direction, and in the vertical direction to the axis of the bone, that is in the Y-direction. Diffusion of force P in the direction of the axes resolves it into its components P_x and P_y. The pressure component P_x is minimal and approaches zero (see the third force parallelogram). Mathematically,

$$P_x = P \cos \alpha$$
$$P_y = P \cos \beta$$

We can say that if α approaches 90°, then β approaches 0. Then $\cos \alpha = 0$ and $\cos \beta = 1$, which are the conditions for the optimal direction of the force and the size of their components. We can then write

$$P_x = 0 \quad \text{and} \quad P_y = P$$

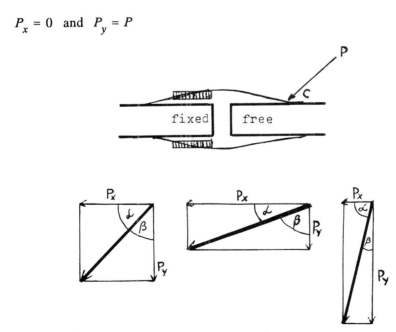

Figure 36.3 Direction of the effect of the force

303

If this presumption is not fulfilled, component P_x has a very negative influence on the mobilization and manipulation action, since it increases the specific force between the two segments and thus makes more difficult the mutual shifting movement of the segments. This is also the cause of difficulties in mobilization and manipulation if force S_x, created by the muscle spasm, comes into play at the same time. The manipulative force must then be directed so as to act against force S_x. The ideal should be $P_x = S_x$ (Figure 36.4). The resulting force, made up of force S_x and P is P_y, which acts in the direction of the y-axis. This type of manipulation with a 'negative directional effect' is difficult; it requires practise and experience. For a better understanding of the problem, intentionally chose the state of an ideally evenly spread muscle spasm. In all other instances, the action is considerably more complicated.

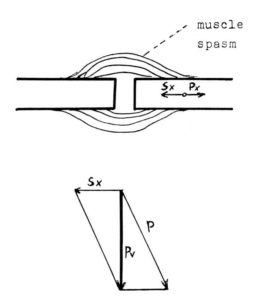

Figure 36.4 Effect on the force of muscle spasm

Theoretically, there is only a very small area of directional diffusion for achieving optimal effects of the acting force combined with an optimal therapeutic effect. That is why two people can do the 'same' and yet the result can be very different.

Many doctors, and especially those who have not undergone any course in manipulation and who proceed only on the basis of what they have observed, are not aware of these facts. An experienced doctor of manual medicine knows from the behaviour and attitude of the patient (conditioned by fear of manipulation and from his own preparation for the manipulation, that the patient has been manipulated by an untrained person. It is interesting that manipulation is carried out even by those doctors who are outstanding specialists in their field and who themselves condemn dilletantism or amateurism.

The conclusion, therefore, is that an optimal technique is a technique that brings results in the optimal direction, place and magnitude. In order for this condition to be met, the physicians carrying out manipulation would have to be of the same size and strength. However, these would not be people but figurines. That is why each physician must develop his own specific technique that is guided by the general principles of the optimal effect of force and is adjusted to the specifics of the person carrying out the manipulation. Proof of the correctness of this thesis is the fact that some colleagues have their own personally adjusted manipulation methods that suit them and are therefore effective. On the other side are those, who, in too slavishly attempting to carry out manipulation by precisely copying their instructor, do not achieve good results because they have not adjusted their methods to their own specific traits and abilities.

37

Non-inflammatory joint pain in rheumatoid arthritis: the diagnostic role of intra-articular anaesthesia in the understanding of brachiogenic shoulder pain

K. HIEMEYER and H. MENNINGER

INTRODUCTION

Patients with rheumatoid arthritis (RA) frequently complain of shoulder pain (SP). Local treatment of the shoulder often shows little effect. In patients with RA shoulder pain is not automatically caused by omarthritis. Nevertheless, two recently published studies[1,2] concerning painful shoulder in patients with RA do not differentiate which mechanism results in SP, and assume a local inflammatory process.

By a detailed mode of clinical examination[3] it is possible to localize shoulder pain exactly into the joint or extra-articular tissues, i.e. tendons, muscles and bursae. If pain is found to be located in tendons or muscles, there need not necessarily exist local damage in this structure. Bruegger[4,5] postulates a functional-regulatory guarding mechanism of the CNS that can result in muscular pain ('reflex tendomyopathy'). Apart from local muscular pain caused by over-use or inflammation (with local irritation of nociceptors), and apart from referred pain, there may exist a third type of pain in the muscular system: reflex tendomyopathy, centrally controlled tendo-muscular pain (CCTMP). This kind of muscular pain seems to be very common. Its function appears to be to protect damaged structures by blocking those movements that would increase irritation of nociceptors in these structures:

- Muscles that increase irritation of nociceptors by contraction become *hypotone* tendomyotic (i.e. painful during contraction – the patient feels painful muscular fatigue);

– Muscles that by contraction diminish this irritation become *hypertone* tendomyotic (i.e. painful while relaxing – the patient feels painful stiffness).

The patient very often suffers mostly from the regulatory painful muscle (efference). For a causal treatment, however, one must look for the site of irritation of nociceptors (afference). The site of painful muscle is very often distant from the site of nociceptor activity. If pain in the efference disappears after anaesthesia in the afference, the functional nature of this pain is proved.

We found in patients with RA that SP often disappeared after local injection of cortisone or after synoviorthese in a wrist joint. A regulatory mechanism could cause the phenomenon. Muscles moving the shoulder have an effect on elbow and wrist as well, and can increase nociceptor activity in these joints. According to the Bruegger theory, the CNS might try to stop movement of the shoulder by making it painful.

In order to verify this theory, and because SP is very common in patients with RA, we wanted to know whether SP is improved by intra-articular anaesthesia of an inflamed distal joint.

METHODS

Patients suffering from RA were selected for this study if they met the following criteria:

– History of painful shoulder for 4 weeks or longer;
– Absence of palpable swelling in painful shoulder;
– Active abduction of shoulder limited to at least 120°;
– Arthritis of ipsilateral wrist or elbow joint.

Examination of the shoulder included palpation, active and passive movement, as well as isometric muscle tests. Subsequently the inflamed ipsilateral wrist or elbow joint was *injected* intra-articularly with 2 ml of 1% mepivacaine. Five minutes after injection *active abduction* was assessed again and improvement was classified as

– Absent: gain in abduction less than 30°;
– Partial: gain in abduction more than 30°;
– Complete: abduction 170° or more.

In addition, subjective improvement of pain in active abduction was evaluated by the patient to be absent, partial or complete.

RESULTS

Forty patients fulfilling the criteria were examined. We found SP to be localized in the supraspinus muscle in 17 patients, in the infraspinus muscle in 5, and in subscapularis or biceps muscle in 1 patient each. After injection 36 patients (90%) showed partial or complete improvement of active abduction and subjective pain:

No pain, abduction completely improved	9	patients
No pain, abduction partially improved	10	patients
Pain partially and elevation completely improved	5	patients
Pain and abduction partially improved	12	patients
No improvement	4	patients

Figure 37.1 shows the active abduction before and after injection of wrist or elbow.

active
abduction
before IA

active
abduction
after IA

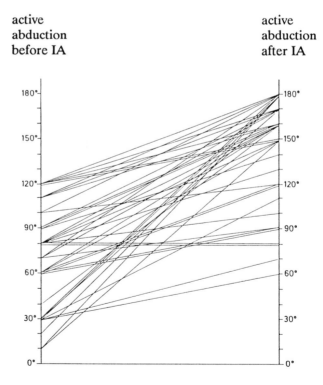

Figure 37.1 Active abduction of shoulder before and after intra-articular anaesthesia (IA) of inflamed wrist or elbow joint in 40 patients with rheumatoid arthritis

DISCUSSION

Shoulder pain in RA is usually believed to result from inflammation, i.e. arthritis in humeroscapular or acromioclavicular joints, inflammatory involvement of the rotatory cuff or tenosynovitis of the biceps tendon[1,2,6]. Our results, however, suggest that SP may very often be localized in muscles and tendons and in a high percentage immediately responds to intra-articular anaesthesia (IA) of a distal inflamed joint. Apparently, anaesthesia stops irritation of nociceptors in these joints (afference) and so the pain in the shoulder (efference) ceases. This would be an explanation for prompt improvement of pain and mobility in the ipsilateral shoulder without local treatment. Shoulder pain is then a centrally controlled tendo-muscular pain (CCTMP) theory described above.

IA of a joint distant to the site of muscular pain is a diagnostic method to prove the reflex nature of a tendomuscular pain syndrome and to identify the supposed site of nociception (afference). The favourable response usually lasts only for several hours. Thus, IA in these cases must be understood as a diagnostic rather than therapeutic tool. IA helps to localize the site of further therapy.

Our results support the hypothesis that there exists CCMP as a common pain mechanism different from local nociceptor pain and from referred pain with a segmental distribution. IA appears to be helpful in characterizing this recently described type of pain[4] and should encourage both clinicians and neuro-physiologists to determine the methods by which it can be clearly recognized.

SUMMARY

We examined 40 patients with rheumatoid arthritis suffering from painful shoulder. While the shoulder itself was not treated, mepivacaine was injected into an arthritic joint of wrist or elbow. In 36 out of 40 patients we achieved full or partial improvement of pain and movement of the shoulder.

We conclude that pain in the shoulder of these patients was caused by a regulatory mechanism, triggered by nociceptors in an arthritic distal joint in order to protect this damaged structure. The therapeutic consequence implies treatment of the distal joint rather than treatment of the painful shoulder itself.

REFERENCES

1. Peterson, C.J. (1986). Painful shoulders in patients with rheumatoid arthritis. *Scand. J. Rheumatol.*, **15**, 275–279
2. Petri, M., Dobrow, R., Neiman, R., O'Keefe, Q.W.S. and Seaman, W.E. (1987) Randomized, double-blind, placebo-controlled study of the treatment of the painful shoulder. *Arthr. Rheum.*, **30**, 1040–1045
3. Cyriax, J. (1982). *Textbook of Orthopaedic Medicine, Volume 1: Diagnosis of Soft Tissue Lesions.*

(London: Bailliere Tindall)
4. Brügger, A. (1980). *Die Erkrankungen des Bewegungsapparates und seines Nervensystems*, 2nd edn. (Stuttgart: Fischer)
5. Brügger, A. (1987). Die Funktionskrankheiten des Bewegungsapparates: Ein neues Konzept für häufige Schmerzsyndrome. *Akt. Rheumatol.*, **12**, 314–319
6. Ennevaara, K. (1967). Painful shoulder joint in rheumatoid arthritis. *Acta Rheumatol. Scand.*, Suppl. II, 10–86
7. Hiemeyer, K., Joist, R. and Menninger, H. (1989). Nachweis der funktionellen Genese von Schulterschmerzen bei chronischer Polyarthritis (CP) durch diagnostische Lokalanästhesie entzündeter distaler Gelenke. Eine Pilot-Studie. *Z. Rheumatol.*, **48**, 139–143

38
The foot and manual medicine

Patrick DEMMA

I here present a new and original technique of podology that we have been practising for the last few years with Dr R.J. Bourdiol. In this technique, the foot is regarded as one of the most essential links of the reflex orthostatic system. The foot is the basis of the somatic edifice. I intend to demonstrate that a manual or reflex orthopaedic treatment of the foot allows somatic modifications.

First, let us examine the high-order control of this reflex system: the cerebellar. Cerebellar control has functions of automatic regulation on equilibration, mobility, coordination of movement, muscular tonus of posture. Also, it regulates orthostatism.

Besides this high-level control, there is local muscular and tendinous control named the 'gamma system'. This is a system in which a proprioceptor is sensitive to muscular extensions – its response to the muscular strain is a muscle contraction. Against this stimulative proprioceptor is opposed an inhibitive proprioceptor set on the tendinous insertion of the same muscle. This inhibitive receptor will short-circuit the muscular contraction induced by the stimulative receptor when the contraction is excessive. The local reflex system is under the control of the cerebellum, spinal cord and the neurovegetative system.

These are the qualities of the stimulative and inhibitive proprioceptors that we shall use for the manual and orthopaedic techniques. Moreover, vertebral manipulations use the inhibitive proprioceptor's relaxing effect. Muscular reconstructions use the stimulative proprioceptor's tonic effect. These two manual techniques also can be used for feet. Regarding orthopaedic techniques it is easily understood that a wedge set under a muscular body (an area where there are only stimulative proprioceptors) will increase the general and podal muscular tonus, whereas a wedge set on a tendinous area where there are only inhibitive proprioceptors will be relaxing for muscle.

Given these considerations, we laid down a protocol of clinical investigation covering measurement, footprints and muscular palpation. Usually, a patient standing in reference posture touches a plumb line in three places: at the occiput, the sacrum and the scapulum, and the interscapulary zone. This plumb line determines the cervical and lumbar lordosis distances that are normal for the adult man: 6 cm for cervical and 4 cm for lumbar. These norms admit

311

physiological variations that we need to know: in children, women and the obese, for example. Other measurements allow us to discover somatic deformations, twisting pelvis, or short leg. Muscular palpation and footprints are also very important in informing us about aetiology and amelioration or aggravation of the pathology.

From the pathological point of view we may sum up neurophysiology as follows. In vertical posture, the cutaneous proprioceptors of pressure and those of the feet muscles inform the cerebellar central control about muscular contraction. The cerebellar control replies immediately to all excitation by general and local muscular tonus adaptation, either by stimulation or inhibition. Thus, we can see that two kinds of syndrome may affect the patients:

– one in which pathology concerns stimulative proprioceptor tonic function: we shall call this hypotonic syndrome or involutional syndrome;
– another in which pathology concerns the inhibitive function of tendinous proprioceptors: we shall call this hypertonic syndrome or allergenic syndrome.

HYPOTONIC OR INVOLUTIONAL SYNDROME

This syndrome will be acquired, affecting a weakened patient, for example during puberty, pregnancy, menopause, nervous breakdown, or infectious diseases. We notice a weakening then a breakdown of the muscular podal and somatic tonus with valgus foot, internal rotation of the legs, hypotonic pelvis, anterior projection of the lumbar rachis and the abdomen, with the principal sign of the scapulum being behind the sacrum. These patients will suffer from mechanical pain because the kinetic muscles have to palliate the static muscles. These patients will suffer from podalgia and also from gonalgia taking a course towards gonarthrocace, lumbago and most of all dorsalgia. These patients often have shoulder pains since their shoulders are not maintained in place by muscles.

All these pains increase with effort and decrease during rest, but no manipulative techniques could cure the dorsalgia or scapulo-humeral periarthritis affecting patients whose shoulders are bending forwards. Such periarthritis is very often attributed to the menopause or to nervous breakdown. This is correct, but it is on account of the disturbance of the tonus posture.

A podological treatment should always be associated with all manual techniques. It will have to be tonic, either manual or with a small wedge set under a podal muscle body. The immediately improved modification of the cervical and lumbar lordoses will indicate the correct area for the wedge.

HYPERTONIC OR ALLERGENIC SYNDROME

This syndrome will be either hereditary or congenital, or sometimes acquired. The patient will suffer from functional locking which will increase. Feet are hollow with external coxal rotation leading to coxarthrosis. There is also muscular hypertonicity with locked pelvis and lumbar rachis, but scapulae and sacrum remain on the same line.

These pains are paradoxical, increasing in rest and improving with mobility. They are alarming, and the patient will not be able exactly to localise them. These pains, at first ameliorated by vertebral manipulations, are later exacerbated by the same manipulation using defective circuits.

The manual treatment of the foot is aimed at obtaining tendinous relaxation and the orthesic treatment will involve setting a small wedge under the tendinous flexors just behind their insertions.

To these two syndromes, we have to add a third one: dysmorphic syndrome.

DYSMORPHIC SYNDROME

Some patients successively present with the two types of syndromes involving an association of somatical deformations. In this case, the right approach is to treat the patient for his immediate suffering and then treat the real causal pathology.

Other patients present simultaneously with two types of syndrome: for instance, a hypotonic patient who incidentally suffers from a sciatica will have a hypertonic syndrome in one foot and a hypotonic syndrome in the other, with a range of pains and somatic modifications.

Finally, other patients present with either one side more hypotonic than the other or one side more hypertonic than the other, involving, once again, somatic modifications. These disorders may induce some pain, which could recur though correctly treated previously. This is because the basis of the edifice, the foot, has not been cured. Here I mean cured by reflex techniques that would have an effect on the cause, affecting central control and therefore the postural edifice.

As we have already seen, results of podological techniques are immediately verifiable and measureable with the equipment we use (stereometer, anthropometric ruler, plumb line). Wedges, although extremely thin (1–3 mm thick) instantaneously improve static disease significantly and often spectacularly. Results are perfectly objective.

Patients no longer suffer and do not have recurrence. This is the reason why more and more patients are conscious of the important role of the foot in statics and consult in a preventive way.

In conclusion, when a patient consults for somatic pains, especially if they are recurring, you must look for static disorders and search for their aetiology. You will then have to practise adequate manipulative treatment, and if our technique has convinced you, you will be able to finish with reflex podological treatment.

39

Frozen wrist: the contribution of thermography

Richard M. ELLIS and Ian SWAIN

INTRODUCTION

The differential diagnosis of pain and restriction of movement at the wrist, without external trauma, is generally considered to be between arthritis of degenerative, inflammatory or infective type, and tenosynovitis and over-use syndromes. The following cases appeared untypical on presentation, and when initial treatment brought no response, thermography was used to differentiate a local condition from a proximal, neurogenic one.

CASE REPORTS

Case 1

A 14-year-old schoolgirl presented with right wrist pain and stiffness with no previous trauma. In the past she had been well apart from one episode of torticollis and one episode of back pain that had cleared without treatment. The wrist stiffness became more severe and involved the fingers, with associated paraesthesia in a median nerve distribution. There were no other symptoms, and in particular no neck symptoms. She held her hand and wrist still with the fingers flexed. Examination showed no heat or swelling, and wrist movement was markedly reduced, with no crepitus. There was marked pain on passive movement of the fingers as well as the wrist.

There was no improvement with local physiotherapy and carpal tunnel injection of steroid during 2 weeks; by 3 weeks there was slight improvement, and by 7 weeks the wrist was almost normal. Nine months later the symptoms recurred. The signs were the same. Investigations comprised X-ray of the wrist and nerve conduction tests, which were normal. Thermography revealed the wrist and forearm to be abnormally cool.

Detailed examination of the neck revealed reduced movement in the lowest cervical joints and the left craniocervical junction. It was demonstrated that relief

314

of wrist pain could be achieved by cervical traction; and the pain, stiffness and other wrist and hand symptoms cleared with treatment to the cervical spine.

Case 2

A 28-year-old nurse related a 6-week history of increasing pain and stiffness in the left wrist, with no neck symptoms. Examination showed less than 10° wrist extension or flexion and marked local tenderness. Blood count, ESR and nerve conduction tests were normal, and thermography showed the left wrist and forearm to be cooler than the right.

Overall cervical movement was normal, but examination of individual segments revealed stiffness of certain left-sided cervical joints. Cervical traction eased the wrist pain and ten treatments allowed a return to normal wrist function.

THERMOGRAPHY

Thermographic assessments were undertaken at an ambient temperature of 23°C ± 1°C, using an Agema 782 shortwave infrared camera. Five standard views were taken of each subject showing back, neck, lateral aspects of both arms and hands and forearms. The subjects were left in the temperature-controlled room for a minimum of 20 minutes prior to recording the images to ensure equilibration. Normal ranges of temperature asymmetry were obtained from a previous study of control subjects. The cases studied in this report showed asymmetry outside the 95% confidence limit of 0.98°C (0.72°C for men).

SUMMARY

The pain and restriction of joint movement was associated with clinical signs of abnormality of cervical joint function in each case, while the thermograph was not consistent with a local inflammatory condition. We considered that the restriction in movement at a peripheral joint, apparently controlled by a proximal abnormality of spinal function, and presumably mediated through the nervous system, superficially mimicked synovitis but was distinguished by thermography.

40

The New Zealand Association of Musculo Skeletal Medicine – postgraduate courses for doctors

D.R. DALLEY

The New Zealand Association of Musculo Skeletal Medicine was inaugurated at a meeting in Rotorua in 1980 following efforts by a group of Auckland doctors who recognized the lack of knowledge and training in musculoskeletal medicine within the medical profession. This deficiency in medical training had been recognized for a long time, but the findings of the Commission of Inquiry into Chiropractic in New Zealand in 1979 emphasized in no uncertain terms the inadequacy of the traditional medical approach as perceived by the public and reported to the Commission. The Government of the day declared that unless the medical profession could substantially improve its image and performance then chiropractors would be given the same privileges and recognition as the medical profession.

Visits to New Zealand by Johannes Fossgreen and Torben Pripp in the mid-1970s had introduced about fifty NZ doctors to the rapidly developing science of manual medicine as practised in Europe at the time. A further visit by Fossgreen accompanied by Torben Rasmussen, later to be followed by Barry Wyke, Robert Burns and Paul Goodley, further developed the interest and expertise of this early group of doctors.

The NZ Association subsequently developed an education programme entitled 'An Introductory Course in Musculo Skeletal Medicine' comprising four days' teaching and practice in elementary examination, mobilization and manipulative techniques. This was well received and over three hundred NZ doctors attended these courses over the years. It soon became apparent, however, that the introductory course led nowhere, and practitioners who found the manual approach so helpful in their everyday clinical practice were requiring additional knowledge and more advanced examination and treatment techniques.

In 1985 Professor Greenman from the College of Osteopathic Medicine at Michigan State University, spent six months in the Department of Medicine at the Christchurch School of Medicine and laid the foundation for a more broadly based and comprehensive education programme to be developed and offered

316

through the University as well as The New Zealand Association of Musculo Skeletal Medicine. However, it was not until 1986, when Dr Jiri Dvorak from Switzerland attended *The Spine in Action Conference* in Christchurch that the detailed basis and structure of the new education programme became established. With this visit and several subsequent visits, Dr Dvorak and a group of more experienced doctors within The NZ Association developed the new programme, which is now produced on a regular basis for NZ doctors, particularly general practitioners.

THE POSTGRADUATE EDUCATION PROGRAMME IN MUSCULOSKELETAL MEDICINE

The programme is based substantially on the structure and experience of the programme offered by the Swiss Manual Medicine Association, but incorporating variations learned from our other visitors. Four courses are produced annually.

Course 1 The Spine – Diagnostic and Examination Techniques
Course 2 The Peripheral Joints – Diagnosis and Manual Therapy
Course 3 The Spine – Mobilization and Neuromuscular Therapy Techniques
Course 4 The Spine – Neuromuscular Therapy and Mobilization with Impulse

Two courses are produced in Auckland and two in Christchurch each year. The courses are structured for 30 participants. Each course spans 5 days and is essentially practical, with hands-on instruction provided by a core of 12 teachers comprising The NZ Teaching Body for The Association. These same teachers also contribute to the Diploma programme at the University, working alongside specialist colleagues from within the University departments appropriate to the Diploma course. Each Association course also features plenary and academic sessions emphasizing and clarifying the essential anatomy, physiology, biomechanics, and neurology. A practical Manual is provided at each course and the Dvorak text books on *Manual Medicine* (1) *Diagnostics*, and (2) *Therapy*, are provided to all participants.

We have now produced at least one of each course, the 1989 Course 2 being conducted by Dr Dvorak. Manuals have been prepared for Courses 1, 3 and 4, with the Course 2 Manual not being required until 1990.

Promotion of the postgraduate courses is on a regular basis utilizing the medical press in NZ and particularly promoting Course 1. Thereafter the Course 1 participants are kept in touch by regular mailing, as well as through the revision course comprising a weekend approximately two months after the main course. Once entering the programme each participant is mailed information concerning the appropriate subsequent course so that their practice plans may be made early. Promotion of the courses is also directed at undergraduates

317

through the University Department of Orthopaedics and Musculo Skeletal Medicine as well as trainee general practitioners comprising approximately one hundred involved in The Family Medicine Training Programme throughout New Zealand.

THE DIPLOMA OF MUSCULO SKELETAL MEDICINE

The University of Otago now offers a Diploma in Musculo Skeletal Medicine through the Christchurch School of Medicine for 30 doctors per year. This is a more broadly based programme than the Association courses and uses pain as its model. By comparison, the Association courses are less broadly based, and use dysfunction as the model. The two programmes complement each other well. Courses 1 and 2 from the Association are taken entirely into the Diploma 'on-campus' programme utilizing Association teachers.

Our programme in postgraduate musculoskeletal training has been enthusiastically received by NZ doctors attending, and we are now very confident that The NZ Association is in a position to offer NZ doctors a postgraduate education in Musculo Skeletal Medicine comparable to the best available anywhere in the world.

41
The nature and significance of trigger points

R.T.D. FITZGERALD

Much discussion and speculation have been expended upon trigger points and fibrositis for over a hundred years, in spite of which no one seems to have any clear idea of what they are, except that they occur together and are in some way related. This confusion is reflected in the terminology used to describe the signs. The Germans use the term *Nervenpunkte*, the French *taches douleureux* and the Americans *trigger points*, which, as I shall show later, seems to be the best term, for these tender spots are the triggers of a great variety of symptoms of which only one is usually recognized and that is fibromyalgia. The problem was increased when Sir William Gowers unfortunately invented the term 'fibrositis' in 1904, since when there has been a fruitless search for the pathology suggested by the name.

It so happens that the answers to these puzzles were published between 1937 and 1945 by Professor Kellgren, James Cyriax and Sir Thomas Lewis in England and Michael Kelly in Australia, but sadly this work has not been recognized as offering such explanations. My own work on spines and trigger points in the past 35 years has helped to clarify the situation still further.

Kellgren's classic experiments on referred pain in 1937 and 1938 and the mapping of dermatomes and myotomes depended upon injections of hypertonic saline to cause foci of irritation which, although they were hardly noticed by the volunteers, did however cause wide areas of referred pain to be produced in the same anatomical segment as the injections. The referred pain could be felt in the skin, muscles, bones or viscera depending on the depth of the injection, and it is the visceral symptoms that have been largely forgotten and neglected but which are perhaps the most important.

In 1938 Cyriax pointed out that injections of hypertonic saline in the suboccipital region caused headache. In 1941 Sir Thomas Lewis, working with Kellgren, found that injections into the upper thoracic interspinous ligaments could cause chest pain that his cardiac patients were unable to distinguish from the pain of angina pectoris. In all cases it was found that the site of the referred pain was specific for the site of the injections and that if the injection site was anaesthetized the referred pain disappeared.

A fact that has escaped notice is that these foci of irritation were in fact artificial trigger points. This experimental work was turned to practical use by Cyriax and Kelly who injected trigger points and their areas of referred pain as a treatment for fibromyalgia. Then in 1983 Janet Travell, making use of this work, published her great book *Myofascial Pain and Dysfunction: The Trigger Point Manual*, which is now the standard work on the subject. But, alas, even Travell failed to realize the true nature of trigger points and fibromyalgia or the myofascial lesion as she called it.

Why has no pathology ever been discovered? Simply because there is no pathology or myofascial lesion, as was shown by Cyriax over 40 years ago when he noticed that areas of both trigger points and fibromyalgia frequently moved following spinal manipulation. If tender spots move they can only have a functional cause and not be due to local pathology. As they are often also palpable, the only possible cause is muscle spasm. If a nodule of muscle spasm is removed it is deprived of its nerve supply and therefore the spasm disappears and only normal muscle tissue remains to be seen under the microscope. However, electron microscopic evidence of ischaemia has recently been observed, which is what one might expect from spasm. If you squeeze a sponge the liquid is expressed.

What other evidence of spasm is there? In 1973 the Magoras and their co-workers in Israel found electromyographic recordings of high potentials in painful neck muscles. Janet Travell had made similar recordings in both tender muscles and trigger points and I have myself made similar recordings on trigger points. Such recordings can only come from muscle activity and indicate that we are dealing with muscle spasm.

It is these high potentials in the trigger points, acting like batteries implanted into muscles and ligaments, that cause symptoms within their own segment: they act as irritants in the same way as Kellgren's injections of hypertonic saline that I have just described as causing artificial trigger points, and therefore we may expect to find similar somatic or visceral symtoms in both situations.

What has previously not been recorded is that the symptoms are not confined to pain but may also be autonomic. The nearest description that I have found to this is a paper of last February in which Professor Yunus noted that fibromyalgia was often associated with tender spots, headache and irritable bowel syndrome. This sounds fanciful but Yunus is quite correct except that he has unfortunately put the cart before the horse. It is the trigger points that cause the fibromyalgia, the headache and the irritable bowel syndrome.

Some of the specific relationships between trigger points and symptoms that have been noticed are as follows:

Level of 2nd cervical spine	recurrent headache of all types
Temporomandibular joint	temporomandibular joint dysfunction pain syndrome
Tip of the mastoid process	vertigo and dysequilibrium
Upper thoracic spine	chest pain

10th thoracic spine	dyspepsia and peptic ulcer
11th and 12th thoracic spines	irritable bowel syndrome and ulcerative colitis
1st lumbar spine	pelvic pain

One of these trigger points, that on or alongside the second cervical spine, is pathognomonic of recurrent headache of all types. Recurrent headache without this sign is due to intracranial causes. Other associations that are very common are the vertigo and dyspepsia trigger points. It is therefore not surprising that all the cases of Meniere's syndrome that I have seen in recent years have had both the headache and vertigo trigger points. As regards other trigger points, I have not seen enough cases to warrant further comment.

Thus far the situation seems fairly logical and compatible with anatomy. I believe that spinal manipulation or traction can have little effect on anything other than intervertebral discs. Disc protrusions can irritate the dura, thus causing symptoms. One pathway is the recurrent meningeal nerves. These nerves innervate the unpaired structures of the spinal canal. They also anastomose with fellows above and below, thus creating a nervous pathway running the length of the spinal canal and therefore an anatomical pathway for extrasegmental symptoms and signs. Among these are trigger points of which the patient is seldom aware: the patient is only aware of the referred symptoms caused by the trigger points, as in Kellgren's experiments.

The big problems arise when one considers the positions occupied by trigger points and the manner in which they move. For here we observe events that are totally missing from current neurological experience.

On spinal manipulation not only do trigger points move as observed by Cyriax 45 years ago but, of course, their referred symptoms move with them. These movements are always across dermatomes and always follow the same pattern by moving towards either the fifth lumbar or sixth cervical spine by the most direct route, and at these points they disappear together with their symptoms. Since the fifth lumbar and sixth cervical spines are the commonest levels at which disc protrusions occur, it is presumed that trigger points invariably move towards the disc lesion that is their cause, and disappear if and when the protrusion is fully reduced. I should add that I can only completely reduce one disc protrusion in three.

Lumbogenic trigger points never occur above the level of the first lumbar spine, whereas cervicogenic trigger points can occur anywhere in the body, even in the feet! From this you will realize that the movement patterns of cervicogenic trigger points are quite non-anatomical and resemble only one thing – a chart of acupuncture meridians. You will also realize that cervicogenic trigger points, by overlapping the lumbogenic area, can cause exactly the same symptoms as lumbogenic trigger points, so that patients with cervical disc protrusions may present with low back pain or even mimic plantar fasciitis! This unfortunately invalidates 25 years of backache records that I made before this observation.

Even more puzzling is the ability of a single disc protrusion to cause multiple trigger points – even as many as a hundred – all of which can move simultaneously with a single manipulation. I would have considered this to be quite impossible had it not been a daily occurrence for me to see such movements of multiple trigger points. I do not often see patients with more than 20 trigger points, but such patients have invariably been referred for psychiatric treatment because of their multiple symptoms which have defied diagnosis.

When there are only one or two trigger points it is easy to reduce the causative disc protrusion, but when there are many trigger points it may be time-consuming and difficult or impossible. Trigger points are therefore of prognostic value in the treatment of disc protrusions and are also a much better guide to the progress of manipulative treatment than the spinal movements, for spinal movements can be very variable and may even become full long before the last trigger point has disappeared, thus leading one to think the patient is cured when in fact this is not so.

In the space available I can only present these brief notes: I could write a book on the subject. I shall have to be content to point out the importance of trigger points not only as a guide to the progress of manipulation but as diagnostic signs, for they can be a cause of symptoms in every part of the body including the viscera, a fact that is not generally appreciated, thus leading many patients to be labelled as having psychosomatic symptoms or to being frankly hysterical because the origin of their genuine symptoms is not recognized.

I would like to conclude with a useful reminder to have framed and hung up in one's consulting room: 'If a symptom, no matter where in the body, cannot be diagnosed or depends upon movement or posture, think of a disc protrusion and look for trigger points'.

42
Low back pain, manipulation and long-term outcome

A.G. CHILA

INTRODUCTION

Low back dysfunction is a very common presenting complaint in physicians' offices. Waddell[1] observed that in Western society, the past thirty years have seen a dramatic increase in low back disability. Industrially related low back dysfunction has a significant impact on the cost of health care. In the United States, for example, compensatable and non-compensatable costs for low back dysfunction approximate 14 billion dollars annually. This represents a major social problem as well as a patient problem[2].

NATURAL HISTORY

Contemporary medical thought offers several observations about low back dysfunction. A very high percentage of patients experiencing low back dysfunction will recover satisfactorily in approximately 3 weeks. Self-limitation as a characteristic of this complaint is also high. Recovery without hospitalization or surgery is extremely high. In terms of percentages, it has been noted that 80% of people may be expected to experience low back dysfunction at some stage of life. Of the at-risk population, 2–5% will seek medical attention while as many as 60% will not necessarily do so. Approximately 80–90% of episodes of low back dysfunction will recover within 6 weeks, regardless of the administration or type of treatment. Variability in the loss of work and the practitioner's appreciation of the subjectivity of pain are not the least important of the considerations of low back dysfunction.

CONSIDERATIONS IN MANAGEMENT BY MANIPULATION

Kirkaldy-Willis[3] emphasized lumbar degenerative dysfunction due to repeated minor trauma. The spectrum of degenerative disease was defined by three phases: dysfunction (decreased movement); instability (increased abnormal movement); stability (stabilization), reflecting progression of the dysfunctional process. The development of a rational treatment plan should consider the implications of this spectrum and should also be individualized. Appropriate intervention in the dysfunctional phase is thought to reverse changes associated with pain due to synovitis, sustained muscle hypertonicity with posterior joint splitting and ischaemic effects resulting in pain and altered muscle metabolism.

Despite a long history of use by orthodox physicians and other health-care providers, manipulation, particularly in the United States, remains controversial. The effectiveness of manipulation has not been the subject of extensive research. Attempts to validate the efficacy of manipulation have been undertaken by a number of researchers during the past decade. Long-term management of low back dysfunction by manipulation has not been a characteristic of studies reported in the literature.

There are several general indications for the use of manipulative treatment. These are: movement of body fluids, modification of somatosomatic, somatovisceral, or viscerosomatic reflex patterns, tonic effects on circulation and general body function; maintenance care. The decision to use manipulative treatment is largely influenced by the ability of the physician. The wide range of indications are readily applicable to each phase of the spectrum of degenerative disease. The appropriate choice of manipulative approaches can provide successful intervention in situations of decreased movement (dysfunction). Selective use of manipulative approaches while additional judgements are being formulated may be appropriate in situations of clinical recurrence (instability). Selective use of manipulative approaches as maintenance may be appropriate in situations that cannot be eliminated (stabilization). In any of these situations, the use of manipulative treatment should be viewed as though the physician were preparing a prescription[4]. In this fashion, thought will be given to consideration of the method to be used, the activating forces to be applied, the amount of treatment and the frequency of application of treatment. Additional considerations would be appropriate as regards the acuteness or chronicity of the problem, the use of adjuncts, and modifications that address the patient's age or health status.

Manipulative procedures are described by a variety of names. In the interest of simplification, three groups may be described: soft-tissue procedures; articulatory procedures; procedures to remove restriction within a specific joint. Empirical observation of clinical responses suggests that a single procedure may effectively resolve a specific dysfunction. It should be noted, however, that combinations of procedures may be appropriate during a single visit. This consideration certainly exists for the use of manipulative procedures over time in the management of low back dysfunction. In dealing with acute clinical manifestations, the use of manipulation seeks to effect a physiological response without undue patient discomfort. In addressing chronic clinical manifestations, the use of manipulation seeks to achieve tissue responses. Examples of such responses include increased joint mobility, vasomotor flush or the relief of pain. While developing a prescription for the use of manipulation for a particular patient, the physician needs to be constantly aware of two factors:

(1)   The manipulative treatment and management of low back dysfunction may need to include procedures in areas of the body other than the low back.
(2)   In any clinical situation, the appropriate use of manipulation seeks to ensure that subsequent treatments are built on documented effects from previous treatments.

LONG-TERM MANIPULATIVE MANAGEMENT OF PATIENTS WITH LOW BACK DYSFUNCTION

Ten patients are presented for discussion. All of these patients have received manipulative treatment in connection with low back injuries incurred while working. Nine of these patients have returned to full-time work in their original occupations; one patient has been declared totally disabled since 1981. The group of patients includes 6 females and 4 males. Multiple manipulative approaches have been employed in the management of these patients. Palpatory diagnostic findings have been recorded at the time of each visit. This sample of patients receives periodic manipulative treatment under the philosophy of chronic management of chronic problems. A synopsis of each patient's history of injury, diagnostic studies and findings, manipulative management plan and complicating factors is presented in Table 42.1.

IMPLICATIONS FOR CLINICAL RESEARCH STUDIES

The contemporary arena for the conducting of research studies generally accepts the randomized controlled trial as the most reliable method of conducting clinical research. According to Pocock the principles of the scientific method may be followed thus[5]:

(1)   Define the purpose of the trial
        (a)   State specific hypothesis

(2)   Design the trial
        (a)   Establish a written protocol

(3)   Conduct the trial
        (a)   Ensure good organization

Table 42.1

Patient	Demographic	Injury	Diagnostic studies	Findings	Manipulative management plan	Complicating factors
T.J.	48:WM	1976	1976–1983			
		Attempted to support a falling weight in excess of 1000 lb	Multiple lumbar X-rays	Negative	Maintenance 2–3 week intervals since 1979	Consultant's comments, 1978: Single root pathology exists on the left side of the L5 root. Under usual circumstances, herniation of L5-S1 will compromise S1. However, if the herniation is lateral, it misses the root of S1 and impinges on the L5 root in an area not visualized in the myelogram. Surgical exploration of the L5 root should be done
			Multiple EMG studies	Negative	Some reduction of symptomatic complaint of pain	
			Myelograms (4)	Negative		
			Hospital-based pain rehabilitation program	No change in complaint	Significant reduction in use of analgesic medication	
			1986: CT Scan	Negative		
			1987: Repeat EMG and myelogram	Negative		Consultant's opinions, 1979 and 1980: No surgery – the patient is malingering. No consultant since 1978 has recommended surgical exploration
J.D.	48:WM	1977	1980: Lumbar X-ray	Residual contrast from myelogram. Otherwise negative	3–4 week intervals since 1979	Continues in physical labour activity. Intermittent left lower extremity radicular complaints
		Thoracolumbar and lumbar strain while attempting to stop a falling vending machine	1985: Lumbar X-ray	Negative		
			1987: Lumbar X-ray	Mild degenerative change, L5-S1		
			1988: Lumbar X-ray	Minimal narrowing, L4-L5, posteriorly. Minute anterior proliferative change		

Patient	Demographic	Injury	Diagnostic studies	Findings	Manipulative management plan	Complicating factors
M.K.	69:WF	1977 Low back strain while lifting	1981: Lumbar X-ray 1988: Lumbar X-ray	Moderate rotatory scoliosis, lumbar spine. Degenerative disc changes, L5-S1 Osteoarthritic changes, apophyseal joints, L4-L5 right and L5-S1. No change. Slight decrease in bone density	Monthly intervals since 1971	Intermittent increase in lumbosacral discomfort
P.T.	42:WF	1980 Slipped on floor at work, stopping fall by grasping railing	1980: Lumbar X-ray 1984: Lumbar X-ray 1988: Lumbar X-ray	Negative Negative Minor degenerative arthritis, L5-S1	3–4 week intervals since 1980	Continues in heavy physical labour activity. Intermittent exacerbations of lumbosacral discomfort
J.Mc.	43:WF	1983 Fall on buttocks	1984: Lumbar X-ray Myelogram CT scan EMG 1985: Lumbar X-ray 1987: Lumbar X-ray 1989: Lumbar X-ray	Negative Lumbar lordotic splinting. Minimal bilateral acetabular hypertrophic reaction Straightening, lumbo-sacral spine. Otherwise normal Negative	2–3 week intervals since 1984	Rt. sphenobasilar SBR strain. Rt. O-A strain. Work-related stress on continuing basis

(continued)

Table 42.1 (*continued*)

Patient	Demographic	Injury	Diagnostic studies	Findings	Manipulative management plan	Complicating factors
M.S.	45:WF	1983 Low back strain while lifting patient	1984: Lumbar X-ray 1989: Lumbar X-ray	Bilateral sacralization, L5. Extensive hypertrophic changes, lumbar vertebrae suggestive of ankylosing spondylitis No change	4–6 week intervals since 1984	MVA Feb. 1989. Compression fx., superior end plate L3
H.E.J.	33:WM	1983 Fall down steps	1983: Lumbar X-ray 1984: Lumbar X-ray 1985: CT scan Myelogram EMG 1989: Lumbar X-ray	Coccygeal fx. Healed coccygeal fx. Herniated disc, L5-S1 No evidence of nerve encroachment Normal Negative	3–4 week intervals since 1984	Work-related stress on continuing basis; duodenal ulcer; duodenitis. Antral gastritis
N.S.	36:WF	1986 Sudden, rotational low back strain while lifting	1986: Lumbar X-ray 1989: Lumbar X-ray	Mild lumbar scoliosis, apex L3 Mild proliferative spurring, L3-L4 right. Slight narrowing, L4-L5 left. Mild degenerative lumbar spine disease	3–4 week intervals since 1986	Intermittent tightness of left leg. Intermittent numbness over medial toes, left foot

Table 42.1 (continued)

Patient	Demographic	Injury	Diagnostic studies	Findings	Manipulative management plan	Complicating factors
S.B.	39:WM	1986 Two-storey fall	1986 (Aug): AP pelvis Lateral hips Lumbar spine	Negative	2–3 week intervals since 1986	Exploratory surgery for spleen injury. Psychological stress factor: released for work in early 1988; job not granted
			1986 (Oct): Lumbar spine	Sacralization, L5. Fracture, left batwing deformity. Old and healed fractures, sublux. L5.		
			1987: CT scan	Negative		
			Myelogram	Asymmetric filling S1 nerve root		
D.J.	52:WF	1987 Low back strain while lifting heavy object	1988: Lumbar X-ray	Negative	1–2 week intervals since 1988	Continues in heavy physical labour activity. Persistent right lumbosacral strain pattern
			1988: Lumbar X-ray	Negative		
			CT scan	Negative		

(4)   Analyse the data
       (a)   Utilize descriptive statistics for the testing of hypotheses

(5)   Draw conclusions
       (a)   Publish results

As applied to studies dealing with manipulation, Tobis and Hoehler[6] described the principles which help to underscore special problems peculiar to such studies:

(1)   Absence of any generally accepted diagnostic criteria defining patients who are appropriate for manipulative therapy.

       (a)   Diagnosis is fundamentally subjective, primarily involving musculo-skeletal rather than objective laboratory measurements.

(2)   Factors predicting the success of manipulation therapy are largely unknown; hence, it is virtually impossible to stratify patients meaningfully. There is also difficulty accounting for variability of response in *post hoc* statistical analyses.

       (a)   This essentially ensures that there will be a large amount of residual variability in the response to treatment. This tends to cloud any assessment of the results of the trial.

(3)   There is disagreement regarding the appropriate manipulative therapy to employ in a trial. The exact form employed will depend on each individual clinician's assessment of each individual patient. Although this variability can be reduced, the cost lies in reducing the generality of the results.

(4)   A serious problem exists with the difficulty involved in the design of an appropriate control group.
       (a)   Placebo control similar to methods used in drug studies cannot be employed.

       (b)   The physician will always be aware of the treatment being delivered.

       (c)   The patient will not easily be deceived.

       (d)   Spurious superiority of manipulative therapy might be concluded if an equivalently enthusiastic 'laying on of hands' is not provided for the control group as well.

(e)   The virtual impossibility of a true placebo control must also affect the final assessment of the results of treatment.

  (i)   The patient's awareness of the nature of treatment might possibly be communicated to the assessor.

  (ii)   If the measure of success is subjective (alleviation of 'pain'), the patient is, in effect, responsible for the assessment of results.

TERMINOLOGY AND INTER-RATER RELIABILITY

Various attitudes toward manipulation are expressed by various groups of practitioners, contributing to a lack of uniform terminology. In the United States, the Educational Council on Osteopathic Principles (ECOP) represents a group of faculties from all of the 15 colleges of osteopathic medicine. This group has compiled a glossary that attempts to standardize the terminology used by the osteopathic profession. The North American Academy of Musculoskeletal Medicine (NAAMM) has developed a glossary of terms that attempts to bridge the views between these two groups. The Scientific Advisory Committee of the International Federation of Manual Medicine (FIMM) attempts to address communication problems within the field and across languages.

Reconciliation of these factors does not appear to be easy with respect to testing the efficacy of manipulative intervention in controlled studies. Johnston[6] offered an alternative strategy, the testing of diagnostic hypothesis rather than alternative forms of treatment. Criteria for diagnostic findings must be clearly established, and patients selected on the basis of presence or absence of those findings. Comparing the results of treatment will have little basis for validity until this is done. The general literature of studies in manipulation appears to have pre-empted the investigation of diagnostic signs.

REFERENCES

1. Waddell, G. (1987). A new clinical model for the treatment of low-back pain. *Spine*, **12**(7), 632–644
2. Snook, S.A. (1982). Epidemiology in low back pain. Presented by Brigham and Women's Hospital and Harvard Medical School, November 29–December 1, 1982
3. Kirkaldy-Willis, W.H. (1983). The three phases of the spectrum of degenerative disease. In Kirkaldy-Willis, W.H. (ed.) *Managing Low Back Pain*, Chap.7. (New York Churchill Livingstone)
4. Kimberly, P.E. (1980). Formulating a prescription for osteopathic manipulative treatment. *J. Am. Osteopath. Assoc.*, 79(8), 506–543
5. Pocock, S.J. (1983). *Clinical Trials – A Practical Approach*. (New York: Wiley)
6. Tobis, J.S. and Hoehler, F. (1986). *Musculoskeletal Manipulation – Evaluation of the Scientific Evidence*. (Springfield, Ill.: Charles C. Thomas)
7. Johnston, W.L. (1985). Inter-rater reliability in the selection of manipulable patients. In Burger, A.A. and Greenman, P.E. (eds.) *Empirical Approaches to the Validation of Spinal Manipulation*, Chap. 8. (Springfield, Ill.: Charles C. Thomas)

43

The computerized documentation of clinical and manual results

M. HANNA, H. TILSCHER and C. WEICH

INTRODUCTION

The computerized documentation of anamnesis facts as well as clinical and manual results should rationalize, improve and economize medical treatment and thus benefit the patient by making treatment more exact.

The time had come to find a way of standardizing the information about a patient, the problem being to adapt in a suitable way the verbal, typed reports made on admission. The patients concerned are mostly people with pain syndrome caused by disturbances in the supporting apparatus and in the locomotor system who have been admitted for diagnostic clarification, therapeutic treatment and the recording of their symptoms to aid rehabilitation because of a long-lasting resistance to therapy, or signs of relapse, or because of the seriousness of the clinical picture.

Figure 43.1 shows schematically the relationship of the system.

QUESTIONNAIRE

The Patient Questionnaire

Each patient is requested to complete a 'Patient Questionnaire' on being admitted to hospital. He is asked about his home circumstances (marital status, children, occupation, hobbies, sport, etc.), his sleeping, eating and drinking habits, previous stays in hospital, therapy already given, allergies and so on.

The summary of the anamnesis

In practice the patients questionnaire is usually completed somewhat subjectively, remaining incomplete in parts. For this reason a form is also completed by the doctor, which clarifies the information given in the patients questionnaire, particularly that describing the main symptoms and their causes.

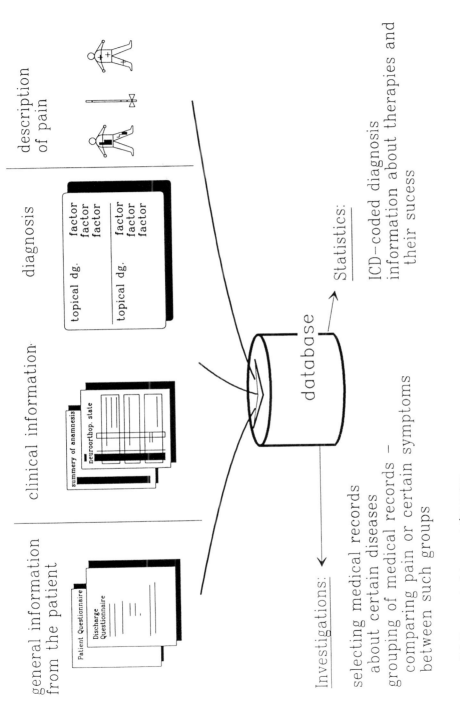

Figure 43.1 Computerized documentation system

333

The Discharge Questionnaire

Before being discharged, the patient completes a 'Discharge Questionnaire' in which he is asked which forms of treatment have improved his condition in his opinion (and to what extent).

Since these questionnaires are standardized, the information thus gained can easily be recorded. The data from the questionnaires is input into the computer point for point. The text that appears on the monitor is as far as possible identical to that on the questionnaire.

NEURO-ORTHOPAEDIC STATUS

The patient is examined in manual-medical, orthopaedic and neurological ways in which a definite sequence is to be followed. Previously the doctor recorded his findings on tape; this was then typed out and added to the case history. This form of documentation is inadequate for a standardized analysis, since symptoms that are obviously not present are neither investigated nor mentioned. It is difficult to distinguish later between 'not investigated' and 'investigated – result normal'. In addition, it is troublesome to sort out the relative facts from a number of case histories.

We have therefore included the majority of investigations on a standard form. Following the normal routine anamnesic procedures, the doctor enters the results (e.g. finger–floor distance, head-rotation capacity). For each test a number of possible results is offered (multiple choice) and the doctor has simply to tick that which is nearest to his findings. He can include additional observations in text form (Figure 43.2). This form also includes manual-medical investigation techniques such as the spine test, the springing test of the iliosacral and Patrick's sign in the classical neuro-orthopaedic examinations.

On the one hand, the doctor should simplify the information as much as possible by ticking in multiple choice possibilities, and on the other hand the most common and the most important results should be given exactly. In order to obtain a progress report on the clinical findings, a neuro-orthopaedic status is established for each patient on admittance and on discharge. Thus, the form is a compromise and makes no claims to completeness. It is not intended to be an alternative but a supplement, giving a general view of the main symptoms.

RECORDING THE SYMPTOMS

For more than 20 years our department has recorded the 'pain illustration' of each patient. It is ascertained before a diagnosis is made, and provides the basis for further investigations. Changes in the referred pain during the patients stay in hospital indicate the effect of therapy. The areas of pain, as described by the patient, are entered on a stylized 'pain figure'.

Neuro–orthopaedic Status

Date:
Doctor:

Patient

Basics

Relieving limp		1 negativ 2 left 3 right
Shortening limp		1 negativ 2 left 3 right
Walking on tip-toe impossible		1 negativ 2 left 3 right 4 both sides
Heel walking impossible		1 negativ 2 left 3 right 4 both sides
others	o o	o o	Swaying upper body deficient background motor system small steps swaying

lumbar pelvic hip area

Iliac crest	1 straight 2 low level left 3 low level right
Low level left	cm
Low level right	cm
Lumb. vert. column lateral list	1 negativ 2 left 3 right 4 both sides
limited	
Lumb. vert. column retroflexion	1 negativ 2 limited
Finger floor space	cm
Bent walk phenomenon	1 negativ 2 left 3 right

Shoulder

Grip behind neck limited	1 negative 2 left 3 right 4 both sides
Grip behind back limeted	1 negative 2 left 3 right 4 both sides
Outer rotation	1 negative 2 left 3 right 4 both sides
Final movement limited	1 negative 2 left 3 right 4 both sides

Cervical vertebral column

Trapezius hypertonus	1 no 2 yes
Chin-jugulum-distance (+1)	1 0 QF 2 1 QF 3 2 QF 4 3 QF 5 more than 3 QF
Head rotation left maximum	
Head rotation right maximum	
Limited rotation head bent	1 negative 2 left 3 right 4 both sides
Limited rotation head forwards	1 negative 2 left 3 right 4 both sides

Charact. muscles weakened

C5 shoulder abduction	1 negative 2 left 3 right 4 both sides
C6 elbow bending	1 negative 2 left 3 right 4 both sides
C7 elbow stretching	1 negative 2 left 3 right 4 both sides
C8 little finger abduction	1 negative 2 left 3 right 4 both sides

Formular: L. Boltzmanninst. für kons. Orthopädie u. Rehabilitation

Figure 43.2 Neuro-orthopaedic status

335

Points of pain palpated by the doctor are also entered. Dysfunctions such as blocking or hypermobility are entered on a schematic illustration of the spinal column at the relevant level. In order to input this data the information is broken down as follows:

- Position of pain (Figures 43.3 and 43.4)
- Dysfunctions (Figure 43.5)
- Palpated painful structures (Figure 43.6)

Position of pain

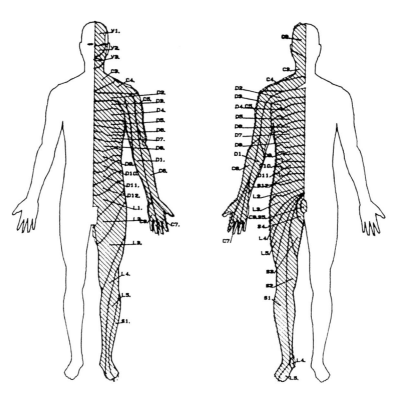

Figure 43.3 Pain referred to dermatomes

The computer 'pain figure' is divided into pain areas, which completely cover it twice. Each of these areas can be described as painful. These are referred to as the dermatome, and the actually painful areas. The one system of painful areas represents the division into dermatome, which can appear as referred pain by disturbances in the function of the spinal column. Our experience is, however, that they seldom appear in this form (Figures 43.3 and 43.4). In order to input pain data as described by the patient there is a second area division, which can readily be combined with that of the dermatome pain. The surface of the body is divided into quadrants which do not represent the anatomical–medical divisions but are based on the language used by the patient, e.g. in the upper extremities:

shoulder
upper arm (four quadrant lengthwise)
elbow
lower arm
wrist
palm (two halves lengthwise)
back of the hand (two halves lengthwise)

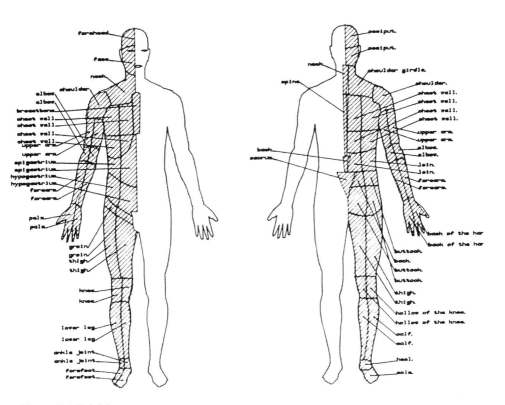

Figure 43.4 Painful areas

This method of recording the pain areas provides the possibility of comparing the input pain illustration with the pain illustration of the referred pain in the dermatome. The computer automatically shows the percentage of dermatome by other input pain illustration.

Disturbances in the functions of the spinal column

The information about eufunction, blocking and hypermobility can be input exactly. For the spinal column, for the costotransversal joint and for the sacroiliac joint, the following data can be input:

- investigated and mobility normal;
- blocked (possibly left/right);
- hypermobile (possibly left/right) (Figure 43.5).

Palpated painful structures

The source of the pain can often be established by palpation. It is possible to record exactly the trigger points (muscular maximum points) and other painful structures such as muscle insertions, ligament insertions and joints. There is an input possible for nearly all points investigated. Since all possible painful points are palpated during the course of the examination, there is no difference here between 'not investigated' and 'investigated – normal'. Thus, a point is marked 'painful' or 'not painful' (Figure 43.6).

THE DIAGNOSIS

The following method has been proved reliable in arriving at the final diagnosis.

A 'topical diagnosis' is made for the patient based on the description of his pain. Further clinical and manual investigations are, as already mentioned, necessary, in order to establish an exact 'structure analysis', namely the type and position of the functional disturbance. A number of topical diagnoses can be input for each patient. To each topical diagnosis is added the structure analysis in the form of several 'factors', disturbances that cause the pain. The relevant ICD-9-Keys are input with the factors, describing or complementing the factor.

Diagnoses and factors are principally input in text form. For a number of syndromes there are set texts that are used whenever possible because their uniformity makes the later evaluation much easier. Only when the set text is inadequate to describe the syndrome can an individual text be used.

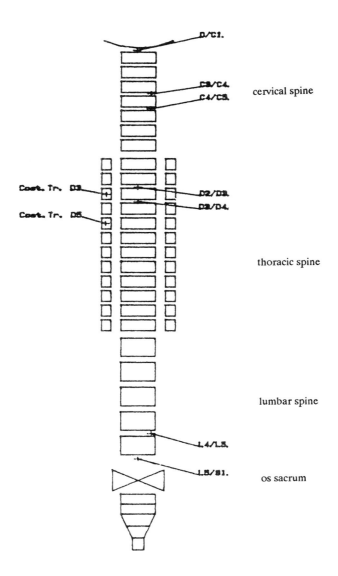

Figure 43.5 Site of somatic dysfunction

339

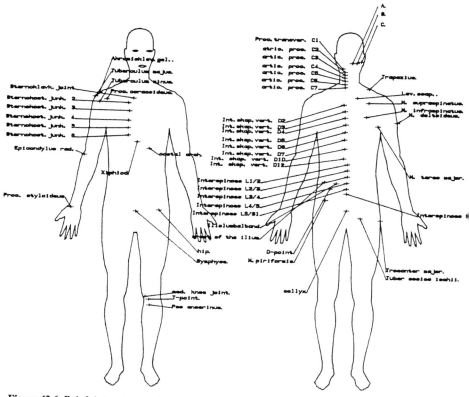

Figure 43.6 Painful structures, trigger points

EVALUATION

The purpose of storing the data described is to investigate the reasons for the occurrence of pain. Thus, for example, a comparison can be made between painful areas and functional disturbances of individual joints. In order to do this a particular painful area is chosen and the distribution of the functional disturbances of those patients who complained of pain in this area is compared with the average of all patients. As many patient groups as desired can be formed by this system. A given factor or a number of factors (pain, living circumstances, etc.) are pin-pointed and all the patients who comply with this are thus formed into a group. The differences within such a group between the pain illustrations, in the results, or in whatever else has been stored, can now be observed and statistically analysed.

As an example, we have charted the painful areas that are most commonly complained of by patients in conjunction with lumbar, calf, or knee pains (Figure 43.7). The second example demonstrates the division into groups: patients who

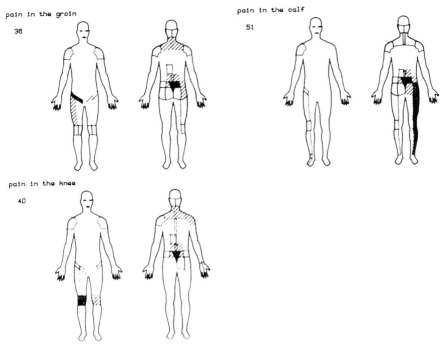

pain in the groin
36

pain in the calf
51

pain in the knee
40

Figure 43.7 Pain topic illustrating areas most often complained of in conjunction with lumbar, calf or knee pains. Solid, > 75%; hatched, > 50%; open, > 25%

have had an intervertebral disc operation at an earlier stage were chosen and divided into three groups – L4/5 operated, L5/S1 operated, and operated on more than once. Between these groups a comparison is made of the finger–floor distance (Figure 43.8).

DISCUSSION

The computerized registration of data of patients admitted to hospital would seem to offer a wealth of advantages. The increasing accuracy of a diagnosis from the pain symptoms shows itself in the departure from purely topical diagnoses to structural analytic statements, whereby it can be seen time and again that a number of structural disturbances, i.e. different interference factors, can result in one clinical picture, which could set in doubt the monotherapy that is demanded by traditional medicine.

The spread of use of computers in registration of in-patients could result in a standardization of medical terms that by no means exists at the moment (terms used in manual medicine, by orthopaedic specialists, by rheumatologists, neurologists, radiologists, etc.).

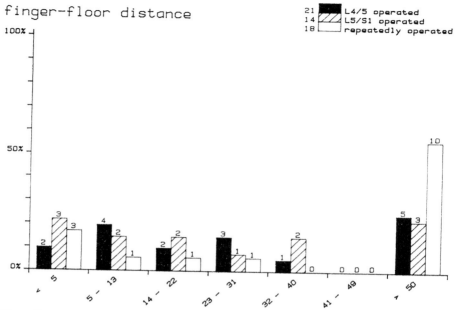

Figure 43.8

Multicentric activities could considerably speed up research into disturbances of the supporting apparatus and locomotor system.

Therapeutic consequences are no longer a matter of the intuition (or even bias) of the doctor, but are standardized, whilst still allowing certain variations.

The standardization of terms also makes possible better communication with non-medical groups, e.g. insurance companies, social insurance contributors, public authorities, etc.

ACKNOWLEDGEMENT

We would like to thank all those who supported this project, and particularly the Austrian National Bank for its generous contribution.

FURTHER READING

Eder, M. and Tilscher, H. (1988). *Chirotherapie*. (Stuttgart: Hippokrates Verlag)

Eder, M. and Tilscher, H. (1988). *Schmerzsyndrome der Wirbelsäule Grundlagen, Diagnostik und Therapie*, 4th edn. (Stuttgart: Hippokrates)

WHO. (1979). Diagnoseschlüssel nach der internationalen Klassifikation der Krankheiten der WHO, ICD 9. Revision. (Aarau: Veska)

Hansen, K. (1952). *Therapeutische Technik für die ärztliche Praxis*. (Stuttgart: Thieme)

Head, H. (1988). *Die Sensibilitätsstörungen der Haut bei Visceral-erkrankungen*. (Berlin: Hirschwald)

Mackenzie, J. (1971). *Krankheitszeichen und ihre Auslegung*. (Wurzburg: Kabitzsch)

Tilscher, H. and Eder, M. (1989). *Reflextherapie*, 2nd edn. (Stuttgart: Hippokrates)

44

Lumbar sciatica – comparison of results 10 years after surgical or conservative treatment

ST. LÖRINCZ, H. TILSCHER and M. HANNA

INTRODUCTION

The medical decision of whether to treat a case of lumbar disc prolapse by the conservative method or by an operation should only be made after due consideration of all relevant information. Signs of a caudal lesion, or unbearable, endless pain with neurological deficits, make the decision to operate easier. The recurring or therapy-resistant pain syndrome, often with unobtrusive neurological deficits, which is termed 'commonplace' lumbar sciatica, gives rise to a confrontation between the group 'surgeons', in particular the neurosurgeons, orthopaedic surgeons and the traumatologists, and the larger, inhomogeneous group 'the conservative therapists'. Included in this group are the general practitioners, the conservative therapist orthopaedic specialists, doctors of physical medicine, rheumatologists, algesiologists, etc., whose methods of treatment are often even more inhomogeneous than the group itself. This confrontation, that is to say the weighing up of the pros and cons, should actually take place within each individual doctor.

The arguments for an operation are, above all, the results of many follow-up examinations[1,2,4,5,8,10,12]. A summary of many of these investigations seems to make an operation obligatory, and to force the conservative therapy into the role of 'calculated risk'. What, then, are the arguments for the vast number of conservative methods applied? Their very non-uniformity, a result of the necessity to take into consideration the individual symptoms of illness, and the variations in medical training, makes scientific investigation difficult. It is doubtless still above all else the fear of an operation, which is not lessened by the absence of a vital indication.

Many methods of conservative therapy have been examined in order to establish their efficiency, but not, however, that method which is chiefly practised, namely polypragmasy; that is the combination of many therapies, based on the topical diagnosis, the empirical and the individual diagnostic and therapeutic possibilities.

343

In the Department of Conservative Orthopaedics and Rehabilitation of the Orthopaedic Hospital, Vienna, 4123 patients were admitted between 1971 and 1985, comprising 1828 sciatica patients with neurological deficits, 1664 without neurological deficits, and 631 intervertebral disc operated with continuing symptoms. Depending on the topicality diagnosis and the structural analysis, most of these cases were treated in a conservative way, that is to say, with drugs, reflex therapy (manual medicine, using therapeutic local anaesthetic and acupuncture), and physically, followed by rehabilitation. In view of the arguments of the surgeons, it now seemed important to establish just how far the therapeutic concept described was justified.

The immediate therapy results are, of course, shown in the results of the patient-discharge questionnaire. However, long-term results are particularly important in orthopaedics, that is to say, the later problems of vertebral patients from the perspective of the given therapy. For this reason, the Department of Conservative Orthopaedic and Rehabilitation collected relevant information via clinical examinations and a standard questionnaire from the patients who had been admitted 10 years previously, the results of which were to be compared with a similar investigation carried out on patients who at the time had had vertebral disc operations.

METHOD

Thirty three patients treated in a conservative way, and 33 patients who had been operated on for lumbar sciatica were included in this investigation. Only patients whose admittance to hospital was at least 10 years prior to this were included. These 66 patients were asked to complete the following questionnaire to establish information about their medical and day-to-day situation.

(1) Since leaving the Orthopaedic Hospital 10 years ago, have you been in hospital again because of your original back/leg problems? If so, how often?

(2) After leaving the hospital 10 years ago, did you still have back problems?

(3) After leaving the hospital 10 years ago, did you still suffer from pain in the same leg?

(4) After leaving the hospital 10 years ago, did you suffer from pain in the other leg?

(5) After leaving hospital 10 years ago, did you have complaints in both legs?

(6) After leaving the hospital 10 years ago, did you suffer from weakness or paralysis in either or both legs?

(7) Did you experience a prickling feeling or numbness in either or both legs, after leaving the hospital 10 years ago?

(8) After leaving hospital 10 years ago, did you have a sensation of coldness in your legs, that is to say in the leg which had suffered pain?

(9)   In comparison to the time prior to your stay in hospital, were the complaints the same, stronger, weaker, or much weaker?

(10)   Have you needed medical treatment since then? If so then as an out-patient (GP, specialist), or were you admitted to hospital?

(11)   Have you had a vertebral disc operation? If 'yes' then please give details.

(12)   Have you been to a sanatorium since then?

(13)   Have you received treatment from a masseur since then?

(14)   What else have you done to alleviate your symptoms – regular exercise, physiotherapy, change of place of work, change of job, early retirement, something else, nothing.

(15)   Did you have to take time off work as a result of your sciatica?

(16)   Did you have to take medicaments for your sciatica?

(17)   Was a 'focal assignation' done?

Patients were also given a clinical examination, aimed at the following evaluations:

(a)   The pain topic;
(b)   The finger–floor distance;
(c)   Lasegue's sign;
(d)   Neurological deficit syndrome of the segment L3 to S1.

The results of the questionnaire, and the results of the clinical tests of those treated in a conservative way, and those operated on, were then compared.

RESULTS

The results of the questionnaire

Thirty three patients who had received conservative treatment were examined, 19 men and 14 women, with an average age of 58.2 years. The anamnesis period in this group was 5.5 years of chronic recurring lumbar syndrome and 8.6 weeks of acute pain. The average time spent in hospital was 30.7 days in this group (Tables 44.1 and 44.2).

Thirty three patients who had been operated on were also examined, 11 men and 22 women, with an average age of 53.2 years. The anamnesis period in this group was 6.6 years of chronic symptoms and an average of 8.4 weeks of acute pain. The average time spent in hospital was 46 days (Tables 44.1 and 44.2). The period of chronic pain was longer in the operated group ($p=0.59$). The difference in the period of acute pain was statistically insignificant ($p=0.3$). The answers to questions 1–8, 12, and 14–17 can be seen in Table 44.3.

Table 44.1 Mean ages

Operative	53.2 years	
Conservative	58.2 years	$p = 0.04$

Table 44.2 Anamnesis period

Chronic	Conservative	5.5 years	
	Operative	6.6 years	$p = 0.59$
Acute	Conservative	8.6 weeks	
	Operative	8.4 weeks	$p = 0.3$

Table 44.3

		Number of 'yes' responses	
Question		Conservative	Operative
1	Hospital	6	5
2	Back pain	26	24
3	Pain in same leg	24	18
4	Pain in other leg	8	8
5	Pain in both legs	6	5
6	Weakness	10	9
7	Paraesthesia	17	22
8	Sensation of coldness	11	22
12	Sanatorium	18	23
14	Change of place of work	3	0
14	Change of job	4	3
14	Early retirement	1	4
15	Loss of worktime	13	10
16	Medicaments	15	14
17	Focal assignation	25	24
Total		187	191

The questions were so phrased that a 'yes' always expressed a negative result, and a 'no' a positive one. On comparing the answers to the 15 different questions, it can be seen that there are 187 'yes' responses in the conservative group, and 191 in the operated group. It is, of course, obvious, that not all symptoms and circumstances can be compared with one another.

Question 9. Comparison of pain after 10 years. In the conservative group 6 patients suffered the same pain, 2 had more pain, 10 had less and 15 had much less pain. In the operated group, 3 suffered the same pain, none had more pain, 12 had less and 16 had much less pain, one patient gave no details, and one patient had no pain at all (Figure 44.1)

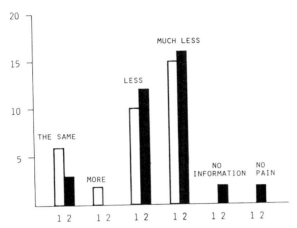

Figure 44.1 Question 9. Comparison of pain with that 10 years before: 1 = conservative; 2 = operative

Question 10. Medical treatment. In the conservative group, 6 received treatment as out-patients, 18 were treated by their GP, 12 by a specialist, and 6 were in hospital. In the operated group, 5 were out-patients, 13 were treated by their GP, 15 by a specialist, and 5 were in hospital (Figure 44.2).

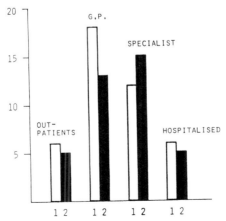

Figure 44.2 Question 10. Where treated: 1 = conservative; 2 = operative

Question 11. Vertebral disc operation. None of the patients had a disc operation after leaving the hospital 10 years before.

Question 13. Masseur. Fourteen patients from each group had regular treatment from a masseur.

Question 14. Three of the points in this question have already been dealt with in Table 44.3. Eighteen patients in the conservative group claimed to experience positive improvement with physiotherapy. The same was claimed by 8 of the operated group.

The consequences in career and working life can be seen in Figure 44.3:

Conservative: 3 changed place of work
                4 changed job
                1 took early retirement

Operated: 0 changed place of work
            3 changed job
            4 early retirement

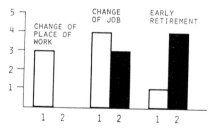

Figure 44.3 Question 14. Consequences in working life: 1 = conservative; 2 = operative

Results of the clinical examination

The pain topic

The pains in back, buttocks (gluteal), leg and foot were assessed. On comparing the conservative group with the operated group it can be seen that with the 'conservatives' 69 painful areas were present on admission, reducing to 43, that is to say 26 fewer. Nine patients were free of pain.

In the operated group there were initially considerably more painful areas for the same number of patients, namely 81, reducing to 36, that is 45 fewer. Fourteen patients had no pain (Table 44.4). In summary, the number of pain topics per patient was reduced from 2.45 to 1.09 ($p = 0.004$) in the operated group, and from 2.09 to 1.39 (p = 0.02) in the conservative group. On comparing these results with the spot-check tests by Wilcoxon, there is no statistical significance (p = 0.28).

Table 44.4 Pain topic

Group	Admission	Check-up	
Conservative	69	43	p = 0.02
Operative	81	36	p = 0.004
Operative to conservative: p = 0.28			

Back pains

Nine patients in the conservative group originally complained of back pains; at the check-up examination it was 20. In the operated group the results were more balanced: 13 patients originally had back pains, and 14 at the check-up examination. There is no statistically significant difference (p = 0.07).

It must be noted that the reasons for the increase in pain in the conservative group, 9 to 20, were not investigated (Table 44.5).

Pain in the buttocks

For pain in the buttocks, a pain reduction from 24 to 13 patients could be seen in the conservative group. In the operated group there was a reduction of 26 to 7 patients. There is no statistically significant difference between these groups (p = 0.25) (Table 44.6).

Pain in the leg

Here the situation was practically identical in both groups. In the conservative group 31 patients complained of leg pains and at the check-up it was 13, in the operated group it was originally 30, going down to 12 at the check-up (p = 0.99) (Table 44.7).

Table 44.5 Pain topic, back

Group	Yes	No	
Conservative			
Before	9	24	
After	20	13	$p = 0.002$
Operative			
Before	13	20	
After	14	19	$p = 0.8$

Operative to conservative: $p = 0.07$

Table 44.6 Pain topic, buttocks

Group	Yes	No	
Conservative			
Before	24	9	
After	13	20	$p = 0.002$
Operative			
Before	26	7	
After	7	16	$p = 0.00005$

Operative to conservative: $p = 0.25$

Table 44.7 Pain topic, leg

Group	Yes	No	
Conservative			
Before	31	2	$p = 0.0001$
After	13	20	
Operative			
Before	30	3	$p = 0.0001$
After	12	21	
	Operative to conservative: $p = 0.99$		

Table 44.8 Pain topic, foot

Group	Yes	No	
Conservative			
Before	5	28	
After	0	33	
Operative			
Before	12	21	$p = 0.07$
After	3	30	

Pain in the foot

Five patients in the conservative group originally complained of pains in the foot, but none at the check-up. In the operated group 12 patients originally had foot pains and at the check-up it was 3. Owing to the 0 in the conservative group it is not possible to perform a statistical comparison here (Table 44.8).

The finger–floor distance

The average finger–floor distance in the conservative group was originally 22.7 cm, and 7.4 cm (p = 0.001) at the check-up. In the operated group the original finger–floor distance was 33.3 cm and improved to 12.0 cm (p = 0.0015). Both groups showed a positive change here; there is no statistically significant difference (Table 44.9).

Table 44.9 Finger–floor distance (cm)

Group	Admission	Check-up	
Conservative	22.7	7.4	p = 0.001
Operative	33.3	12.0	p = 0.0015

Lasegue's sign

Lasegue's sign was to be seen at an average of 74.1° positive originally and at 89.1° at the check-up (p = 0.0003) in the conservative group. In the operated group it was 49.3° and 90.2° at the check-up (p = 0.0015). Thus, an obvious improvement was present in both groups, although the initial situations varied (that of the conservative group being more favourable), but the results are the same in both groups (Table 44.10).

Table 44.10 Lasegue's sign (degrees)

Group	Admission	Check-up	
Conservative	74.1	89.1	p = 0.0003
Operative	49.3	90.2	p = 0.0015

Neurological deficits

In the conservative group a radicular lesion L4 was found to be present in 3 patients on admission. These were not present at the check-up. In the operated group there was none with L4 signs. Of the 10 patients with L5 sign, 4 could be seen at the check-up. Of those operated it was originally 6 and was 4 at the check-up. Of the 20 conservative patients with S1 lesions, 17 still had deficits at the check-up. Of the 25 operated patients with S1 signs, 17 still had neurological deficits. Identical results could be seen in both groups at the check-up (Table 44.11).

Table 44.11 Neurological deficits, conservative group

Group	Admission	Check-up
Conservative		
L4	3	0
L5	10	4
S1	20	17
0	–	12
Operative		
L4	0	0
L5	6	4
S1	25	17
0	2	12

DISCUSSION

A comparison was made of the therapeutic effect on 33 conservatively treated patients and 33 operated on patients suffering from sciatica, whose treatment took place 10 years before, via questionnaire and check-up examinations. The mathematical evaluation was done by Professor Schreiber (Institute of Medical Statistik, Vienna) and was purely exploratory. No direct comparisons were made between the two groups, it was simply an attempt at establishing a tendency to improvement and changes in individual results within the groups. The original condition and changes following treatment were statistically examined in both groups. There are:

- Clear differences in the original condition by Lasegue's sign and the finger–floor distance;
- No noticeable differences in the anamnesis period.

There was a distinct reduction in the pain topic in both groups, particularly for back pains. The operated patients came out best here. Lastly, noticeable changes took place in both groups over the 10 years, and the conservative group showed slightly less improvement. The final results are very similar. The poorer admission examination results of the operated group had two different consequences:

(1) A statistical consequence, since in both groups the choice of patients was not a matter of coincidence.

(2) The consequence that, from the number of pain topics, from the positiveness of Lasegue's sign, and the noticeably reduced finger–floor distance, a considerably more intensive pain syndrome can be presumed in the operated group. The conservative group did not have to show as much improvement in order to achieve the same results as the operated group.

On studying the points of the questionnaire, it can be seen that the questions, and answers given to them, in Table 44.3 are relatively balanced. The comparison of present pain with that of 10 years before showed more favourable tendencies in the operated group. The 'career-life consequences' shown in Figure 44.3 cannot be adequately interpreted owing to the low number of cases. However, the fact that four of the operated patients and only one of the conservative patients entered early retirement gives rise to thought.

What conclusions can be drawn as a result of this investigation by the practising doctor with regard to the treatment of his patient, this being the main point of interest of all medical scientific investigations? It would appear that the conservative method is to be recommended for all lumbar sciatica with discrete neurological lesions, including those of longer duration. The control over the dominant symptoms, above all the pain, must be closely supervised. If neurological deficits increase or if a caudal symptom develops, then the absolute indication to operate is given. An operation is also to be considered if therapy shows no sign of improvement after 2–3 weeks of intensive treatment.

On the grounds of this investigation, the results of operative treatment would appear positive, although the fact that 631 disc-operated patients had to be re-admitted to hospital casts a shadow on this optimism. Pain as a subjective phenomenon is confirmed by clinical results. It is, therefore, an important indication for a disc operation for the so-called 'commonplace lumbar sciatica'.

Thus, conservative therapy is not a calculated risk nor is the indication to operate to be seen as a therapeutic defeat.

REFERENCES AND FURTHER READING

1. Biederst, S., Reuther, R. and Winter, R. (1984). Zur konservativen Behandlung des lateralen lumbalen Bandscheibenvorfalles mit segmentalen motorischen Ausfällen. In Hohmann, Kügelgen, Liebig and Schirmer (eds.) *Neuroorthopädie 2*, pp. 448–450. (Berlin: Springer Verlag)
2. Bischoff, H.P. (1984). Vertebrale Syndrome nach Bandscheibenoperationen Ihre Beurteilung und Behandelbarkeit. In Hohmann, Küglegen, Liebig and Schirmer (eds.) *Neuroorthopädie 2*, pp. 422–426. (Berlin: Springer Verlag)

3. Bogner, G. and Tilscher, H. (1979). Zur Differentialdiagnose der Bandscheibendegeneration. Round-Table-Diskussion, Rehab.-Zentrum Bad Schallerbach. In *Die Bandscheibendegeneration und ihre Behandlung*, pp. 24–25. (Wien: Hrsg PVArb. u. Heilmittelwerke)
4. Bösch, J. (1974). Indikationsstellung aus der Erfahrung von 1506 Bandscheibenoperationen. *Z. Orthop.*, **112**, 796–797
5. Ebeling, U., Reichenbach, W. and Reulen, H.J. (1984). Ergebnisse der mikrochirurgischen lumbalen Bandscheibenoperation. In Hohmann, Kügelgen, Liebig and Schirmer (eds.) *Neuroorthopädie 2*, pp. 399–403. (Berlin: Springer-Verlag)
6. Eder, M. and Tilscher, H. (1988). Schmerzsyndrome der Wirbelsäule Grundlagen. *Diagnostik und Therapie, 4th edn.* (Stuttgart: Hippokrates)
7. Landsiedl, F., Bogner, G. and Tilscher, H. (1978). Spondylodiszitis nach Bandscheibenoperationen. *Orthopädische Praxis*, 9/XIV, 706–707
8. Leblhuber, F., Witzmann, A. and Reisecker, F. (1984). Verlaufsbeobachtung bei operierten und nicht operierten nachgewiesenen lumbalen Bandscheibenläsionen. In Hohmann, kügelgen, Liebig and Schirmer (eds.) *Neuroorthopädie 2*, pp. 444–447. (Berlin: Springer-Verlag)
9. Mumenthaler, M. (1979). *Neurologie*, 6th edn. (Stuttgart: Thieme)
10. Schmitt, O., Fritsch, E., Hassinger, M. and Schmitt, E. (1984). Epikritische Langzeitergebnisstudie nach lumbalen Bandscheibenoperationen. In Hohmann, Kügelgen, Liebig and Schirmer (eds.) *Neuroorthopädie 2*, pp. 410–416. (Berlin: Springer-Verlag)
11. Tempelhoff, W.v. and Maxon, H. (1984). Katamnestische Untersuchungen bei 55 Patienten nach einer lumbalen Bandscheibenoperaton Misserfolge in Abhängigkeit von psychogenen Einflüssen. In Hohmann, kügelgen, Liebig and Schirmer (eds.) *Neuroorthopädie 2*, pp. 417–421 (Berlin: Springer-Verlag)
12. Thomalske, G., Galow, W. and Ploke, G. (1977). Operationsergebnisse bei 2000 Fällen lumbaler Bandscheibenläsionen. *Münch. Med. Wochens.*, **36**, 119
13. Tilscher, H. and Eder, M. (1989). Reflextherapie, 2nd edn. (Stuttgart: Hippokrates)
14. Tilscher, H., Friedrich, M., Bogner, G. and Landsiedl, F. (1980). Ursachen für rezidivierende Schmerzzustände nach lumbalen Bandscheibenoperationen. *Orthop. Praxis*, **16**, 24–28

45

A study to evaluate the outcome of acute backache with drug therapy and manipulation

M.R. SHAH

INTRODUCTION

Backache is an important problem both to the individual and to the community. It emerged as the third most frequently experienced symptom (after headache and tiredness) in Morrell and Wade's study[1]. Each year, 2.2 million individuals consult their GP for backache, three times the number relating to coronary heart disease. The condition incurs considerable expense to the National Health Service, accounting for 2.6% of GPs' workload and a total cost of £156.1 million (1982). DHSS figures for 1982/3 estimate 33.3 million days of certified incapacity due to backache.

Various therapies are employed to deal with backache and these include oral drugs, physical measures (rest, manipulation, traction, massage), surgical, injected drugs, counter-stimulation, biofeedback and behaviour therapy. The effect of special manipulation on the outcome of an episode of backache has been compared with other therapeutic measures/placebos in several studies. However, there are scanty references to comparison of manipulation with non-steroid anti-inflammatory drugs (NSAIDs). The aim of this study is to compare the outcome of an episode of acute backache treated with either manipulation or a non-steroidal anti-inflammatory drug (Naprosyn). Both these measures can be employed as therapeutic tools in the community.

METHOD

The study was based in a general practice in a Health Centre in Walthamstow, London. The practice consists of five partners and two trainees, with all seven participating in the study. One of the partners has special training in manipulation and performed all manipulation.

356

Two criteria were used to identify those patients who would be included in the study:

Inclusion

(i) Pain onset, 4 weeks or less
(ii) Age, 16–55 years

Exclusion

(i)   Established spinal disorder
(ii)   Pregnancy
(iii) Known hypersensitivity
(iv)   On long-term NSAID, steroid or anticoagulant therapy
(v)   Significant renal, haematological or hepatic disorder
(vi)   History of peptic ulcer disease
(vii) Evidence of superficial muscle or ligament injury
(viii) Evidence of spinal pathology, e.g. tumour, infection
(ix)   Psychiatric history
(x)   History of asthma

All patients were asked to complete questionnaires (Appendices A and B) at the initial consultation. Patients were subsequently allocated randomly to one of the treatment groups and the appropriate therapy commenced. All patients were requested to complete the questionnaires at the following intervals:

Questionnaire A: After 1 and 4 weeks
Questionnaire B: Daily for the initial 7 days

The questionnaires are a slight modification of those devised by Roland and Morris[4].

RESULTS

A total of 17 people were eligible for inclusion in the study, of which 16 were entered and one declined to take part. Those who entered included 14 males and 2 females. The subject who declined to enter was male. The 16 subjects in the study were allocated to treatment groups as follows: manipulation, 10; Naprosyn, 6. Completed questionnaires were received as follows:

Set 1 (Pretreatment)	Set 2 (After 1 week)	Set 3 (After 4 weeks)
16	16	10 (Manipulation, 5; Naprosyn, 5)

357

The mean duration prior to seeking treatment was 15.7 days (range 3–35 days).

Table 45.1 Changes within each treatment group at day 3 and day 7. Figures in brackets represent percentage of total subjects for that group

	Manipulation Days		Naprosyn Days	
	0–3	0–7	0–3	0–7
Improvement	4 (40)	5 (50)	4 (66)	5 (83)
No change	3 (30)	1 (10)	1 (16)	0
Deterioration	3 (30)	2 (20)	0	0
No response	0	2 (20)	1 (16)	1 (16)
Total	10 (100)	10 (100)	6 (100)	6 (100)

Table 45.1 shows changes within each group at days 3 and 7. Table 45.2 shows the median values for each group and Figure 45.1 shows changes in median values over the first 7 days.

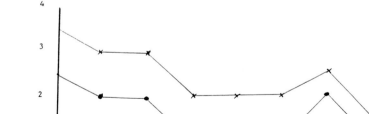

Figure 45.1 Changes in median values for the two groups over the first 7 days. × manipulation group, • Naprosyn group

Table 45.2 Median values for the two groups

	Day							
	0	1	2	3	4	5	6	7
Manipulation	3.5	3	3	2	2	2	2.5	1.5
Naprosyn	2.5	2	2	1	1	1	2	1

STATISTICAL ANALYSIS

Analysis was by the Wilcoxon Rank Sum test on unpaired samples.

Days 0 to 3: results not significant at both 5% and 1% critical values.
Days 0 to 7: results not significant at both 5% and 1% critical values.

CONCLUSIONS

The results show a good response in the return of questionnaires at the end of the first week (100%) but a less enthusiastic response at the end of the fourth week (68.8%). Of those who failed to respond, 40% were from the manipulation group and 17% from the drug treatment group. It is postulated that at the end of the four weeks, the majority of patients would have a reduced severity or absence of symptoms. In the case of manipulation, which usually involves a single episode of treatment, the chances of forgetting to complete the questionnaires are higher than for those on drug treatment, which is usually taken over a longer period.

Referring to the results for days 0 to 7, the baseline for the median values of the drug therapy group is lower than that for the manipulation group (see Figure 45.1). The durations of symptoms (in days) prior to the initial consultation are:

	Mean	Median
Drug group	11.8	14
Manipulation group	18	17

N.B. One source of error is the inclusion of a patient with duration of symptoms of 35 days.

Both the above observations are difficult to explain because:

(i)   All patients completed the initial questionnaire prior to either the doctor or patient being aware of their treatment allocation.

(ii)   All patients were randomly allocated to the treatment group.

Considering the individual results and referring to Table 45.1, the drug therapy group shows a greater proportion exhibiting improvement at both days 3 and 7.

ACKNOWLEDGEMENT

I am grateful to the staff of the Department of Clinical Epidemiology and General Practice, The Royal Free Hospital School of Medicine, London; the trustees of the Claire Ward Fund of the British Medical Association; and Dr F.H. Arustu, principal and GP trainer at St. James Health Centre, London.

REFERENCES

1. Morrell, D.C. and Wade, C.J. (1976) *J. R. Coll. Gen. Prac.*, **26**, 398–403
2. OHE (1985). *Back Pain*, 5. (London: HMSO)
3. Department of Health and Social Security. (1979). Report of the Working Group on Back Pain. (London: HMSO)
4. Roland, M. and Morris, R. (1983). A study of the natural history of back pain. *Spine*, **8**, 141–143

DRUG THERAPY AND MANIPULATION IN ACUTE BACKACHE

APPENDIX A

Please complete this Form ONE WEEK and FOUR WEEKS after your initial appointment

SURNAME:
FORENAME:
ADDRESS:
TELEPHONE NO: HOME   WORK
DATE COMPLETED:

When your back hurts, you may find it difficult to do some of the things you normally do.
This list contains some sentences that people have used to describe themselves when they have back pain. When you read them, you may find that some stand out because they describe you today. As you read the list, think of yourself today. When you read a sentence that describes you today, put a tick against it. If the sentence does not describe you, then leave the space blank and go on to the next one. Remember, only tick the sentence if you are sure that it describes you today.

Please <u>complete the questionnaires at home</u>, before going to see the doctor.

DISABILITY QUESTIONNAIRE

Please tick as appropriate   <u>Yes</u>   <u>No</u>

1. I stay at home most of the time because of my back   ....
2. I change position frequently to try and get my back comfortable   ....
3. I walk more slowly than usual because of my back   ....
4. Because of my back I am not doing any of the jobs that I usually do around the house   ....
5. Because of my back I use a handrail to get upstairs   ....
6. Because of my back I lie down to rest more often   ....
7. Because of my back I have to hold on to something to get out of an easy chair   ....
8. Because of my back I try to get other people to do things for me   ....
9. I get dressed more slowly than usual because of my back   ....
10. I only stand up for short periods of time because of my back   ....
11. Because of my back I try not to bend or kneel down   ....
12. I find it difficult to get out of a chair because of my back   ....
13. My back is painful almost all the time   ....
14. I find it difficult to turn over in bed because of my back   ....
15. My appetite is not very good because of my back pain   ....
16. I have trouble putting on my socks (or stockings) because of the pain in my back   ....
17. I only walk short distances because of my back pain   ....
18. I sleep less well because of my back   ....
19. Because of my back pain, I get dressed with help from someone else   ....
20. I sit down for most of the day because of my back   ....
21. I avoid heavy jobs around the house because of my back   ....
22. Because of my back, I am more irritable and bad tempered with people than usual   ....
23. Because of my back, I go upstairs more slowly than usual   ....
24. I stay in bed most of the time because of my back   ....
25. Have you consulted any other member of the health profession regarding your present back problem?   ....
26. If you are currently in employment, since what date have you been absent from work as a result of your back pain?   ....

Date returned to work.

361

APPENDIX B

SURNAME:
FORENAME:
DATE COMPLETED:

Please complete this form <u>EVERY DAY</u> for <u>SEVEN MORE DAYS</u>

<u>PAIN RATING SCALE</u>

Now we want you to give us an idea of just how bad your back pain is at the moment.
    Here is a thermometer with various grades of pain from 'no pain at all' at the bottom to 'the pain almost unbearable' at the top. We want you to put a cross by the words that describe your pain best. Remember, we want to know how bad your pain is at the moment.

<u>PAIN RATING SCALE</u>

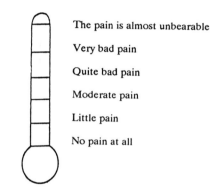

The pain is almost unbearable

Very bad pain

Quite bad pain

Moderate pain

Little pain

No pain at all

Please return after completion to:

Dr M R Shah
St James Health Centre
St James Street
London
E17 7NH

Tel: 01-520 0921

46

Dorso-lumbar junction: biomechanical role of mamillaris processus and transversospinales muscles

G. PIGANIOL, P. TROUILLOUD, G. BERLINSON and J.-Y. CORNU

The dorso-lumbar junction is a very important limit between areas where vertebrae have very different morphology and therefore function. Everyone stresses the shape and the orientation of articular faces in the dorsal and lumbar spine. In the dorsal spine, the instant rotation centres of the articular processes are in the middle of the intervertebral disc, which makes rotation easier. At the lumbar level, the instant rotation centres project themselves on the spinous process more or less near its extremity. In the lumbar moving segments there are thus two rotation centres, the first corresponding to discal rotation, the second to rotation of articular facets. Rotation is only possible by a clipping movement inside the disc. However, the lumbar spine is the privileged site of flexion extension, due to the thickness of the disc being greater at this level. The morphological transition may be only on one vertebra, usually T12, or on two or three.

We wanted to study another characteristic of this area, the existence of which classical authors consider as a characteristic of lumbar vertebrae up to T12. In fact, the mamillaris processus or Owen metapophysis is characteristic of the dorso-lumbar junction. They exist from the last thoracic vertebrae to the diaphragmatic vertebra according to H.V.Vallois and on the first lumbar vertebrae. We wanted to verify their exact settling site in humans and their morphology in elucidating their biomechanical role.

We studied more than 50 dry complete spines from dissected fresh bodies and the results from 50 spines were:
- 2 spines did not present any mamillaris processus;
- 26 spines only presented mamillaris processus on one level and in two thirds of cases on T12;
- 21 spines presented mamillaris processus on two levels, most often on T11 and T12;
- 1 spine presented mamillaris processus on three levels.

Concerning the role of mamillaris processus:

- 12 spines out of 50 had only small processus, less than 4 mm long and 4 mm wide;
- 34 spines out of 50 had one or several processus of a great length on T10, T11, T12 or on the first lumbar vertebra.

The length is much more important than usually appreciated; it ranges between 5 and 11 mm, with an average value of 7 mm. The highest frequency of a long mamillaris processus occurs on T12 (8 cases from 10), then on T11 (4 cases from 10). Globally, in more than half of the spines studied, the size of the mamillaris processus of T12 exceeded 4 mm.

These results illustrate the frequency and the importance of these processus, but it was necessary to try to discover their relationship with the area's muscles. Valois points out the role of the mamillaris processus in mammals and about their role as inserts for longissimus and transversospinalis muscles. In the cetaceans which have no multifidus, the processus migrates out of the transverse processes. The multifidus muscles were first described by Virchow and the works of Trollard and those of Winckler gave a systematic description of them as superposed chevrons, muscles rotatores, brevis and longi. They considered that the muscles present variations all along the spine.

In fact, our dissections showed quite a different situation. At the level where the mamillaris processus is more developed, the multifidus presents itself as a fusiform body muscle, voluminous (7–8 cm long and 2–3 cm wide), inserted on the two or three spinous processes of the upper levels and ending on the largest mamillaris processus. The morphological quality of the muscles in this area corresponds to special physiological value.

When the two multifidus muscles contract simultaneously on both sides, they have an important part in spinal erection. Unilateral contraction leads to a lateral bending and rotation. The multifidus mamillaris processus pairs have very particular function in rotational movement. The maximal axial rotation range in the dorso-lumbar spine occurs in T10, T11, T12 and L1. A third of the range of average rotation occurs at this level, according to the observations of Gregersen. Mechanically this involvement in rotation is possible because of the shape of the articular process of T12, owing to the existence of floating ribs that do not limit rotation and mechanical play of the multifidus, which our dissections showed to be very different and much more developed than the corresponding muscles of lower and upper levels. Longitudinally, this muscle disappeared nearly completely to be replaced by very thin muscular fasciculus as the rotators become thicker.

The particular physiology of this area explains the frequency of diseases at this level; segmental dysfunctions are very frequent and it is one of the privileged areas of disease which react well on vertebral manipulation.

364

FURTHER READING

1. Evans, H.E. and Christensen, G.C. (1984). *Anatomy of the Dog*. (London: W.B. Saunders)
2. Gegenbaur, C. (1899). *Lehrbuch der Anatomie des Menschen*. (Leipzig: Wilheim Engelmann)
3. Gregersen, G.G. and Lucas, D.B. (1967). An in vivo study of the axial rotation of the human thoracolumbar spine. *J. Bone Joint Surg.*, **49A**, 247–263
4. Odgers, P.N.B. (1933). The lumbar and lumbo-sacral diarthrodial joints. *J. Anat.* (London), **67**, 301–317
5. Piganiol, G. *et al.* (1987). *Les Manipulations Vertébrales. Bases Théoriques, Cliniques et Biomécaniques*. (Dijon: GEMABFC)
6. Poirier, P. and Charpy, P. (1912). Muscles spinaux du trone. *Anatomie Humaine*, Vol.2. (Paris: Masson)
7. Vallois, H.V. (1920). La signification des apophyses mamillaires et accessoires des vertèbres lombaires. *Extrait des C.R. des séances de la Société de Biologie*, **83**, 113–115
8. Vallois, H.V. (1921). La vertèbre diaphragmatique et la séparation des colonnes dorsale et lombaire chez les mammifères. *C.R. de l'Association des Anatomistes*, **2**, 974–975
9. Vallois, H.V. (1921). La valeur morphologique des muscles spinaux. *C.R. de l'Académie des Sciences et nombreuses communications dans le Bull. de la Soc. des Sc. Méd. et Biol.*, **1**, 235–240
10. Vanneuville, G. (1980). Eléments de biomécanique du rachis. *63ème Congrès de l'Association des Anatomistes*. Clermont Ferrand 1980 Livre du C.R. du Congrès
11. White, A. and Panjabi, M. (1974). Clinical biomechanics of the spine. (Philadelphia: Lippincot)
12. Xash, C.L. and Moe, J.H. (1969). A study of vertebral rotation. *Case Western Reserve University School of Medicine*, **51A**(2)

47

Skin rolling in the treatment of chronic pain

S. KARAGOZIAN and J.-P. DUIVON

Many authors have described reflex dermalgias, painful subcutaneous areas in the connective tissue, arising from chronic pain states. The main authors are Head, Mackenzie, Wetterwald, Dicke, Jarricot, Bagot and Maigne. In 1932, Jarricot described reflex dermalgia as a modification of subcutaneous tissue; such dermalgia is often spontaneously muted. Clinically the dermalgia is defined by one sign – cellulocutaneous denseness or thickness – and one symptom – the exquisit pain triggered by the key manoeuvre of skin rolling.

The skin rolling manoeuvre was described by Wetterwald in 1912 in the practice book of kinesitherapy Alcan. It is a technique of superficial skin petrissage with rolling movement of the skin fold. In Roscoff, Bagot uses the technique and is at the forefront of skin rolling. In 1953, Bagot began to treat chronic pain states in his institute of thalassotherapy known as 'Roc-Kroum'. To complete skin rolling treatment, he uses balneotherapy.

THE TECHNIQUE OF SKIN ROLLING

Bagot describes three steps:

- formation of the skin fold;
- rolling movement of the skin fold;
- massage.

First the formation of the skin fold is done by the thumbs staying in the same line, and the other fingers folding the skin over the thumbs, the thumbs themselves dipping into the fold of skin. The rolling movement is done without pinching the skin. The thumb moves forward at the skin fold base, and the other fingers bring the skin onto the thumb, with a flexion-extension movement of the phalanges joints, like 'a galloping horse'. The skin fold is rolled 'as one rolls a cigarette'.

The pressure must be adjusted to the thickness of the dermalgia without pinching skin, to keep all the sensitivity of the finger pulps. The fingers are rubbing, massaging the internal parts of the skin fold in an alternating massage.

What are we looking for in the examination of the dermatalgia?

- a tension state of the skin stuck to the connective tissue;
- a thickened congestive and turgescent tissue;
- large folds, or tender ryzoid nodules in the subcutaneous tissue;
- the skin temperature, always lower than the standard skin temperature;
- the exquisite characteristic pain response during skin rolling.

LOCALIZATION OF THE DERMALGIA

These cutaneous tender infiltrations are located close to a joint, a tendon, or a muscle, and often show a distribution following the metamere, a radiculalgia, and the posterior branch of the spinal nerve (Maigne).

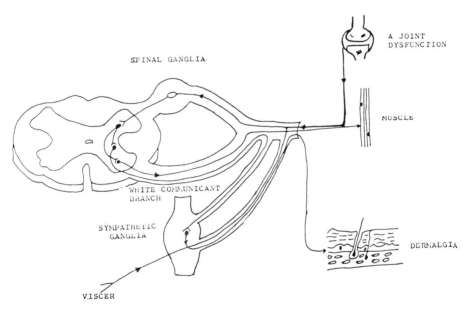

Figure 47.1

Today, we know that the dermalgia is the direct consequence of a modification in the skin vasomotricity, probably a blood vessel spasm set in motion by a reflex mechanism of the sympathetic nervous system.

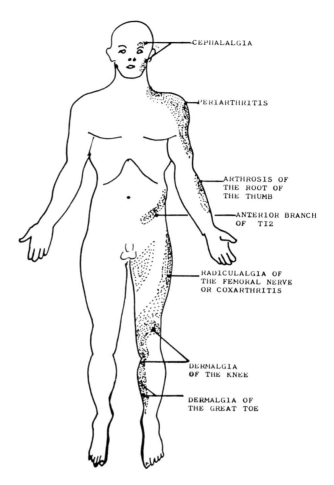

Figure 47.2 Anterior dermalgias

The nociceptive reflex coming from the skin, from the joint, the muscle or the viscera is through the posterior nerve root, or the cranial nerves, to the posterior horn of the spinal cord (Figure 47.1). This nociceptive reflex involves not only the cerebrospinal system, but also the orthosympathetic nervous system. These orthosympathetic nervous system mechanisms explain microcirculation disorders, giving objective and palpable skin modifications: dermatalgia or cellulalgia. This is why the localization of the dermalgia is often not metameric, but diffuses over one radicular area.

Firstly, skin rolling is a diagnosis technique. Secondly, it is a treatment of the dermalgia, and therefore of the chronic pain.

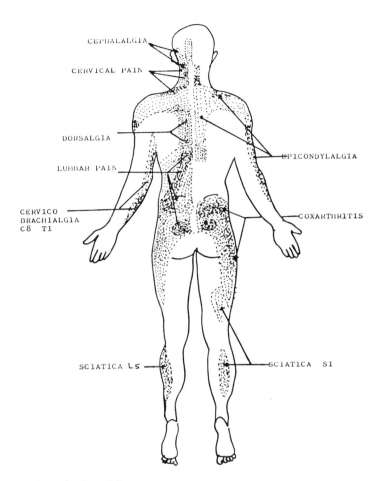

Figure 47.3 Posterior dermalgias

With Bagot's experience, supported by more than a thousand cases, and our own experience, we can describe the main areas of the dermalgias we observe in manual medicine. Figures 47.2 to 47.5 show the localizations of these chronic states. Six to twelve treatments bring good results.

CONCLUSION

Skin rolling is an original therapy that should be part of manual-medical technique. Skin rolling is a simple therapy, but the localization of dermalgias has to be investigated carefully for an effective treatment.

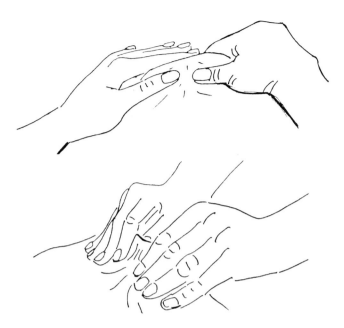

Figure 47.4

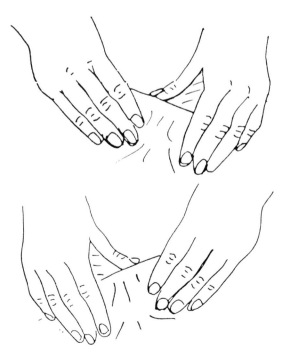

Figure 47.5

FURTHER READING

Auge, R. (1986). Le massage. *Encycl. Méd. Chir.* (Paris)

Auge, R. (1986). *Kinésithérapie*, 26100 A 10, 4.11.04, 4 p.

Aumjaud, (1984). Thalassothérapie et masser-rouler. Thesis, Faculté d' Angers.

Bagot, R. (1949). Une grande méconnue: La cellulite. *Rev. de Rheumatol. d'Aix les Bains*

Bagot, R. (1963). La place du massage en thalassothérapie. *L'Ouest Medical*, **16**, (no. 6; 25 Mars) 303–306

Bagot, R. (1982). La place du massage en thalassothérapie. *Ann. Méd. Phys.*, 5(3), 1.6

Bagot, R. (1963). Le rhumatisme chronique dégénératif. Technique de cure à l'Institut marin de Roscoff. *Congrés International de Thalassothérapie*, Venise)

Barczewski, B. (1911). *Hand und Lehrbuch meiner reflex massage für den Arzt.* (Berlin: Goldschmidt-Verlag)

Bossy, J. (1978). *Bases Neurobiologiques des Réflexothérapies*, 2nd edn. (Paris: Masson)

Bourdiol, J. (1983). *Réflexothérapie Somatique.* (Paris: Maisonneuve)

Daniaud-Turpin Rotival, J. (1964). *Stimulothérapie Cutanée* (Paris: Maloine)

Duivon, J.P. (1973). *La dorsalgie bénigne de la femme jeune et son traitment en milieu Marin,* Mémoire CES de rhumatologie. (Lyon: CES)

Gybels, J. (1976). Stimulation cutanée et gate control. *Kinésithérapie scientifique*, Paris)

Hansen, Schliack H. (1962). *Segmentale Innervation, ihre Bedentung für Klinik und Praxis,* (Stuttgart: Thieme Verlag)

Head, H. (1983). On disturbance of sensation with especial references to the pain of visceral disease. *Brain*, **16**, 1–133

Hendrickx, A. (1981). *Les Massages Réflexes, Étude Comparative.* (Paris: Masson)

Jarricot, H. (1932). Sur certains états douloureux: viscéralgies, dermalgies réflexes, cellulies et quelques phénomènes réflexes d'origine thérapeutique. Essai clinique et thérapeutique. Thesis, Lyon.

Jarricot, H. (1971). Séméiologie viscérocutanée. *Cahiers de Biothérapie*, **8**, (31)

Jarricot, H. (1980). Dermalgies réflexes viscérocutanées postérieures et organisation nouvelle du méridien principal de la vessie. *Méridiens*, no. 51–52, pp.169–179

Lazorthes, G. (1981). Les douleurs rapportées, quelques exemples dans le domaine oto-neuro-ophtalmoligique. *Rev. d'Otorhinophtalmol.*, **53**, 145–150

Lazorthess, G. and Zadeh, J. (1987). Constitution et territoire cutané des branches postérieures des nerfs rachidiens. *Rev. Méd. Orthop.*, **53**, np. 10, 5–9

Maigne, R. (1974). Origine dorso-lombaire de certaines lombalgies basses. *Rev. Rhum.*, **41**(12), 781–789

Maigne, R. (1977). *Douleurs d'Origine Vertébrale et Traitement par Manipulation.* (Paris: Expansion)

Mrejen, D. (1987). *Mésothérapie Ponctuelle Systématisée.* (Paris: Mediffusion)

Teirich-Leube, H. (1957). *Grundriss der Bindegewebsmassage*, 1st edn. (Stuttgart: Fischer Verlag)

Teirich-Leube, H. (1972). *Bindegewebsmassage. Massage du Tissu Conjonctif dans les Zones Réflexes.* (Strasbourg: Edition Apell)

48

The importance of patient selection and imaging techniques in the success of chemonucleolysis

Peyto SLATTER

Chemonucleolysis is dissolution of the nucleus pulposus of an intervertebral disc by the injection of the specific enzyme chymopapain into the centre of the nucleus; the subsequent chemical destruction causes a reduction in intradiscal pressure and bulk[19]. The usual recommended criteria for the use of such treatment is that it shall be used only in cases of lumbar disc herniated nucleus pulposus (HNP), where all conservative methods of treatment have failed and where some form of intervention is indicated[14].

One is constantly reminded of the poor results likely to have been obtained in earlier years, mostly owing to poor patient selection[7,10,14,16]. Whilst it is appreciated that operating technique and the handling of recovery and rehabilitation can also influence the figures, this paper explores the procedures leading to that final selection or rejection, describing the place of current imaging techniques and the use of discometry. It could be regarded by some as a centralization of ideas in the form of a 'cook book'. They could be right, but the aim is to equal published success rates and there is no harm in so doing; this sort of procedure is equally applicable when aiming to succeed in flying aeroplanes or playing golf[2,7,8,10]!

THE IMPORTANCE OF DIAGNOSIS

Attempts to list the primary causes of low back pain become infinite and can vary between malaria and tonsillitis. It goes without saying that to reach that small group of mechanical conditions responsible for locomotor problems in the area of the low back requires a complete history and physical examination accompanied by other necessary screening tests.

When discussing the orthopaedic medical approach to the diagnosis of low back pain, Barbor lists the most common diagnoses under the heading 'Lumbar instability':

- Ligamentous insufficiency;
- + or – Sacroiliac joint subluxation;
- Facet joint jamming;
- Spondylolysis/spondylolisthesis;
- Lumbar disc protrusion of the annulus and of the nucleus (HNP).

For treatment by chemonucleolysis we are only interested in the last, and both Barbour and Cyriax[6], in particular have described in detail the pertinent points arising in the history and examination to reach such a clinical diagnosis.

SYMPTOMS AND SIGNS OF HNP

(1) The low back and/or leg pain is of gradual onset.
(2) Increase in low back stiffness.
(3) Pain increases on:
   - loading
   - getting in and out of a chair
   - coughing and sneezing or impulse

(4) Lumbar movements are decreased and the pain increases on:
   - forward bending in the back/limb
   - backward bending in the limb
   - sideways bending towards the painful side

(5) Straight leg raising is decreased on the painful side and may also demonstrate:
   - positive nerve root stretch signs
   - positive 'bow string'
   - contralateral pain distribution
   - neurological deficit

In addition, McCulloch and Macnab[14] list their specific signs of HNP required for chemonucleolysis. The patient needs to qualify in two or more out of the following five groups:

(1) Leg pain greater than back pain
(2) Specific paraesthesia
(3) Straight leg raising
   - less than 50%
   - and/or 'crossover' (cross leg pain)
   - and/or 'bow string'

(4) Neurological (at least two or more out of the following four):
  – diminished reflexes
  – muscle wasting
  – muscle weakness
  – sensory loss
(5) Imaging: positive magnetic resonance imaging and/or computer tomographic scan.

However, despite these signs, those who are pregnant, who are grossly obese, who have neurological disease or whose routine lumbar spine X-rays demonstrate a spondylolisthesis of Grade 2 or more cannot be considered[14].
Again, to qualify for intervention the patient must fail a regime of conservative treatment which, within the armoury of the orthopaedic physician, would include, progressively[6]:

– Manipulation – aiming at reducing the disc protrusion, although this is unlikely to be effective
– Sustained lumbar traction – in the absence of neurological deficit
– Epidural infiltration
– Sinuvertebral block

Even at this stage, should the possible diagnosis be that of an adherent nerve root rather than HNP, Stoddard[20] recommends a specific manipulation that he has developed and carries out under general anaesthesia, with maximum relaxation. This manipulation is contraindicated where the straight-leg-raising test is less than 30° and would only be advised where pain had been present for more than 2 months. In 50 cases, he reports significant reduction of pain in 72% 2 weeks after treatment, with no change in 24%, and 4% of patients temporarily worse.
If conservative treatment has failed and intervention (chemonucleolysis or surgery) is to be considered, accurate imaging of the HNP must be achieved[15,18]. The choice rests between myelography, magnetic resonance imaging (MRI) and computer tomographic scanning (CT). Modic[17] and his colleagues examined all three modes and reported their accuracy in agreeing with surgical findings as follows:

Myelography	71.8%
MRI	82.6%
CT	83.0%
Myelography + CT	89.4%
MRI + CT	92.5%

He concluded that MRI was acceptable as an alternative procedure to myelography. We therefore use both MRI and CT in all cases, thus avoiding an invasive procedure with known morbidity that is unpleasant to the patient, and avoiding hospitalization.

Perhaps a pause is appropriate here to consider collecting evidence to eliminate patients for whom chemonucleolysis is contraindicated or where surgery could be considered the preferred primary treatment.

Contraindications: Apart from those already mentioned, if CT demonstrates a central disc protrusion of such magnitude that it flattens the normally circular spinal bundle, this would represent a disqualification. Injection of such a disc with the normal 2.0 ml of enzyme could increase the protrusion sufficiently to cause a cauda equina syndrome. A history of previous disc surgery at the offending level would also disqualify the patient[14].

Surgery: This should be considered if imaging has demonstrated a large central disc protrusion, particularly if there is any S3 or S4 nerve root involvement. This also applies if the disc is sequestrated or ruptured, in many cases MRI and CT demonstrate this well[14]. Chymopapain is only effective on the nuclear material and cannot have any effect on a hard sequestrated fragment or annulus. The combination of a ruptured disc plus a sequestrated fragment, possibly adherent to the dura with a possible cerebrospinal fluid leak (extremely rare), could provide a scenario for the passage of chymopapain into the subarachnoid space via the nucleus. This could be disastrous. Severe degenerative disc disease, significant apophyseal joint arthropathy or spinal canal stenosis call for consideration of surgery[14].

It would be hoped at this stage that all evidence shows an HNP at a single level matching the clinical findings and imaged clearly by both MRI and CT. But what if all the evidence collected does not point with certainty to a clear non-ruptured HNP matching the clinical levels? There could be:

- Clinically a clear HNP but negative imaging;
- Alternatively, positive imaging at a different level or two levels;
- A positive MRI but negative CT scan, or vice versa;
- Disc degeneration without extrusion at the appropriate level – sufficient to negate treatment by discolysis;
- Doubt as to which level is responsible for the patient's pain.

Discography could be used for further assessment of the severity of disc degeneration, at the same time demonstrating any leak of the nucleus into the epidural space and whether this should exclude the patient[1,15]. It is suggested that this is the only excuse for using radio-opaque material in view of adverse reactions, particularly when used in association with chymopapain[14]. To obtain maximum benefit from the treatment, chymopapain should not be injected into a 'dirty' disc; thus, if discography has been performed, actual treatment should be delayed by 48 hours or more.

If there is doubt concerning the correct disc level responsible for the patient's pain, this can best be confirmed by carrying out discometry at the suspect levels.

The simple injection of the nucleus pulposus with normal saline can be very informative[11]:

- If it reproduces the patient's pain – this identifies the correct disc space.
- If there is a firm 'end point' after injecting about 2.0 ml – the nucleus is intact and the disc is not ruptured.
- If two levels tested reproduce pain – only then would treatment be considered at both levels.

I quote again from McCulloch and Macnab[14]: 'If there is a normal disc at discometry – firm end point and *no* response from the patient – any deficit on imaging can be set aside as a false positive'.

Manometric pressure readings, taken through the injection needle, can also aid in the assessment of the degree of degeneration or the presence of disc rupture[1,4,11].

An interesting case was that of a 36-year-old male executive, travelling long distances by car daily. He complained, initially, of severe low back pain following a heavy lift. After 24 hours the pain started to radiate into the full length of his right leg to include the little toe. His back pain disappeared. After 2 weeks, his signs were classically that of a soft lumbar disc protrusion on the right side with an S1 nerve root palsy. He failed to respond to two epidural injections. MRI indicated 'a large right-sided disc with probable sequestration at L5/S1'. CT reported 'a disc protrusion at L5/S1, mainly on the right-side and obliterating the nerve root with sequestration of the disc itself'. Discolysis was felt to be inappropriate and discometry was bypassed in favour of a neurosurgical opinion. Microdiscectomy was decided on, but on inspection with a very clear view it showed no evidence of any lumbar disc protrusion at either L5/S1 or L4/L5. At the L5 space there were small adhesions around the S1 nerve root and it was tight in the bony canal; this was freed. Postoperatively, the patient's leg pain disappeared completely in one week and his S1 palsy recovered in 2 months.

At this stage, completion of the Macnab diagnostic score card is extremely useful; the total points giving a forecast on the results of treatment, and often helpful to the enquiring patient. Negative points are awarded for evidence of poor psychological background, long absences from work and, above all, pending litigation.

Javid[10] has shown in a study of 214 patients an overall success rate, after 1 year, of 84.6%. In 172 patients, *not* receiving workmen's compensation, this rises to 90.7%. However, in the 42 patients drawing workmen's compensation, the success rate falls to 59.5%.

Our experience comparing patients in the private sector (a high percentage of which are self-employed), with those in the National Health Service shows evidence of a similar disproportion. In the latter case most patients are drawing sickness benefit and in many cases it is possible to make a secondary diagnosis of superadded 'compensitis'. Graham[8] from Sydney, Australia, states that in his experience such cases, unless circumstances are exceptional, do not warrant treatment by chemonucleolysis as the results are so poor.

At this stage we are on the 'launch pad' and ready for final 'count down'. Bearing in mind that in the past the major complication was cogent anaphylaxis occurring in 0.3% of patients, skin testing would be carried out immediately prior to the procedure, and one would rely on a negative response[3-5]. Subsequent discolysis at a different level can be carried out as long as 12 months have elapsed from the first injection and the skin test remains negative. It has been reported that a patient's sensitization following the first injection rapidly decreases after 9 months. There have been no reports of severe anaphylaxis occurring in patients with a negative skin test. Patients with positive skin tests would always be rejected[5,8,12,13].

So now – with a well-identified, intact, painful HNP in a patient negative to skin testing – discolysis using chymopapain can proceed.

However, how does one maintain a high success rate during treatment, recovery and rehabilitation? That is another story!

REFERENCES

1. Adams, M.A. et al. (1986). The stages of disc degeneration as revealed by discograms. *J. Bone Joint Surg.*, **68B**(1), 36–41
2. Benoist, M., Bouillet, R. and Mullholland, R. (1983). Chemonucleolysis: results of a European survey. *Acta Orthop. Belg.*, **49**, 32–47
3. Bernstein, D. and Bernstein, I. (1986). Chymopapain induced allergic reactions. *Clin. Rev. Allergy*, **4**, 201–213
4. Brock, M. (1987). Chemonucleolysis – has it come and gone? *J. Orthop. Med.*, **2**, 31
5. Cogen, F., Goldstein, M. and Zweiman, B. (1985). Skin testing in chymopapain anaphylaxis. *J. Allergy Clin. Immunol.*, **75**, 728–730
6. Cyriax, J. (1975). *Textbook of Orthopaedic Medicine*, 6th edn., Vol. 1. (London: Ballière Tindall)
7. Fraser, R.D. (1984). Chymopapain for the treatment of intervertebral disc herniation: the final report of a double blind study. *Spine*, **9**, 815–818
8. Graham, C.E. (1988). Chemonucleolysis: the recipient's verdict. *J. Bone Joint Surg.*, **70**, 166
9. Heinz-Michael, M. et al. (1986). Skin testing for chymopapain allergy in chemonucleolysis. *Surg. Neurol.*, **25**, 283
10. Javid, M.J. (1988). Signs and symptoms after chemonucleolysis. A detailed evaluation of 214 worker's compensations and noncompensation patients. *Spine*, **12**, 1428–1437
11. Lavignolle, B. et al. (1989). Prospective evaluation of correlation between discometry and MR imaging data. *J. Orthop. Med.*, **1**, 14
12. Mayer, H.M. et al. (1986). Skin testing for chymopapain allergy in chemonucleolysis. *Surg. Neurol.*, **25**, 285–289
13. McCulloch, J. (1985). Thoughts on skin testing. *Altern. Spinal Surg.*, **2**, 12
14. McCulloch, J.A. and Macnab, I. (1983). *Sciatica and Chymopapain*, 1st edn. (Baltimore: Williams & Wilkins)
15. McCulloch, J. and Waddell, G. (1978). Lateral lumbar discography. *Br. J. Radiol.*, **51**, 498–502
16. Merz, B. (1986). The honeymoon is over: spinal surgeons begin to divorce themselves from chemonucleolysis. **286**(3), 318
17. Modic, M.J. et al. (1986). Lumbar herniated disc disease and canal stenosis – prospective evaluation by surface coil MR, CT and myelography. *Am. J. Radiol.*, **147**, 757–765
18. Schipper, J. (1987). Lumbar disc herniation: diagnosis with CT or myelography? *Radiology*, **165**, 227–231
19. Smith, L. et al. (1963). Enzyme dissolution of the nucleus pulposus. *Nature*, **198**, 1311–1312
20. Stoddard, A. (1983). *Manual of Osteopathic Practice*, 2nd edn., p.184. (London: Hutchinson Medical)

49

Radiofrequency denervation of the zygapophyseal joint nerve supply

David George VIVIAN

INTRODUCTION

The use of radiofrequency denervation to treat pain of zygapophyseal joint or posterior spinal compartment origin has been gaining in interest since studies showed that heat lesions selectively block smaller fibres in a nerve – the pain-conducting A-δ and C fibres[10] and also since the resurrection of the concept that chronic pain can derive from these posterior structures.

THE ZYGAPOPHYSEAL JOINT NERVE SUPPLY – THE DORSAL RAMI

The zygapophyseal joints receive their nerve supply from the medial branches of the dorsal rami. The L1–L4 dorsal rami are different from the L5 dorsal ramus[2].

L1–L4

These dorsal rami are short (5 mm). They divide in the intertransverse space, usually into three branches – the medial, intermediate and lateral – and sometimes into two branches.

The medial branch runs in a groove between the root of the transverse process and the superior articular process in a postero-medial direction, and then through a groove between the mamillary process and the accessory process, covered by the mamillo-accessory ligament. Branches then arise to the corresponding superior and inferior zygapophyseal joint, and the nerve terminates in multifidus and the interspinous region. The fibres do not become cutaneous.

The intermediate branch supplies longissimus thoracis pars lumborum. Communication occurs between the intermediate branches at different levels.

The lateral branch crosses the transverse process lateral to the accessory process, goes through iliocostalis lumborum, and the L1-L3 branches are cutaneous over the iliac crest.

L5

This nerve is longer, and divides into two, the medial and intermediate. The medial branch supplies the lumbo-sacral zygapophyseal joint and the fibres of multifidus arising from the L5 spinous process. The intermediate branch supplies longissimus and communicates with branches from S1[2].

AGE AND TRAUMA CHANGES IN THE ZYGAPOPHYSEAL JOINT

The term 'posterior marginal damage' has been coined in recent studies to describe changes seen in the lower quarter of the zygapophyseal joint. The changes include:

- Stretching and tearing of the joint capsule;
- Articular cartilage tears;
- Articular cartilage separation from subchondral bone plate;
- Incongruity of the bony margin at the articular cartilage/subchondral bone plate interface;
- joint instability[12].

These changes are seen both in middle or later life and in younger spines as a result of acute trauma. In a study of 204 lumbar spines of all ages, there was a group of 31 lumbar spines that had been involved in a violent event that had led to death. Lateral and antero–posterior X-rays did not reveal evidence of injury to the zygapophyseal joints. Post-mortem studies of up to three joints were made (L1–L2, L3–L4 and L4–L5). Of these 31 spines, only two were clear of zygapophyseal damage. Eleven had evidence of bony injury, six having fractures of the subchondral bone plate, the rest having central infractions of the subchondral bone plate. Soft-tissue injuries occurred in 26 of these lumbar spines. The changes included posterior marginal damage, with capsular tears, articular cartilage splits or separation from the subchondral bone plate[12].

The age changes that appear are accelerated and aggravated by instability of a motion segment. These changes can cause potent stimulation of the nociceptive fibres in the zygapophyseal capsule, and can produce pain.

DIAGNOSTIC PROCEDURES

Local anaesthetic blocks have been used to delineate pain of possible zygapophyseal joint origin. Two methods can be used.

(1)   *Zygapophyseal block.* In this procedure one or more zygapophyseal joints are visualized under fluoroscopic control. Bupivacaine 0.5% (Marcain) 0.5 ml and methylprednisolone 20 mg are injected into each joint.

(2)   *Dorsal ramus block.* In this procedure the expected site of the dorsal ramus branches are injected at each level under fluroscopic control with bupivacaine.

Prior to the procedure, the movement patterns with pain response are recorded. Five minutes after the procedures, the movements are re-tested. If the pain is eliminated and the movements are now full, the posterior structures including the zygapophyseal joints are likely to be contributing to the patient's pain.

The patient is given a pain chart to fill in for the 6 hours after the procedure. He is required to record range of movements and pain response, and is also required to report on pain response to the usual aggravating activities, e.g. gardening, driving, sitting, etc. With bupivacaine, pain relief of about 4 hours is expected. Shorter-acting anaesthetics can be used.

In order to implicate the posterior structures as a possible source of pain, the majority of pain must be eliminated in movement tests and in performing tasks that usually aggravate the patient's pain.

Sometimes these procedures can produce a therapeutic effect. Radio-frequency denervation of the posterior structures is used as a treatment if:

(1)   The posterior structures have been implicated as a source of pain by zygapophyseal joint or dorsal ramus block;
(2)   The therapeutic effect of the block has subsided.

The problem with diagnostic procedures for detecting pain of posterior compartment origin is that local anaesthetic leaks prominently into other areas. It has been demonstrated in our procedures that the injected material often leaks into the epidural space. Profound examples of this occur in the case of spondylolysis where the material often leaks into the opposite joint, and sometimes even into the joint above or below. It is probable that, even with low doses of anaesthetic, blockade occurs at many areas, and in fact there may be segmental blockade to the innervation to the disc, the spinal canal and other zygapophyseal joints. Thus, it is probable that the diagnostic test lacks specificity. Perhaps a better indicator of a zygapophyseal joint as a source of pain is a therapeutic response from a joint injection.

Because of this difficulty I have tended to abandon diagnostic blocks as a procedure, and tend to do radiofrequency denervation on clinical grounds.

RADIOFREQUENCY DENERVATION

The patient is admitted to hospital in which the following facilities are available:

(1)   X-ray screening table;
(2)   Image intensifier with C arm;

(3)   Radionics radiofrequency lesion generator system;
(4)   Anaesthetic and resuscitation equipment.

The patient lies prone on the table. The lumbar lordosis is maintained to some extent if possible to facilitate needle placement. A more vertical needle entry can then be made to enable the needle tip to run as parallel as possible with the dorsal ramus branches[1].

A light general anaesthetic and analgesic is given to the patient, who remains conscious and moderately alert if possible during the procedure.

The target points are identified on the image intensifier using a direct postero-anterior screen, and these points are marked on the skin. Needle entry points are selected, taking into consideration that the needle tip needs to run as parallel as possible to the target nerve.

The skin is sterilized and draped; the surgeon gloves. The stimulator needle is connected to the generator system, and the circuit is completed with a diathermy pad attached to the patient's leg.

The needle is inserted onto the target point, always onto bone. The stimulation system is used. A positive stimulation response is with pain reproduction, particularly distal referred pain. A lesion is then applied, usually for 1 minute. The rate of stimulation is set at 50, and about 30 volts is used. If the procedure is too painful, local anaesthetic is injected at the needle tip.

As there is communication between adjacent dorsal rami, and because of the dual nerve supply to the joints, two or more dorsal rami are stimulated and denervated on one or both sides.

RESULTS

At this stage there have not been any controlled studies of radiofrequency procedures. There have been favourable reports in long-term follow up.

The reports of results usually designate good, fair or poor as the response, with good being 50% improved or better. The patient groups are frequently divided into unoperated and operated groups.

Published results

Shealy reported on 380 patients who had radiofrequency denervation in the lumbar spine. Good results were quoted in 80% of unoperated cases, 40% of operated (non-fusion) cases, and 29% of fusion operations[11].

Lora and Long reported on 149 patients who had spinal radiofrequency denervation. Good results were obtained in 61% of unoperated cases, 27.5% of patients who had one operation and 0% in patients who had more than one operation[6].

Rashbaum reported on more than 100 patients, and described 82% good relief at one year, and 68% sustained relief. He noted that the procedure did help in patients with chronic backache after successful surgery for radicular pain, but that it was ineffective in patients with multiple surgery even if the diagnostic blocks were positive, and in spondylolisthesis[8].

Oudenhoven reported on 801 patients at six months. Of the 603 who had not had surgery, 57% reported excellent relief, 26% good relief, and 17% were failures. Of the 198 who had previous surgery, 25% reported excellent relief, 32% good relief and 43% were failures[7].

Lavignolle and Senegar reported on 352 patients at 1 year and then 3 years. In the unoperated group, 70% reported good results at 1 year[4].

Ray reported on 1020 patients, stating that 65–80% had a good immediate result, and 50% had a permanently good result[9].

Katz and Savitz reported on 115 patients. They did not perform diagnostic blocks and reported good results in 66% of all patients (75% in the unoperated group and 58% in the operated group)[3].

Most recently, Rossi and Pernak reported on 3000 cases of which 55% were in the lumbar region. Overall they reported good results in 60–80% of cases at 3–6 months, and 50% in the longer term. They reported good results in less than 30% of operated cases, and noted that the worst results were in patients who had a fusion operation. They achieved best results in cervical radiofrequency[10].

CONCLUSIONS

It is my opinion that radiofrequency denervation does have a part to play in the management of pain of musculo-skeletal origin when the pain is derived from the zygapophyseal joint. It should be emphasized that this procedure does not produce a cure. It denervates these structures, and if the injured structures recover in the period when the denervation is active, then there will be no further pain. If the injury does not recover, there will be reactivation of pain when the denervation wears off (this is in about 1 year) and the procedure may need to be repeated.

If it is clear that one joint is involved, future treatment options could include synovectomy or capsulectomy of the appropriate zygapophyseal joint. Other options include fusion at that level to stop movement occurring at the joint.

From preliminary results, it appears that the procedure is best used in the following patients:

(1)　Those who have been involved in trauma, e.g. motor car accidents; direct trauma where there has been a blow to the back or they have fallen hitting an object; hyperextension injuries.

(2)　Where there is a referred pain pattern. It does not appear at all useful where there is neurogenic pain, but is useful in somatic referred pain.

(3) It is not indicated when a disc prolapse is clinically evident.
(4) If disc injury is suggested by the history, e.g. particularly in lifting incidents, or where there is insidious onset of pain, then it is unlikely that the zygapophyseal joints are the source of pain. In these cases radiofrequency denervation is destined to failure.
(5) Recurrent pain after spinal operation. If pain begins some months or years after a successful operation, and the pain is in a referred pattern with tenderness over the posterior structures, then radiofrequency denervation can often control this pain. The pain in these cases can of course be due to zygapophyseal joint osteoarthritis, but could also be discogenic in nature. A radiofrequency denervation will often settle the issue, but in these cases it is likely that continual procedures over the years will be necessary.
(6) Spondylolisthesis. I have performed denervations in five patients with this condition, and the indication has been backache and/or leg pain. Four of the five have reported 3 months after the procedure that it has enabled them to function much better. They had all had pain for more than 3 years. Three of the five had been out of work for periods greater than 12 months prior to the procedure; and 3 months after the procedure, two of them were back working.

SUMMARY

In summary, it does appear that there is a group of patients in whom radiofrequency denervation of the dorsal rami branches provides some pain relief. At this stage it does not appear that any particular physical or radiological findings are relevant in predicting which patients will benefit. Radiofrequency denervations cannot be used to treat radicular pain.

I select patients on the basis that they have chronic pain, whether it be localized to the low back or referred into the legs, even as far as the foot, and that they have tried physical therapy, exercises, ergonomics and other conservative regimes without long-standing success.

The procedure is safe and significant side-effects do not appear in the literature. The coagulation of the nerve does not involve transection, and so the nerves will recover slowly. During this period of restoration of the nerve function, further spinal education and management is undertaken.

The reported results so far have lacked objectivity; in the future, results will need to be established by an outside observer.

Now that the method of needle alignment in relation to the medial branch has been elucidated, better results should follow[1].

REFERENCES

1. Bogduk, N., Macintosh, J. and Marsland, A. (1987). Technical limitations to the efficacy of radiofrequency neurotomy for spinal pain. *Neurosurgery*, **20**, 529–535
2. Bogduk, N., Wilson, A. and Tynan, W. (1982). The human lumbar dorsal rami. *J. Anat.*, **134**, 383–397
3. Katz, S.S. and Savitz, M.H. (1986). *Mt. Sinai J. Med.*, **53**, 523–525
4. Lavignolle, B. and Senegar, J. (1985). Rhizolysis: results in Europe. *The First International Symposium on Alternatives in Spinal Surgery*, Paris
5. Letcher, F.X. and Goldring, S. (1968). The effect of radio frequency current and heat on peripheral nerve action potential in the cat. *J. Neurosurg.*, **29**, 42–47
6. Lora, J. and Long, D. (1976). So-called facet denervation in the management of intractable back pain. *Spine*, **1**, 121–126
7. Oudenhoven, R. (1981). Facet rhizotomy – an obvious misnomer – general information. Presented at the *7th Meeting of the International Study of Lumbar Spine*, Paris
8. Rashbaum, R. (1983). Radio frequency facet denervation – a treatment alternative in refractory low back pain with or without leg pain. *Orthop. Clin. N. Am.*, **3**, 569–575
9. Ray, C.D. (1985). Presented at the *First International Symposium of Alternatives in Spinal Surgery*, Paris
10. Rossi, U. and Pernak, J. (1988). The facet syndrome. Presented at *The Pain Clinic*, Florence (Proceedings in press)
11. Shealey, C.N. (1976). Percutaneous radio frequency denervation of spinal facets. *J. Neurosurg.*, **43**, 448–451
12. Twomey, L.T. and Taylor, J.R. (1987). Zygapophyseal joints of the lumbar spine: current research. *Proceedings of the Fifth Biennial Conference, Manipulative Therapists Association of Australia*, pp. 389–398

50

Manipulative medicine and sports injuries

Franco COMBI and Ivano COLOMBO

It is a well-known fact that sporting activity can cause vertebral conflict leading to a complex and varied symptomatology, often not easy to identify. Our aim here is to describe unclear, symptomatological cases that are sometimes difficult to define, with a certain vertebral origin, which are all too often incorrectly diagnosed so that an inattentive doctor wastes time with inappropriate treatment. The aim is to entreat sports doctors to be aware of this possibility and not to underestimate a thorough examination of the spine, according to Maigne's method, when examining the injured athlete.

We are convinced that many leg mialgias and pubic pains are referred, caused by minor intervertebral conflict, DIM type (minor intervertebral disturbances), in the thoracic-lumbar region. We are also convinced that muscle pain due to contracture (which we would prefer to define 'dysfunctional contractive myalgia', even if it is not treated, will heal spontaneously within 2–3 weeks. All of the myalgias that last for longer are due to damage to the muscle structure (muscle fibrosis due to a trauma), or insertion enthesitis or referred pain from the spine due to irritation of the posterior branch of the spinal nerve in the thoracic-lumbar region.

We intend to deal with this last nosological aspect, as the others are not difficult to identify and diagnose using ultrasonography (scan) that is easily carried out.

On the basis of our experience we are convinced that when examining an athlete with muscle pain in his lower abdomen, pubis, leg adductors, or legs one should not undermine the importance of a detailed examination of the spine to look for painful areas, cellulalgias or pain on passive mobilization of each vertebral and costal articulation (central and lateral pressure, pressure on the interspinal ligament and on the spinal processus). By omitting this examination one runs the risk of an incorrect diagnosis and consequently wasting precious time on symptomatic treatment, often ineffective.

We have obtained excellent results in the treatment of cases that had persisted for several months, using our scheme and indicated treatment.

CASES

During the 1987/88 period we have seen 105 athletes; 80 males, aged between 18 and 29 years, and 25 females, aged between 17 and 26 years. Their events were:

Athletics	35
Football	45
Volleyball	4
Basketball	10
Judo	1
Golf	5
Tennis	5
Total	105

All had suffered musculotendinous pain for more than 2 months and had undergone local treatment (cortisone injection, non-steroidal anti-inflammatory drugs, and various physiotherapies: ultrasound, ionotherapy, massage, analgesic ultrasound, laser-treatment).

In these patients a detailed examination of the spinal column showed vertebral conflict, so they underwent specific manipulation, followed by stretching exercises and strengthening isometric exercises after resolution of the painful symptoms. In all of the patients treated, the symptoms were resolved. In 4 cases the symptoms returned after a period of 2–3 months.

51
T3 syndrome

Donald M. FRASER

A syndrome is described consisting of upper back pain associated with an area of muscle hypertonicity at the thoracic 3 (T3) spinal level; loss of joint play at this level (thoracic disc derangement) and autonomic nervous system changes in the upper extremity which may include paresthesias, muscle weakness and vasomotor responses in a non-dermatomal pattern.

The 'T3 syndrome' may be mistaken for brachial plexus injury, cervical disc syndromes, thoracic outlet syndromes, carpal tunnel syndrome, Raynaud's phenomenon, cardiac or chest pathology. This segmental dysfunction can be treated with manipulative reduction at the T3 spinal segment and, if recognized early, may preclude unnecessary and expensive diagnostic studies and untoward delay in treatment.

CASE STUDY 1

This condition was brought to my attention by this case. A 32-year-old female injured her neck, upper and lower back in a motor vehicle accident and presented with signs of sacroiliac joint torsion. A prominent part of her symptom complex was pain in her upper back; palpable muscle hypertonus at T2, T3 and T4 in her paraspinae muscles. She also complained of difficulty with her hands, more marked on the left than on the right. The left middle and ring fingers were white and swollen (middle finger, distal from the interphalangeal joint and distal segment of the ring finger). An atypical Raynaud's phenomenon was suspected. Manipulation of the T2, T3 and T4 levels was performed using techniques described by Bourdillon[1]. This produced immediate return of colour and warmth to the affected fingers and a beginning of clearing of the hand swelling. Since that initial episode, on recurrence of symptoms and signs not related to temperature change (hot or cold) return to normal function can be achieved by manipulative treatment at the T3 (or appropriate) level.

A second case served to amplify the symptoms associated with this syndrome.

CASE STUDY 2

A male weight-lifter complained of easy fatiguability of his right arm on repetitive bench pressing. The cardiovascular system was normal; testing against resistance showed no loss of muscle strength on either side. Historically, he could perform 25 repetitions without difficulty on the left side. In contrast, the right side, historically 'wore out' with 4–5 repetitions. Physical examination revealed sacroiliac torsion from an old injury and an area of muscular hypertonus at T3 with joint dysfunction (thoracic disc derangement) on the right side. He was pain free before examination, so the results of manipulative reduction to T3 and the sacroiliac joints could not be established immediately as usually happens. He reported full function and power within 24 hours. This made the connection with power loss as part of the 'T3 syndrome'.

DISCUSSION

These cases and subsequently others have caused me to postulate a 'T3 syndrome'. This is similar to the T12 or thoraco-lumbar syndrome described by Robert Maigne[2].

Anatomy

According to the dermatone charts of the *Textbook of Orthopaedic Medicine*[3], there is a small segment of T3 along the axillary area of the arm, but not extending far enough distally to account for the findings that appear to be vasomotor-related. The thoracic segments connect liberally with the sympathetic ganglion at T2 and the sympathetic chains and may be the source of the signs and symptoms.

Presenting problem

There is a history of trauma; often a motor-vehicle accident of the rear-end impact type; a fall on the tucked-in shoulder or a direct blow to the shoulder and upper thorax (anteriorally or posteriorally). The complaints are some or all of the following:

- Pins and needles in some or all 5 fingers;
- Swelling of all or some of the finger or hand (rings are tight);
- Aching deep in upper arm, forearm, wrist or thumb, anterior chest;
- Color changes in hand and/or fingers;
- Weakness or easy fatiguability of muscles of shoulder, forearm or hand;

Loss of active and passive extension of shoulder with inability to reach above head or behind back (cannot fasten brassière at back);
Unable to lie flat on back (shoulder is forward and clavicle prominent);
Aching down arm with restricted range of movement of shoulder joint (a secondary capsulitis of gleno-homeral and/or acromio-clavicular joint).

CLINICAL FINDINGS

1) All six active movements of head and neck do not produce or aggravate the symptoms.

2) All tests for acromio-clavicular and glenohomeral joint are non-capsular or equivocal.

3) Tender paraspinae areas of muscular hypertonus at one or more levels T2, T3 or T4, sometimes associated with areas of muscular hypertonus over the costo-transverse junctions at the same levels.

(4) Tenderness and sometimes palpable displacement of the rib of the same segment anteriorly. This finding often results in an expensive, intensive and negative investigation.

(5) Observable swelling and colour changes on affected limb or hand (fingers).

(6) Weakness on resisted testing of more than one muscle and dermatomal origin, i.e. supraspinatus (C5), biceps (C5, 6), triceps (C7), abductor pollicis (C8) (grip-strength); it is necessary to rule out a brachial plexus lesion.

(7) Non-capsular pattern of restricted passive movement − gleno-humeral joint, i.e. abduction 90°, lateral rotation 90° and medial rotation 50°.

(8) All other arm tests negative.

(9) May or may not have sacroiliac torsion.

TREATMENT

Manipulation of the detected lesion , i.e. T2 and/or T3 and/or T4, results in a dramatic and rapid clearance of signs and symptoms and return of power and improved range of movements in gleno-humeral joint. If there is residual

capsular pattern of joint arthritis (arthrosis), it must be treated in the usu
orthopaedic medicine[3] protocol. If a costo-transverse junction dysfunction
present, it too responds to manipulative reduction described by Bourdillon. Th
fulcrum is moved laterally over the area of hypertonus; it can also I
manipulated and reduced using an anterior approach. If marked ligament laxi
is present with recurrences of the problem due to the joint instability, it
necessary to include ligament-strengthening injections, i.e. sclerothera
(prolotherapy in the United States).

PROGNOSIS

Prevention of recurrence is difficult owing to the nature of the affected levels
and the pull of the arm muscles on the ribs. The ligaments are often stretch
and lax owing to the trauma and aggravated by imprecise therapy before t
diagnosis is made.

REVIEW OF LITERATURE

A review of the literature revealed that this phenomenon was reported by Jo
Bourdillon, in 1985[4] and in addition, under the direction of Robert Kappler,
the Chicago College of Osteopathic Medicine, thermographic studies of the
area and the secondary vasomotor effects are showing early correlation[5].

REFERENCES

1. Bourdillon, J.F. (1982). *Spinal Manipulation* 3rd edn. (New York: Appleton-Century-Crofts)
2. Maigne, R. (1981). Le syndrome de la chaniere dorsolumaire (the thoracolumbar juncti
   syndrome: low back pain, pseudo-visceral pain, pseudo-hip pain and pubalgia. *Sem. Hosp. Pa*
   57, 11
3. Cyriax, J. (1978). *Textbook of Orthopaedic Medicine, Vol. 1, Diagnosis of Soft Tissue Lesions (*
   edn.). (London: Baillière Tindall)
4. Bourdillon, J.F. (1985). *Proceedings of the Annual Meeting of the International Federation
   Manipulative Therapists*, Vancouver, British Columbia, Canada
5. Kelso, A.F. (1985). Recent research in thermography. Paper presented at the *Annual Meeting
   the North American Academy of Manipulative Medicine*, Edmonton, Alberta, Canada

52
Radiographic signs of the function of the intrinsic muscles of the cervical spine

Jan JIROUT

Of the intrinsic spinal muscles, the morphology and function of those located within the dynamic segment (for instance mm. rotatores breves) are least known. According to the anatomical findings, they are represented by separate muscle elements dispersed in the mesh of collagen tissue that connects two neighbouring vertebrae. They cannot be examined by electromyography, but, paradoxically, we can obtain some information on their function by simple X-ray examination.

The following features seem to be associated with the function of these muscle elements:

(1)   By examination of the cervical spine in neutral position and on maximum lateral inclination, we have found that on deep inspiration the lordotic curvature of the cervical spine frequently becomes straightened, the vertebrae are tilted in the sagittal plane, mostly ventrally, and the cervical spine is elongated. On deep expiration the lordosis is usually accentuated; the spine becomes shorter as mostly the upper cervical vertebrae are tilted dorsally and the lower ones ventrally. There is a direct proportion between the degree of tilting and the change in length of the cervical spine. In our opinion these postural changes, synchronous with respiration, are due to the contraction and decontraction of the multisegmental system of the intrasegmental muscle elements.

(2)   This musculature acts as stabilizer and moderator in the dynamics of the spine. Owing to its contraction, a unilateral stress, such as lifting a load or pressing of the head to one side, does not elicit an appropriate degree of scoliosis, but, rather, a reaction in the horizontal and sagittal plane, i.e. rotation or sagittal tilting of vertebrae.

(3)   Similarly, the increased segmental tilting, a segmental hypermobility, can be observed paradoxically with higher percentage on bilateral caudad pressure of both upper extremities than on bilateral lifting of a weight, in

spite of the fact, that on caudad pressure those muscles are activated tha are not attached on the spine.

(4) The sudden decontraction of these muscle elements in multiple segmen associated with manual abolition of blockage can be attributed to th reflex release of their spasm.

(5) It seems that the action of these muscle elements, which otherwise are nc subject to our will, can be triggered by imagined, but not actual performed, changes in the shape of the cervical spine. The subjects wer instructed to concentrate mentally on their cervical spine and to imagin that they were forcing the accentuation of the cervical lordosis – or th reverse, from lordosis to kyphosis. The cervical spine remained in th neutral upright position, the head and shoulders immobilized, supporte by the vertical table of the X-ray machine. On observations, the head an neck exhibited no visible movement. Nevertheless, in a group of 12 persons, a response by vertebrae, namely ventral and dorsal tiltings in th sagittal plane, could be registered on A–P X-ray pictures in about 2/3 vertebrae. Considering that not all subjects could be expected to follo our instructions precisely, the percentage of reacting vertebrae relatively high. It was expected that the mental picture of active, volunta enhancement of cervical lordosis or kyphotization of the cervical spir would lead to actual lordotization or kyphotization of the spine. Thi however, proved to be an extremely rare occurrence.

Generally, the tendency for lordotization prevailed; however som times kyphotization appeared, even while enhancement of lordosis wa being imagined. We observed similar reactions in anticipatory stres when the patient was expecting an impact on the head.

The irregularity of responses, the lack of definite pattern in a larg percentage of cases and the prevailing tendency towards lordotizatic seem to indicate that the intrasegmental muscle elements might play significant role in the dynamics of the phenomenon described.

These features cannot be related to the action of the long, extravertebr muscles. It appears that the contraction of the intrasegmental muscle elements synchronous with respiration and that these elements react to reflex contractic on the segmental blockage. They constitute a polymetameric, polysegment system that exhibits polysegmental reflex reactions. They are not subject to o will; however their contraction can be triggered by mental impulses, while at th same time they exhibit a great deal of autonomy.

It is felt that this muscle system has hitherto been grossly neglected. Th appropriate procedures and training might lead to improvement in o endeavour to prevent relapses of segmental blockage and to manage path logical spinal hypermotility.

53

Radio-functional analysis of the cervical region of the spinal column according to Arlen in post-traumatic syndrome

M. KRAEMER and A. PATRIS

INTRODUCTION

Clinical disorders encountered in post-traumatic syndromes, protean as they may be, are nevertheless often stereotyped. The original nature of each case is due to the association of various symptoms in differing proportions. Barre[7] had already suspected that the sympathetic nervous system was linked to those symptoms qualified as subjective, and had suggested radiography of the cervical region of the spinal column in profile in three positions.

There are numerous descriptions of techniques of radiological investigation into post-traumatic cervical lesions in works by such authors as de Seze et al.[13], Jirout[8] and Wackenheim[14] who describe methods of analysing the mobility of the spine at the cervical level.

CERVICAL RADIO-FUNCTIONAL ANALYSIS ACCORDING TO ARLEN

The radiological diagnosis of dysfunctions of the cervical region of the spinal column is one method of analysing intervertebral cervical dysfunctions[3] in flexion–extension movements. As a simple, but reliable and repeatable method it has been used at the Centre de Cure in Munster since 1960. It has already been the subject of several publications[4,5,6] and is used by certain medical experts – mostly German – in cases of post-traumatic cervico-encephalic syndrome, often in forensic medicine[1,12,15]. It consists of measuring the mobility of each cervical vertebra in relation to its overlying vertebra using radiographs of the spine in profile in the relaxed, flexion and extension positions. The measurment is done on these three radiographs, which calls for particular care when taking the shot.

The results of this study of radiographs lend a dynamic aspect to cervical function that can be transferred to a diagram to facilitate any evolutive comparisons.

The repeatability of the results obtained with the same patient thanks to the use of identical anatomical reference points enables evolutive monitoring supervision during treatment. The advantage of this method, apart from it being very easy to use, is that it is possible to visualize vertebral dysfunctions that are the causes of symptoms encountered in post-traumatic syndromes[11].

METHODOLOGY

Populations studied

We studied 241 patients who had been victims of cervical or cranio-cervical injury without peripheral or central neurological lesion. We avoided including in this group serious injuries that had led to fractures and cervical dislocations. Minor injuries were included, however, even if there was no longer any sign of symptoms.

We compared this group with 240 patients who complained of no cervical pathology and who, on questioning, revealed no past history of cranio-cervical injury. The subjects in the reference group were chosen in such a way that they resembled the other group as closely as possible in age and sex.

The values of the basic angles (Figure 53.1) of each vertebra were noted for each subject according to the radio-functional technique described by Arlen[2,4]. These values were fed into a database (DBASE III+R) where a program calculated the intervertebral angles and the intervertebral mobility in each position (Figure 53.2).

At a second stage the file was processed by statistical software (LOGIST R). Data processing used comparisons of averages (Fischer and Student test) and a two-factor variance analysis.

Composition of the groups (Table 53.1)

The reference group compromised 240 subjects of an average age of 41.0 years (± 13.0), with extreme ages from 11 to 77. This group was composed of 142 women (62%) and 98 men (38%). The group of injured subjects compromised 241 subjects of an average age of 40.8 years (± 13.6), with extreme ages from 8 to 77. This group was composed of 149 women (59%) and 92 men (41%).

We are aware that an individual's range of flexion–extension decreases with age and that it varies considerably with regard to sex[9]. We therefore set up groups who were similar to each other, as far as possible, in age and sex. Owing to the relatively small number of subjects taking part in the study, only two groups were made up (Table 53.1): 39 years and under, 40 years and over.

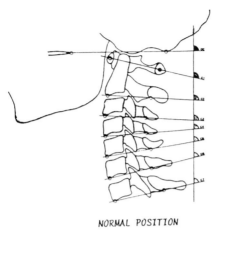

NORMAL POSITION

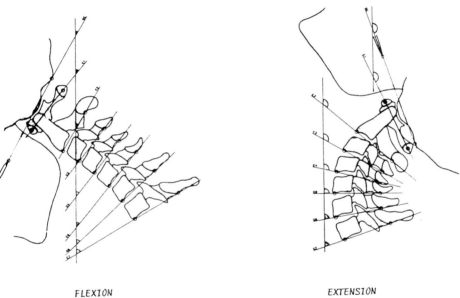

FLEXION   EXTENSION

Figure 53.1 Drawings from radiographs of a patient in profile in the three positions. (From ref. 3)

Comparisons were made of:
- Values of mobility in flexion and extension at each level, and in the overall range between the two groups;
- The differences in mobility in extension, flexion and in the overall range of the spinal column;

- The ranges of movement between two, three, four, five or six adjacent levels in flexion and extension;
- The number of levels where mobility is low (chosen in an arbitrary fashion as less than 4°) or very low (less than 2°).

| | STATIQUE | | | | | | DYNAMIQUE | | | | | DIAGRAMME de MOBILITE | |
| | Angles de base | | | Angles inter-vert. | | | Mobilité inter-vertébrale | | | | | Flexion | Extension |
	Flex.	Norm.	Ext.	Flex.	Norm.	Ext.	Norm Flex.	Norm Ext.	Flex. Ext.	F%			
OC	29	89	161				60	72	132		$OC/C1$		
C1	38	103	154	+ 9	+14	– 7	– 5	21	16				
C2	30	93	130	– 8	–10	–24	2	14	16	13	$C1/C2$		
C3	37	92	120	+ 7	– 1	–10	8	9	17	47	$C2/C3$		
C4	37	84	103	0	– 8	–17	8	9	17	47	$C3/C4$		
C5	38	80	90	+ 1	– 4	–13	5	9	14	36	$C4/C5$		
C6	47	76	79	+ 9	– 4	–11	13	7	20	65			
C7	59	78	71	+12	+ 2	– 8	10	10	20	50	$C5/C6$		
							41	79	120		$C6/C7$		
				$C^2/6$ –17									
									T %	43			

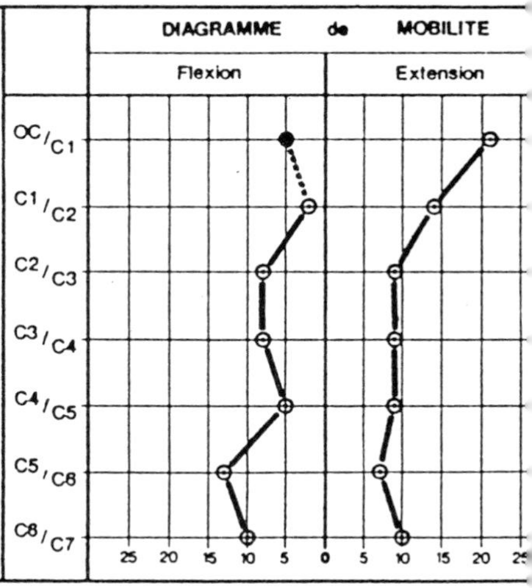

Figure 53.2 Radio-functional analysis of the cervical spine in profile: method of calculation and diagram. (From ref. 3)

OVERALL RESULTS

Total range of movement of the spine at the cervical level

If we consider the total range of mobility without taking into account the age or sex of the subjects, we obtain the results shown in Table 53.2. The total range in extension is significantly reduced in the group of injured subjects ($p=0.0001$, Fischer test). However, the overall range of flexion in the cervical region of the spinal column is identical in the reference group and in the injured group ($p=0.5898$). The overall range is thus significantly reduced ($p=0.0008$ with the Fischer test) in the injured group by the reduction in the range of extension.

As far as the range in the MacGregor line is concerned, the difference is as significant in extension ($p=0.0003$) as in its total range ($p=0.007$). However, no difference was recorded in flexion ($p=0.6916$).

Lordosis remains unchanged in the two groups. The influence of the age factor no doubt weighs heavily on this value[9].

Table 53.1 Amplitudes according to age (in degrees). Reference population ($n = 240$), Injured population ($n = 241$)

	Age range (years)			
	Reference population		After traumatism	
	0 – 39	40 – 80	0 – 39	40 – 80
Men (total 190)	56	42	44	48
Women (total 291)	56	86	68	81

	Age range (years)							
	<10	10–19	20–29	30–39	40–49	50–59	60–69	70–79
Injured population								
Men (total 92)	0	3	21	20	25	19	3	1
Women (total 149)	2	3	31	32	36	32	11	2
Reference population								
Men (total 98)	0	6	14	36	19	16	6	1
Women (total 142)	0	3	18	35	43	33	8	2

Mobility at the various fossae

An overall comparison of the averages for the two groups studied shows the following significant differences (Fischer test of comparisons of averages). *In flexion* the range at C2 increases in the injured group ($p = 0.027$), whereas the range at C3 decreases ($p = 0.007$). *In extension* the range at C4 ($p = 0.05$) and C6 ($p = 0.01$) decreases.

The comparison of the average range of the sum of several successive levels does not provide us with any new facts. The differences are significant in flexion, where calculation includes C3 but excludes C2, and in extension, where C4 and/or C6 are included.

In all calculations there is greater significance as the number of successive levels increases.

Table 53.2 Radio-functional analysis of the cervical spine. Mean values (± 6) according to level

	Flexion			Extension	
Level	Reference pop.	Injured pop.		Reference pop.	Injured pop.
MAC-G	58.55 ± 9.89	58.16 ± 11.71		54.40 ± 11.68	49.93 ± 15.01[a]
OC/C1	−1.67 ± 4.67	−1.09 ± 5.47		14.33 ± 6.52	13.18 ± 6.97[b]
C1/C2	5.87 ± 4.55	6.82 ± 4.74[a]		5.61 ± 4.59	4.92 ± 3.84
C2/C3	5.24 ± 2.64	4.51 ± 3.30[a]		4.61 ± 3.03	4.62 ± 3.10
C3/C4	7.28 ± 3.32	6.87 ± 3.95		7.30 ± 4.00	6.56 ± 4.31[b]
C4/C5	7.10 ± 3.58	6.60 ± 3.52		9.49 ± 4.22	9.11 ± 5.10
C5/C6	7.65 ± 3.91	7.60 ± 3.91		9.20 ± 4.87	8.04 ± 4.82[a]
C6/C7	8.96 ± 3.96	9.25 ± 4.69		5.14 ± 4.03	4.47 ± 5.16
C1/C7	41.50 ± 12.51	42.17 ± 10.21		57.94 ± 13.56	51.60 ± 16.14

[a] Significant difference 1%
[b] Significant difference 5%

Consideration of other factors that influence range of mobility

The age factor has the effect of progressively reducing range of movement in flexion and extension[9]. The sex factor has a less determined effect of increasing certain values while reducing others, which renders statistical study difficult.

Age

A comparison of the average ranges in each of the 'young–old' subgroups does not lead to any obvious differences. Any significant differences in certain values between the injured and the reference group are obviously noted. Among the 'young' injured subjects a significant increase in flexion at C2 ($p=0.01$) was noted as well as a reduction in extension at C2 ($p=0.0155$) and C7 ($p=0.0275$). The least significant reductions in flexion ($p=0.0825$) at C3 and in extension ($p=0.0829$) at C4 were noted for this same group. Among the older subjects an increase in flexion ($p=0.0356$) at C3 and in extension ($p=0.0006$) was noted.

In order to improve the study, we applied a two-factor variance analysis to the subjects. The statistical differences that became apparent are as follows.

The age factor exerts a decisive influence on the values of ranges of mobility at all levels ($p=0.002$ on average) in the reference group as well as the injured group. For the injured group, in the two subgroups divided according to age a significant difference is noted at the following levels compared with the reference group:

- *In flexion* – the range at C2 increases ($p=0.025$) and that at C3 decreases ($p=0.007$);
- *In extension* – the ranges decrease at C1 ($p=0.006$), C2 ($p=0.070$), C4 ($p=0.050$) and C6 ($p=0.008$).

As far as the overall range per fossa is concerned (from extension to total flexion) a two-factor variance analysis of levels C2 to C7 provides us with new elements. The two factors used are age and the existence of post-traumatic syndrome. Injury at the cervical level has a significant effect on levels C3 ($p=0.0070$), C4 ($p=0.0029$), C5 ($p=0.0358$) and C6 ($p=0.0272$).

Table 53.3 Two-factor variance analysis according to age and to sex

According to age				According to sex			
Flexion		*Extension*		*Flexion*		*Extension*	
Levels	*p*	*Levels*	*p*	*Levels*	*p*	*Levels*	*p*
		(C1	0.060)			(C1	0.060)
C2	0.025	(C2	0.070)	C2	0.030		
C3	0.007			C3	0.007		
C5	N.S.			C5	N.S.		
		C4	0.050			C4	0.050
		C6	0.008			C6	0.005

N.S. = not significant

Sex

Significant differences exist between these two subpopulations for some of the levels studied, especially as far as the reference population is concerned:

- A more limited range of flexion at C2 ($p=0.0002$) in men and at C5 and C6 ($p<0.0001$) in women;
- A greater mobility in extension at C4 ($p=0.0147$), C5 ($p=0.0002$) and C6 ($p<0.0001$) in women.

As for the atlas, the range of paradoxical tilt is greater in men than in women, which has been confirmed by other studies[10].

In the injured population, the difference between the two sexes is observed in extension at C3 ($p=0.0035$), C5 ($p<0.0001$) and C6 ($p=0.0001$), with women having greater mobility.

A two-factor variance analysis confirms the predominant influence exerted by the sex factor. No general tendency, however, can be defined on studying the data. Significant differences are noted at levels C2, C3 in flexion and levels C1, C4, C6 in extension.

The MacGregor line case also analysed in this way confirms the fact that the differences in flexion are insignificant, whereas injury leads to a significant reduction in the range of extension ($p = 0.0001$ for the interaction age–injury and $p = 0.0002$ for the interaction sex–injury).

STUDY OF DYSFUNCTIONS AND MOBILITY CORRELATIONS

Dysfunctions

We studied the frequency of very reduced mobility (seizures) whose upper limit was fixed at 2°, and of reduced mobility whose limits were fixed at intervals of 2° exclusive and 5° inclusive.

The χ^2 test illustrates the fact that the frequency of seizures is significantly greater in the injured population ($p = 0.0001$) in extension and flexion. However, hypomobility is about the same in the two groups. If different fossae are considered, the frequency of seizures is significantly greater at C2 in flexion ($p < 0.001$) and C6 in extension ($p = 0.009$).

Correlations between mobility at the different fossae

The study of correlations between mobility at the different fossae in flexion or extension illustrates variations between the two groups studied. Positive correlations correspond to an increase in the range of a given fossa for an increase in range of another fossa. Negative correlations, on the other hand, correspond to a decrease in range at one level at the same time as another level sees its range increase. They can be divided into:

- 'horizontal' compensations that involve the same level;
- 'vertical' compensations that involve two different levels in the same direction of movement;
- 'crossed' compensations that involve two different levels in opposite directions of movement.

Negative correlations

If we take into consideration only the flexion–extension correlations, we notice that the normal subject is likely to compensate for eventual deficiencies by hypermobility in the opposite direction at the same level or at an adjacent level. These compensations are grouped around the levels C2 to C6 ($p < 0.001$). In the case of hypomobility, compensation at the same level and at levels immediately above and below is less common after injury, the latter therefore causing the loss of a part of the spine's capacity to adapt.

Positive correlations

As far as positive correlations are concerned, there are no differences between the two populations in vertical compensations either in flexion or in extension. However, the crossed compensations are clearly influenced by injury. Indeed, compensations at C1 and C7 in flexion occur by extension at C3 ($p=0.001$), C4 ($p=0.001$) and C6 ($p=0.002$). Furthermore, compensations in flexion at C2 by the extension at C3 to C6 noted in the reference population disappear.

To quantify the kind of reduction of mobility, comparisons are made between the two groups with regard to the sum of 2 and 3 successive levels from C2 to C7 in flexion and in extension. For two successive levels, a significantly reduced mobility is found in the injured group in extension ($p=0.016$). There is no difference in comparison with the reference group in flexion. For three successive levels, there is a difference between the two groups, which tends to diminution in the injured group but is not statistically significant ($p=0.069$). No difference is found in flexion. Thus, the injured subject presents two or even three successive levels of reduced mobility in extension with a tight aspect in the part of the diagram concerned, especially between C3 and C6.

CONCLUSION

Injury of the spinal column at the cervical level leads to modifications in the radio-functional analysis according to Arlen:

(1) Decrease in the range of flexion and extension on the tracings;
(2) Reduction in the range of flexion at C3
(3) Reduction in the range of extension at C1, C4 and C6;
(4) Increase in the range of flexion at C2;
(5) Reduced possibilities for the cervical spine to adapt in terms of horizontal, vertical and crossed compensations;
(6) Two or three successive levels of hypomobility in extension.

It is therefore possible to propose a synthesis of the modifications that affect the mobility in the cervical region of the spinal column in flexion–extension after indirect injury (Figure 53.3)

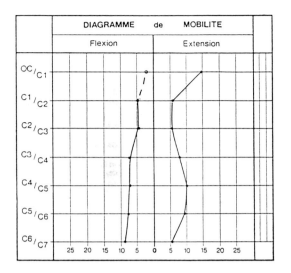

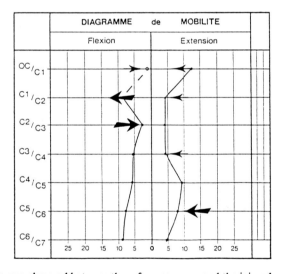

Figure 53.3 Differences observed between the reference group and the injured group

REFERENCES

1. Aeckerle, J. and Teusch, K.H. (1985). Der Roentgenologische Nachweis klinisch diagnostizierter Blockierungen der HWS. *Manuelle Med.*, **23**(2), 33–37.
2. Arlen, A. (1977). Die 'parodoxe Kippbewegung des Atlas' in der Funktionsdiagnostik der Halswirbelsäule. *Manuelle Med.*, **15**(2), 16–23

3. Arlen, A. (1979). Messverfahren zur Erfassung von Statik und Dynamik der Halswirbelsäule in der sagittalen Ebene. *Manuelle Med.*, 17(2), 24–32
4. Arlen, A. (1979). Biometrische Roentgen-Funktionsdiagnostik der HWS. In *Schriftenreihe Manuelle Medizin* Vol. 5. (Heidelberg: Fischer)
5. Arlen, A. (1981). Biometrische Roentgenfunktionsdiagnostik der Halswirbelsäule. *Z. Orthop.*, 119(6), 577–582
6. Arlen, A. and Kraemer, M. (1986). Le diagnostic radiologique des troubles fonctionnels cervicaux. *Rev. Readapt. Fonct. Prof. Soc.*, 15, 42–45
7. Barre, J.A. (1926). Sur un syndrome sympathique cervical postérieur et sa cause fréquente: l'arthrite cervicale. *Rev. Neurol.*, 33, 1246–1240
8. Jirout, J. (1969). Roentgenbewegungsdiagnostik der HWS und der Kopfgelenke. *Manuelle Med.*, 7(6), 121–128
9. Kraemer, M. and Patris, A. (1989). Radio-functional analysis of the cervical spine using the Arlen method – A study of 699 subjects. Part I: Methodology. *J. Neuro-radiol.*, 16, 48–64
10. Kraemer, M. and Patris, A. (1989). Radio-functional analysis of the cervical spine using the Arlen method – A study of 699 subjects. Part II: The parodoxal tilting of the atlas. *J. Neuro-radiol.*, 16, 65–74
11. Lazorthes, G., Gouaze, A. and Salamon, G. (1978). *Vascularisation et circulation de l'encéphale, Vol. 2, Physiologie, exploration angiographie*. (Paris: Masson)
12. Lindner, H.(1983). Die biometrische Roentgen-Funktionsdiagnostik der HWS nach Arlen in der praxis des niedergelassenen Arztes. *Manuelle Med.*, 21(5), 123–125
13. de Seze, S., Djian, A. and Abdelmoula, M. (1951). Etude radiologique de la dynamique dans le plan sagittal. *Rev. de Rhum.*, 18, 111–116
14. Wackenheim, A. (1975). Une méthode de notation de l'épreuve radio-dynamique de flexion-extension cervicale. *J. Méd. Strasbourg*, 6(1), 25–29
15. Zenner, P. (1985). Das posttraumatische zervikookzipitale Syndrom unter besonderer Berücksichtigung von Begutachtungsproblemen. In *Neuro-orthopädie III*, pp. 536–548. (Berlin: Springer Verlag)

54

Therapy of the atlas compared with traditional manipulation in sacroiliac dysfunction

K.J. EIDEN

In daily medical work it is often very difficult to treat patients having a sacroiliac dysfunction and its typical symptomatic pain. The same applies to old patients as well as to patients having osteoporosis or total hip prosthesis, suffering from sacroiliac dysfunction. In the latter cases, local treatment under classical manipulative medicine is contraindicated.

Therapy by manipulative medicine, distant from the area of pain, should be applied to the problems described above. Atlas therapy according to Arlen is an alternative method of treatment in such cases[1,4-6,8,9,15]. I report here first results of a method using atlas therapy to influence the sacroiliac joint. For comparison purposes, two groups of 25 patients each were formed.

The decision who should be treated with which method was made on an *ad hoc* and random basis. The first group was treated with the traditional manipulative medicine according to Sell. The method of Arlen – impulse to the transverse process of the atlas – was applied to the second group. The diagnosis and the treatment were performed during the normal orthopaedic consultation hours. For this reason, only a short time was available for diagnosis.

The following methods were used to test the sacroiliac joint for dysfunction.

(1)   The so-called 'Vorlaufphänomen' as a sign of sacroiliac joint tilting. The posterior-superior iliac spine is palpated with both thumbs from below. If there is tilting on both sides, both thumbs will move. If there is tilting on one side only, the dysfunctional side will move upwards – the posterior-superior iliac spine is pulled upwards together with the sacrum. Asymmetry of the pelvis as well as hip disease must be excluded before performing this test[2,3,8,13,14].

(2)   In case of an unclear result, the test of Kubis and Patrick, a hyperabduction test, was additionally performed. The missing movement of the sacroiliac joint causes greater distances from the knees to the

surface the patient lies on. This test is invalid for patients with arthrosis of the hip joint[2,3,8,13,14].

(3)   The next step was a neurological examination, with test of reflexes and other functions. Patients with neurological diseases were excluded from this study.

(4)   An X-ray of the lumbar spine, imaging the sacroiliac joint, was made to exclude tumorous, metastatic and inflammatory processes. Patients with results of this type were also excluded from the study.

The diagnosis of both groups with sacroiliac joint dysfunction was performed in the same way. A palpatory and (partial) X-ray diagnosis of the atlas situation (anterior, posterior, lateral, normal) was additionally performed in the group for therapy according to Arlen[1,7,10]. Subsequently a functional examination of the cervical spine was performed with inclincation, reclination, axial rotation in medium position, extension and flexion and lateral bending, followed by a reflex examination of the upper extremities.
    Patient group characteristics were:

Group 1:   Therapy according to Sell   25 patients
             Age between 16 and 69 years,
             average 42 years.

Group 2:   Therapy according to Arlen   25 patients
             Aged between 22 and 73 years,
             average 46 years.

Both groups had – by chance – the same number of male (7) and female (18) members.

THERAPY

Group 1: Traditional manipulative technique according to Sell with the so-called *Erlösergriff* or *Panthersprung*[2,11,15]. This technique was performed with 90% tension and only 10% impulse.
Group 2: Therapeutic impulse with the middle finger against the transverse process of the atlas, depending on the diagnosis of its situation[1,10].

The success of the therapy was assessed:
(1)   immediately after the manipulative treatment;
(2)   after 1 week;
(3)   after 2–3 weeks, if necessary.

DIAGNOSTIC RESULTS

Group 1: 14 left-side dysfunctions
    11 right-side dysfunctions of the sacroiliac joint.
Group 2: 12 left-side dysfunctions
    13 right-side dysfunctions of the sacroiliac joint.

Atlas situation diagnosis: LNRP 3
          LLRN 8
          LARN 8
          LNRA 2
          LPRP 1
          LNRL 2
          LARA 1

RESULTS

See Figures 54.1, 54.2 and 54.3.

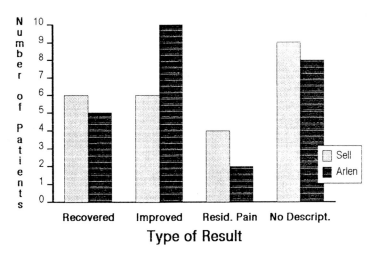

Figure 54.1 Results of both types of therapy immediately after treatment

Group 1 (Sell): Immediately after the manipulative treatment:

– 6 patients had completely recovered;
– 6 patients were improved but still had a positive 'Vorlauf' phenomenon;
– 4 patients still suffered from complaints.

The rest of the patients were unable to describe their situation, which is not unusual after manipulative treatment.

One week after treatment:

- 9 patients had completely recovered;
- 10 had complaints with residual pain in muscles.

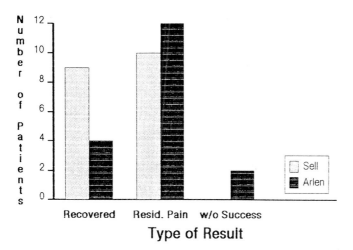

Figure 54.2 Results of both types of therapy after 1 week

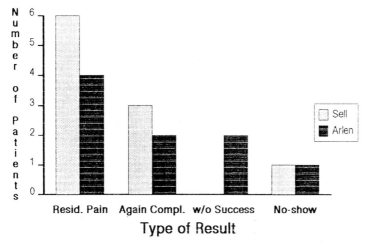

Figure 54.3 Results of both types of therapy after 2–3 weeks

Two to three weeks after the treatment:

- 6 patients had complaints in muscles of the calves;
- 3 patients had been completely without complaints in the meantime, but complaints had arisen again;
- 1 patient did not show up.

Group 2 (Arlen): Immediately after the manipulative treatment:

- 5 patients had completely recovered;
- 10 patients were improved;
- 2 patients had residual pain;
- 8 patients were unable to describe their situation.

One week after the treatment:

- 4 patients had recovered;
- 12 patients had residual pain;
- 2 patients were without therapeutic success.

Two to three weeks after the treatment:

- 2 patients were without therapeutic sucess (1 was an insurance event);
- 4 patients still suffered from pain and had a numb feeling;
- 2 patients had been completely without complaints in the meantime, but then complaints had arisen again;
- 1 patient did not show up.

Summing up, I can say that both methods of treatment showed similar rates of success. About 40% of the patients had to be treated a second or third time. The remainder, about 30%, could not be influenced by either one of the therapeutic methods[3].

Both methods are evidently of equal value, especially for old people and for patients with contraindications for traditional manipulative technique. The atlas impulse according to Arlen is considered to be a suitable alternative[4].

REFERENCES

1. Arlen, A. (1979). Biometrische Röntgenfunktionsdiagnostik der Halswirbelsäule. *Schriftenreihe Manuelle Medizin*, Vol. 5. (Heidelberg; Fischer-Verlag)
2. Bischoff, H.P. (1983). Segmentale Diagnostik an der Wirbelsäule als Voraussetzung der gezielten Manipulationstherapie-Grundlagen der Ausbildung des Dr.-Karl-Sell-Ärzteseminars Neutrauchburg. In Frisch, H. (ed.) *Manuelle Medizin*. (Berlin: Springer-Verlag)
3. Dvorak, J. and Dvorak, V. (1988). Untersuchung: Vorlaufphänomen, Nutation im ISG. In von Dvorak, J. and Dvorak, V. (eds.) *Manuelle Medizin*. (Stuttgart: Thieme)

4. Gutmann, G. (1981). Dokumentation funktionsanalytischer Röntgenbefunde unter besonderer Berückssichtigung der Kopfgelenke im Sinne der H.I.O.-Technik. In *Funktionelle Pathologie und Klinik der Wirbelsäule, Vol. 1, Die Halswirbelsäule*. (Stuttgart: Fischer-Verlag)

5. Gutmann, G. and Biedermann, H. (1984). Afferenzen des Kopfgelenksbereiches und Gleichgewichtsystem. In Gutmann, G. (ed.) *Funktionelle Pathologie und Klinik der Wirbelsäule, Vol. 1, Die Halswirbelsäule*, Part 2, Allgemeine funktionelle Pathologie und Klinische Syndrome (Stuttgart: Fischer-Verlag) ·

6. Hülse, M. (1983). *Die zervikalen Gleichgewichtsstörungen*. (Berlin: Springer-Verlag)

7. Huguenin, F. (1988). Untersuchung des zerviko-okzipitalen Überganges. *Manuelle Med.*, 26, 9–11

8. Lewit, K. (1978). *Manuelle Medizin im Rahmen der medizinischen Rehabilitation*. (München: Urban and Schwarzenberg)

9. Lewit, K. (1989). Manipulation: Reflextherapie und/oder eine Therapie zur Wiederherstellung von Funktionsstörungen im Bewegungssystem. *Manuelle Med.*, 26, 95–96

10. Lohse-Busch, H. (1989). Prinzipien der Metamermedizin Ein Denkmodell. *Manuelle Med.*, 27, 4–7

11. Schneider, W., Dvorak, J., Dvorak, V. and Tritschler, T. (1983). Ausbildungskonzept für manuelle Medizin in der Schweiz. In Frisch, H. (ed.) *Manuelle Medizin*. (Berlin: Springer-Verlag)

12. Tilscher, H. (1983). Indikationen und Erfolgsaussicht der Manualtherapie bei pseudoradikulären Syndromen im Bereich der Halswirbelsäule. In *Neuroorthopädie 1, Halswirbelsäulenerkrankungen mit Beteiligung des Nervensystems*. (Berlin: Springer-Verlag)

13. Tilscher, H. (1984). Zweckmässiger Aufbau des klinischen Untersuchungsganges bei neuroorthopädischen Erkrankungen im Bereiche der Lenden-Becken-Hüftregion. In *Neuroorthopädie 2, Lendenwirbelsäulenerkrankungen mit Beteiligung des Nervensystems*. (Berlin: Springer-Verlag)

14. Tilscher, H. and Eder, M. (1983). *Die Rehabilitation von Wirbelsäulengestörten*. (Berlin: Springer-Verlag)

15. Wolff, H.-D. (1983). Neurophysiologische Aspekte der Blockierung. In *Neurophysiologische Aspekte der manuellen Medizin*. (Berlin: Springer-Verlag)

55
Atlas therapy and neuromuscular diseases

H. LOHSE-BUSCH

Introduction

The only possibility of lightening the burden of neuromuscular diseases today is through muscular training: a causal treatment does not exist. Each of these diseases runs a definite course. One can regularly find muscle shortening, however, in the autochthonous muscles of the spine and in peripheral musculature in all dystrophic and atrophic diseases as well. Muscle shortening is a severe obstacle for training as we know from working with high-performance sportsmen.

Metameric dysfunction always corresponds to the muscle group involved. Spinal muscular atrophy (SMA) shows a diffuse shortening; Duchenne muscular dystrophy (DMD) shows a well-related muscular dysfunction in the involved myotomes. The phenomenon is palpable in the autochthonous muscle system of the spine.

Since Arlen's atlas therapy is able to diminish symptoms of such muscular dysfunction, these findings led to a first attempt to treat the symptomatic signs of neuromuscular disease.

METHOD AND CASE MATERIAL

For the technique of metameric examination and atlas therapy, see Arlen's contribution to this volume.

From September 1985 until May 1989, the following diseases have been treated.

Myogenic muscular dystrophies	10 cases
Facioscapulo-humeral dystrophy (FSH)	2 cases
Becker's muscular dystrophy (BMD)	3 cases
Limb girdle dystrophy (LGD)	2 cases
Emery–Dreifuss' dystrophy (EDD)	1 case
Duchenne's muscular dystrophy (DMD)	2 cases

Neurogenic muscular atrophies	9 cases
Spinal muscular atrophy (SMA) Werdnig–Hoffman II	2 cases
Amyotrophic lateral sclerosis (ALS)	2 cases
SMA Vulpian Bernhard	1 case
SMA Kugelberg–Welander	3 cases
Other neuromuscular diseases	9 cases
Pareses because of poliomyelitis	3 cases
Charcot–Marie–Tooth disease	2 cases
Steinert's myotonia	1 case
Thomsen's myotonia	1 case
Kearns–Sayre–Shy syndrome	2 cases

All patients have been undergoing Arlen's atlas therapy for 3 weeks once to twice a day. The treatment has been completed by Arlen's metameric gymnastics and metameric massage once a day. Types of physiotherapeutics the patients had applied before starting atlas therapy were continued to avoid any possible influence of these therapies on the result of this study.

After 3 weeks of daily intensive treatment, the intervals between treatments were lengthened to one atlas therapy a week, then up to one treatment every 4 weeks, depending on the pathological potential of the different diseases; a SMA Werdnig–Hoffmann II has to be treated once a week; with a SMA Kugelberg–Welander it is sufficient to treat every 4 weeks. Sometimes the individual suddenly experiences a decrease of strength, indicating to the patient himself the necessary rhythm of treatment.

To work out a test programme for each patient individually was indispensable because of the different extents of the diseases and pareses. In these inhomogeneous cases it is impossible to set up a trial design permitting statistical analysis. The number of patients is not high enough and individual physical abilities are too different. Therefore, this pilot study can only offer reports of some cases that represent the different groups of neuromuscular diseases mentioned above.

The age of the patients was between 3.2 and 73 years. The duration of observation and treatment is between 6 and 45 months.

The following parameters were assessed according to the physical ability of the patient.

1) Chronometric measurements
   To stand up five times from a stool of 40 cm height;
   To walk 10 metres;
   To mount 5 steps;
   To mount 20 steps;
   To lift 5 times with stretched arm 500 g in the hand up to 90° in abduction or extension.

(2)   Angles in degrees
        To lift extremities against gravitation.

(3)   Spirographic parameters

(4)   Creatine phosphokinase

RESULTS AND CASE REPORTS

Dystrophy group

(1)   H.A.A., female, 36 years old; FSH-dystrophy with affected peroneal
        nerves on both sides; first clinical appearance at 18 years; beginning of
        atlas therapy in September 1985; duration of treatment up to May 1989,
        45 months. Physical condition:

	Sept 85	Sept 86	Sept 87	Sept 88	May 1989
Flexion of right hip (degrees)	25	70	110	110	110
Abduction of right arm (degrees)	25	60	65	75	100
5 × with 500 g (seconds)			6.3	5.8	4.5
10 m walking (seconds)			10.3	9.8	9.2
Rising from a stool 5x (seconds)			21.9	21.5	15.2
5 steps upstairs (seconds)			7.8	7.0	5.3
Max walking distance (km)	0.3	10	10	12	16

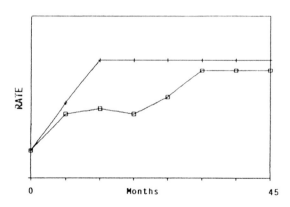

Figure 55.1 H.A.A.: +, flexion of right hip; □, abduction of right arm

412

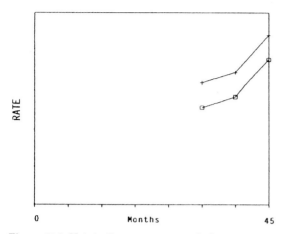

Figure 55.2 H.A.A., first measurements in September 1987: +, 5 times abduction of right arm with 500 g in hand (seconds); □ steps up stairs (seconds)

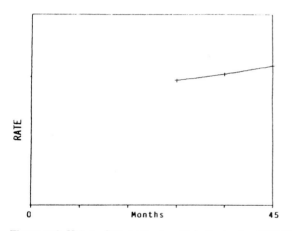

Figure 55.3 H.A.A., first measurements in September 1987: 10 m walking (seconds)

In September 1985 she was not able to comb her hair, had problems with care of the body, walked very sluggishly with a crutch, was unable to mount stairs, and had to hold herself on walls.

In September 1986 she made walking tours longer than 10 km without a crutch, mounted stairs without help, undertook hygiene and body care without help, and worked half a day as physician in hospital. In May 1989 there was no reduction of physical ability.

The patient showed no pathological alteration of blood parameters.

413

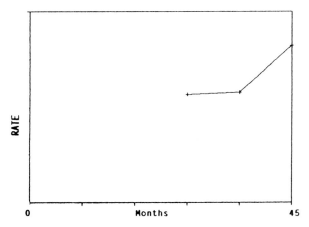

RATE

0   Months   45

Figure 55.4 H.A.A., first measurements in September 1987: 5 times rising from a stool of 40 cm height (seconds)

(2)   S.C.H., male, 11 years old; DMD; atlas therapy from July 1988 to May 1989, 11 months of treatment.

Physical condition in July 1988 before treatment: wheelchair for 2 years; contractures of extremity joints of different degrees; scoliosis; inability to raise his hands to his mouth or to turn himself in bed; bare ability to sit freely.

In this advanced case, chronometric or simple ergometric measurements were not possible. Only spirometric parameters and the values of creatin-phosphokinase (CPK) are available:

	July 88	*May 89*
FVC	1.84	2.09
FEV 1	1.77	2.02
Peak-flow expiration	3.77	4.83
Peak-flow inspiration	2.99	3.20

CPK before atlas therapy		*CPK during atlas therapy*	
Jan 87	1871	July 88	1020
Mar 88	2615	Sept 88	945
Apr 88	2587	Mar 89	656

Physical condition in May 1989: only the regained abilities are mentioned. The boy is able to turn himself round in bed without help. He grips light objects right over the desk. He raises his head when lying in a lateral position. He raises his right arm to 180°. He eats with fork, spoon and knife. He reaches his ears with both hands while sitting in an upright position. Despite his knee and hip contracture he stands on his feet leaning against the wall for 25 minutes while catching and throwing balloons. The scoliosis is actively more upright and can be held for several minutes in this position. The improvement of the erector sacrospinalis is visible, as is the better shape of arm and abdominal muscles. The symptomatic improvement of muscular function by atlas therapy finds expression in spirometric parameters. The decrease of CPK has to be interpreted with caution. The same decrease of CPK has been seen in one case of FSH, LGD, BMD, and the other case of DMD. On the other hand, a disturbance of health such as respiratory or urinary infection leads to CPK increase again.

SMA group

F.R.I., female, 64 years old; SMA Kugelberg–Welander, beginning of clinical appearance at 45 years; atlas therapy from February 1988; duration of treatment to May 1989, 15 months.

	Feb 88	Nov 88	Apr 89
Physical condition:			
5 steps upstairs (seconds)	11.0	7.6	6.8
5 × rising from a stool (seconds)	28.3	16.8	14.9
Flexion of right hip (degrees)	40	90	90
Flexion of left hip (degrees)	45	90	90
10 m distance walking (seconds)	13.4	8.8	8.8
Spirometric parameters:			
FVC	3.72		3.96
FEV 1	3.26		3.51
Peak flow expiration	5.22		7.24
Peak flow inspiration	4.57		6.23

There was no pathological alteration of blood parameters.

The clinical picture of development during atlas therapy seemed to be the same with two other SMA Kugelberg–Welander patients and one SMA Vulpian–Bernhard patient. Two cases of SMA Werdnig–Hoffmann II reacted in principle in the same way, yet in the case treated longest (12 months), physical ability seemed to decrease after the typical improvement at the beginning. But one year later the muscular strength seemed to be still better than before atlas

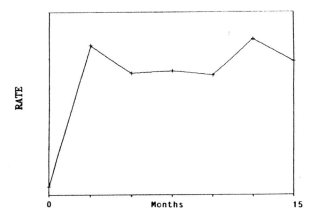

Figure 55.5 F.R.I.: 5 steps up stairs (seconds)

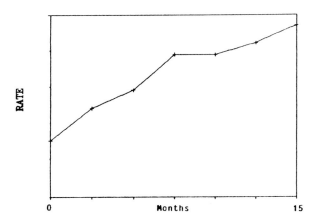

Figure 55.6 F.R.I.: 5 times rising from a stool of 40 cm height (seconds)

therapy. One could therefore presume that the pathological potential of the disease (SMA Werdnig–Hoffmann is more malignant than SMA Kugelberg–Welander) might be in relation to the time the symptomatic improvement lasts. It should be mentioned also that in every case of SMA the sometimes severe disturbances of neurological coordination came nearer to normality. Patients felt surer when walking and fell less often.

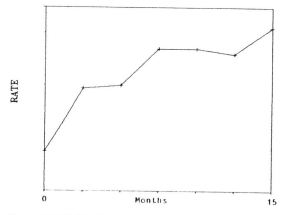

Figure 55.7 F.R.I.: 10 m walking (seconds)

ALS group

F.I.S., 73 years old; female; ALS; beginning of clinical appearance, December 1988; atlas therapy from January 1988 to April 1988; died 20 June 1988 of pneumonia, respiratory insufficiency, and stress ulcer of stomach.

Physical condition:

	14 Jan 88	6 Feb 88	3 April 88
5× abduction right arm with 500 g (seconds)	7.8	5.2	7.0
5× abduction left arm with 500 g (seconds)	6.9	4.8	7.2
5× extension right arm with 500 g (seconds)	6.7	4.3	7.6
5× extension left arm with 500 g (seconds)	6.3	4.1	7.4
20 steps upstairs (seconds)	16.3	8.5	14.6
10 m distance walking (seconds)	10.1	6.9	9.5

January 1988: unable to write because of muscular fibrillation and cramps; walked with crutches; maximum walking distance 150 m; light dysarthria.

February 1988: no cramps; less fibrillation; able to write; walking distance several kilometres without rest; walks without crutches; clear speech.

April 1988: weeping and laughing spasms with urinary incontinence; heavy dysarthria and increase of other bulbar symptoms; maximum walking distance 150 m with crutches.

Katamnesis: increasing bulbar symptoms; confined to bed last week of May; painful lancinating spasms; generalized incontinence; marasmus; hypostatic pneumonia; died June 20 of respiratory insufficiency and copious haemorrhage of a stress ulcer of stomach.

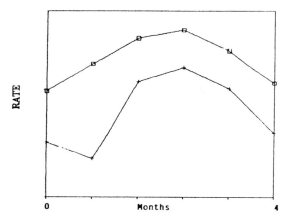

Figure 55.8 F.I.S.: 5 times abduction of right (+) and left (□) arm to 90° with 500 g in hand (seconds)

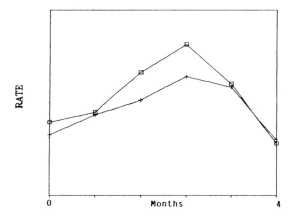

Figure 55.9 F.I.S.: 5 times extension of right (+) and left (□) arm to 90° with 500 g in hand (seconds)

Three cases of ALS were treated. The improvement of strength and physical ability lasted only several weeks. After that time, strength and neurological symptoms became worse. It seems that there is no way of influencing this clinical picture with efficiency by atlas therapy. ALS is different from other SMA. With ALS the first and second motoneurones degenerate. With other kinds of SMA only the second motoneurone is affected. One could suppose that the speed of development and the pathological potential itself is too high in ALS for this form of treatment.

State after poliomyelitis

DEQ, female, 57 years old; poliomyelitis in 1938; paresis of shoulder girdle and pelvic girdle. Beginning of atlas therapy, August 1988; duration of treatment to May 1989, 10 months.

Physical condition: walked sluggishly and weakly with crutch, hands reached just the mouth for eating, problems with body care.

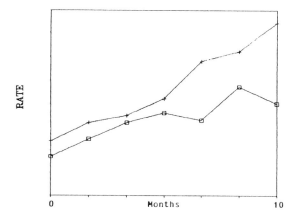

Figure 55.10 DEQ: □, 20 steps upstairs (seconds); +, 10 m walking (seconds)

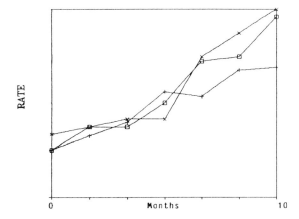

Figure 55.11 DEQ: +, 5 times rising from a stool of 40 cm height (seconds); □, abduction of stretched right arm against gravity (degrees); ×, extension of stretched right arm against gravity (degrees)

419

	Aug 88	Dec 88	May 89
Physical condition:			
20 steps upstairs (seconds)	21.3	13.0	14.2
5× rising from a stool (seconds)	19.8	9.9	9.7
Abduction of right arm (degrees)	50	110	135
Abduction of left arm (degrees)	70	110	135
Extension of right arm (degrees)	60	125	140
Extension of left arm (degrees)	55	115	135
10 m distance walking (seconds)	18.5	11.4	9.6
Spirometric parameters:			
FVC	2.62		2.58
FEV 1	2.05		2.38
Peak flow expiration	3.8		5.16
Peak flow inspiration	1.98		3.05

Since September 1988 she has walked without a crutch and put on her clothes without help, combed her hair, and has no more problems with body care.

Two other cases of poliomyelitis reacted in the same way. The improvement of strength is perceptible and measurable. All depends on whether functions are disturbed or destroyed.

Myotonia

The case of Steinert's myotonia shows a considerable increase of strength and neurological coordination. The 29-year-old female patient was treated until May 1989 for 8 months. After 6 weeks she was able to stand up from a chair and to walk in familiar environments without help. After 8 weeks she was able again to put on her clothes by herself.

The case of Thomsen's myotonia showed a total loss of muscular stiffness with free ability to move for only one or at most two days. Therefore, atlas therapy does not seem to be appropriate for this clinical picture if it is justified to judge from one case only.

Charcot–Marie–Tooth disease

The two cases of this neuromuscular disease, treated up to May 1989 for respectively 10 and 4 months, were 48 and 32 years old. Both were female. They reacted in the same way. Pain due to the disease itself and to secondary orthopaedic problems disappeared within 14 days. There was considerable increase of physical ability (maximum walking distance) and harmony of movements, and decreases of disturbance of neurological coordination were remarkable.

Kearns–Sayre–Shy syndrome

The two cases – brother and sister – are affected by myosis, pareses of musculature of eye, general decrease of strength, and symmetrical polyneuropathy of legs. The reduction of sensible polyneuropathy lasted only for several days after treatment. Strength, however, increased considerably. The myosis and pareses abated. Both patients started to drive a car again.

DISCUSSION

This pilot study suffers from the small number of cases. It was carried out under the inadequate conditions of a common re-education centre. It follows that many parameters that ought to have been measured were not recorded. The results obtained however, suggest the following line of reasoning despite the obstacles mentioned.

It seems that atlas therapy mitigates the symptoms of most of the neuromuscular diseases. The extent of its effect depends on the pathological potential of the treated diseases and the speed of their development. All treated cases showed a considerable improvement of strength and decrease of symptoms caused by neurological discoordination. A phase of relatively steep growth of strength during the first three or four weeks of treatment is followed by a period of slower increasing abilities. The third period seems to be a steady state of variable duration. An explanation may be a synchronization of α-motoneurones during the first period and a training effect during the second period. With regard to SMA Werdnig–Hoffmann and ALS, a fourth period must be postulated. It seems evident that the symptomatic improvement will be overwhelmed by the individual evolution and the pathological potential of these diseases.

The similar results of atlas therapy in the different groups of neuromuscular diseases and the long-lasting effects make a placebo effect improbable.

The conclusions of this study are the subject of a controlled study in a centre of neuromuscular diseases.

ACKNOWLEDGEMENTS

This study was supported by the generosity of Mr Roederer as Director of IPRIAL, Strasbourg. I also want to thank Dr Kraemer, Centre de Cure, Munster-France for his computer designs.

Index